Physical Activity Instruction of Older Adults

Physical Activity Instruction of Older Adults

C. Jessie Jones, PhD
California State University at Fullerton

Debra J. Rose, PhD
California State University at Fullerton

EDITORS

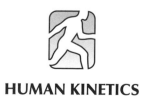

HUMAN KINETICS

Library of Congress Cataloging-in-Publication Data

Jones, C. Jessie.
    Physical activity instruction of older adults / C. Jessie Jones, Debra Rose.
       p. cm.
    Includes bibliographical references and index.
    ISBN 0-7360-4513-9 (hard cover)
    1. Physical education for older people. 2. Aging--Physiological aspects. I. Rose, Debra. II. Title.
    GV447.J66 2004
    613.7'0446--dc22

                                            2004013539

ISBN: 0-7360-4513-9

The Web addresses cited in this text were current as of July 19, 2004, unless otherwise noted.

Acquisitions Editor: Judy Patterson Wright, PhD; **Developmental Editor:** D.K. Bihler; **Assistant Editors:** Amanda S. Ewing, Lee Alexander, and Carla Zych; **Copyeditor:** Karen Bojda; **Proofreader:** Erin Cler; **Indexer:** Swanson Indexing Services; **Permission Manager:** Dalene Reeder; **Graphic Designer:** Robert Reuther; **Graphic Artist:** Dawn Sills; **Photo Manager:** Kareema McLendon; **Cover Designer:** Jack. W. Davis; **Photographer (cover):** C. Jessie Jones; **Art Manager:** Kelly Hendren; **Illustrator:** Tim Offenstein; **Printer:** Sheridan Books

Printed in the United States of America   10   9   8   7   6   5   4   3   2   1

Human Kinetics
Web site: www.HumanKinetics.com

United States: Human Kinetics
P.O. Box 5076
Champaign, IL 61825-5076
800-747-4457
e-mail: humank@hkusa.com

Canada: Human Kinetics
475 Devonshire Road Unit 100
Windsor, ON N8Y 2L5
800-465-7301 (in Canada only)
e-mail: orders@hkcanada.com

Europe: Human Kinetics
107 Bradford Road
Stanningley
Leeds LS28 6AT, United Kingdom
+44 (0) 113 255 5665
e-mail: hk@hkeurope.com

Australia: Human Kinetics
57A Price Avenue
Lower Mitcham, South Australia 5062
08 8277 1555
e-mail: liaw@hkaustralia.com

New Zealand: Human Kinetics
Division of Sports Distributors NZ Ltd.
P.O. Box 300 226 Albany
North Shore City
Auckland
0064 9 448 1207
e-mail: blairc@hknewz.com

Dedicated to the memory of D.K. Bihler. Her gentle spirit
and masterful editing helped us produce a higher quality book.

Contents

PART V   Program Design, Leadership, and Risk Management   280

Contributors

Ken Alan, BS
Ken Alan Associates, Los Angeles

Joan Virginia Allen, JD, CSCS, AS
Valencia, California

Marybeth Brown, PT, PhD, FACSM
University of Missouri, Columbia

Wojtek J. Chodzko-Zajko, PhD, FACSM
University of Illinois, Urbana-Champaign

Janie T. Clark, MA
American Senior Fitness Association, New Smyrna Beach, Florida

Susie Dinan, MS
Royal Free and University College London Medical School, United Kingdom

Duncan N. French, PhD
Northumbria University, United Kingdom

Dawn E. Gillis, MS
University of California, San Francisco

Janene M. Grodesky, MS
Louisiana State University, Baton Rouge

Steven A. Hawkins, PhD, FACSM
California State University, Los Angeles

Gareth R. Jones, PhD
Canadian Centre for Activity and Aging, London, Ontario

Abby C. King, PhD, FACSM
Stanford University, Palo Alto, California

William J. Kraemer, PhD, FACSM
University of Connecticut, Storrs
Adjunct-Edith Cowan University, Australia

Ralph La Forge, MS
Duke University Medical Center, Durham, North Carolina

Richard A. Magill, PhD
Louisiana State University, Baton Rouge

Katie Malbut, PhD
Royal Free and University College London Medical School, United Kingdom

A. Paige Morgenthal, DC, MS
Southern California University of Health Sciences, Whittier

Thomas J. Overend, PhD
Canadian Centre for Activity and Aging, London, Ontario

Roberta E. Rikli, PhD, FACSM
California State University, Fullerton

James H. Rimmer, PhD
University of Illinois, Chicago

Michael E. Rogers, PhD, CSCS, FACSM
Wichita State University, Wichita, Kansas

Roy J. Shephard, MD, PhD, DPE, FACSM
University of Toronto

Dawn Skelton, PhD
University of Manchester, United Kingdom

Ruth Sova, MS
Aquatic Therapy and Rehabilitation Institute, Port Washington, Wisconsin

Anita L. Stewart, PhD
University of California, San Francisco

Anthony A. Vandervoort, PhD
Canadian Centre for Activity and Aging, London, Ontario

Kay Van Norman, MS
Seniors Unlimited, Bozeman, Montana

Sara Wilcox, PhD
University of South Carolina, Columbia

Preface

Identifying ways to promote active life expectancy and reduce the onset of physical frailty has become a major focus for gerontology researchers and physical activity instructors throughout the world. In 1994 there were 357 million people aged 65 and older, a figure that is expected to double between now and the year 2025. Moreover, in the industrialized countries of the world, 20 to 25 percent of all adults will be over the age of 65 by the year 2020, with the fastest-growing segment of that population being people aged 80 or older. This surge in the older adult population brings with it many serious challenges, but it also presents numerous opportunities for those in the field of fitness and health promotion.

The recognized value of physical activity in preserving functional capacity and reducing physical frailty in later years has resulted in numerous physical activity programs for older adults being developed in facilities around the world. Providing safe and effective exercise programs for this population, however, requires specialized knowledge and practical training, particularly because chronic medical conditions are likely to alter the older adult's need for and response to exercise. The need for curriculum materials to train physical activity instructors of older adults at the international level led to a coalition of members from 13 countries and a committee of experts from the United States. These members reviewed and critiqued a set of curriculum standards for preparing physical activity instructors of older adults first published in the *Journal of Aging and Physical Activity* (Jones & Clark, 1998) and a similar set of international curriculum guidelines developed in 2004. The training modules that comprise the agreed upon guidelines are shown in the figure on page xiv. The nine training modules are considered to cover the essential knowledge and skills that should be included in training programs for entry-level physical activity instructors of older adults. The final consensus document, *International Curriculum Guidelines for Preparing Physical Activity Instructors of Older Adults,* was published in the *Journal of Aging and Physical Activity* in October of 2004 (Ecclestone & Jones, 2004). See appendix A for a more detailed description of each training module.

The Purpose of This Book

Physical Activity Instruction of Older Adults represents the first collaborative effort to provide a comprehensive textbook that addresses each of the nine international curriculum guideline training modules. Written for entry-level instructors, undergraduate students, and instructors preparing for certification as well as personal trainers, activity directors and assistants, therapeutic recreation specialists, and group exercise leaders already working with older adults, this book provides the fundamental knowledge and skills recommended in each of the nine training modules. According to training module 4, for example, it is recommended that instructor training programs include information about how to use results obtained from screening, assessment, and client goal-setting activities to make appropriate decisions regarding individual and group physical activity/exercise program design and management. Training module 5 recommends areas of study that provide information on common medical conditions of older adults, signs and symptoms associated with medication-related negative interactions during activity, how to adapt exercise for clients with different fitness levels, and stable medical conditions to help prevent injury and other emergency situations. In addition to addressing each of the nine curriculum training modules

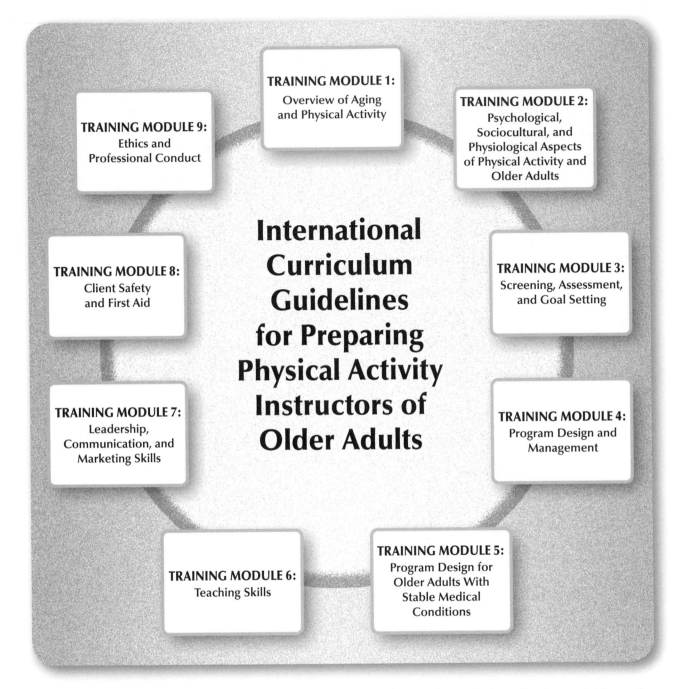

in detail, *Physical Activity Instruction of Older Adults* provides additional knowledge and skills needed for training master athletes.

This book also provides some unique features to enhance understanding and learning retention. At the start of each chapter a list of objectives familiarizes readers with the key concepts they will learn, and each chapter concludes with useful summaries and recommended readings. Terms that are key to learning are highlighted throughout each chapter, as are key points to focus on. Students, instructors, and professionals in training will also find the study questions and practical application activities at the end of each chapter particularly useful for reviewing important topics and applying knowledge to practice.

All these features are provided to meet the overarching goal of this book, namely, to provide the fundamental knowledge and skills needed to lead safe and effective exercises classes or personal training sessions for older adults with diverse functional capabilities. This book should also prepare you to pursue advanced certification training programs now offered by a number of national and international organizations, including the American College of Sports Medicine (ACSM), American Council on Exercise, and the American Senior Fitness Association.

How This Book Is Organized

This textbook is divided into five parts, each of which addresses one or more of the training modules that comprise the international curriculum guidelines. To present the information needed to develop safe and effective physical activity programs for older adults in the most logical and understandable way, the training modules are not addressed in numerical order, and some chapters address more than one module. The best way to read this book is sequentially, in the order that the chapters are presented.

Part I, "Overview of Aging and Physical Activity," begins with the overview in chapter 1 of the demographics and definitions of aging, followed by an introduction to a new field of study: *gerokinesiology*. In chapter 2, C.J. Jones describes successful aging and summarizes its predictors. This is followed by an in-depth discussion of how physical activity affects mind, body, and spirit. In chapter 3, Chodzko-Zajko describes the role of physical activity in the aging process and highlights the psychosocial and cognitive benefits derived from regular physical activity. In chapter 4, Morgenthal and Shephard describe physiological aspects of aging and the functional implications of these changes.

Part II of the book, "Screening, Assessment, and Goal Setting," provides the knowledge and skills needed to conduct thorough preexercise and health screenings and assessments, provide meaningful feedback to clients, evaluate program outcomes, and help clients develop short- and long-term behavioral goals. In chapter 5, Rogers presents preexercise screening tools for determining the general health, physical activity level, and disabilities of older adult participants and explains how to administer and interpret them and share results with participants. In chapter 6, C.J. Jones and Rikli describe field-based assessment tools used to measure physical impairments and functional limitations in the older adult population. Chapter 7, by G.R. Jones, Vandervoort, and Overend, describes laboratory assessments of cardiorespiratory function, muscle strength, body composition, and bal-

ance. Information on how and when to administer these tests and how to interpret the results is also provided in chapters 6 and 7. Finally, in chapter 8, Wilcox and King explain the major personal, environmental, and program-related factors that influence the initiation and maintenance of physical activity by older adults. They also address important theories of behavioral change and cognitive and behavioral strategies that can be used to motivate older adults in group and individual settings.

Part III, "Core Program Principles and Training Methods," delves further into programming, focusing on the core principles and training methods for exercise programs for older adults. Chapter 9, by Gillis and Stewart, discusses the potential functional benefits of the different types of physical activities that should be included in all well-rounded physical activity programs for older adults. This chapter also addresses how to apply several exercise principles for effective program design. In chapter 10, Van Norman describes the warm-up and cool-down components of an exercise program, including specific activities to engage older adults mentally, emotionally, socially, and spiritually. In chapter 11, Brown and Rose describe age-associated changes in joint and muscle flexibility, including the effects of these changes on the basic activities of daily living. They present dynamic and static flexibility exercises that address every major muscle group and joint in the body. In chapter 12, Kraemer and French introduce the resistance-training variables that improve muscular strength, endurance, and power (e.g., resistance, exercise order, repetitions) and provide the skills needed to design a safe and effective resistance-training component for older adults. Chapter 13, by Dinan, Skelton, and Malbut, presents an overview of the critical principles and variables for designing aerobic endurance programs for older adults, including accommodating different fitness levels and functional abilities. In the last chapter of part III, Rose explains how age-associated physiological changes can affect balance and mobility and provides progressive balance and mobility exercises.

Part IV, "Specialty Programs and Training Methods," is devoted to three special topics in physical activity programming for older adults: mind–body exercise, aquatics, and master athletes. In chapter 15, La Forge discusses two mindful exercise forms, yoga and tai chi, and presents strategies and movement sequences to incorporate mind–body exercise into physical activity programming for older adults.

In chapter 16, Sova presents the benefits of aquatic exercise for older adults and offers specific considerations and safety precautions for teaching aquatic exercise to older adults with common age-related disorders. In the final chapter of part IV, Hawkins discusses training that addresses the specific goals of older master athletes, including how to develop sport-specific programs and strategies to prevent overtraining and injury.

Part V, "Program Design, Leadership, and Risk Management," completes the book by focusing on the essential skills and knowledge necessary for creating an effective and safe physical activity program for older adults. In chapter 18, Magill and Grodesky present the key motor learning principles that guide effective skill teaching, including demonstrations and verbal cues, structuring the practice environment, introducing new skills, and providing feedback. In chapter 19, Alan and C.J. Jones discuss leadership skills to enhance teaching effectiveness, including motivation and communication strategies. In chapter 20, Clark discusses specifics of group leadership and management, including effective ways to market a group exercise program for older adults and principles of group dynamics to promote successful learning. Chapter 21, by Rimmer, describes the major disabling conditions that affect older adults and how to modify exercises to enhance safe participation and reduce injury among older adults with specific medical conditions. In the final chapter of the book, Allen discusses several pertinent legal issues and guidelines for developing a risk management plan. She ends the chapter with a discussion of professional ethics.

Putting Knowledge Into Practice

The authors who have contributed to *Physical Activity Instruction of Older Adults* are all highly respected experts in their disciplines. They have repeatedly demonstrated their ability to translate cutting-edge theoretical concepts into meaningful guidelines for effective practice. After you read this book and complete the thought-provoking study questions and practical application activities at the end of each chapter, you will have a solid grasp of the essential knowledge and skills for designing and implementing an effective physical activity program that addresses the needs and interests of *all* older adults. As a result of acquiring the skills needed to appropriately select, administer, and interpret preexercise health and activity screening tests, you will also be able to demonstrate the effectiveness of your program and thereby foster higher participation and retention rates among the older adult community.

Together, we will raise the professional standards for all physical activity instructors of older adults and also address one of the most critical worldwide health issues: improving the quality of life in later years.

Acknowledgments

First, we want to express our deepest appreciation to each of our contributing authors for their dedication to the arduous task of writing for the first edited textbook in the field of gerokinesiology. The journey has been a long but hopefully rewarding one.

Our sincere gratitude also is extended to the numerous professionals throughout the world who since 1974 have contributed to the development of the *International Curriculum Guidelines for Preparing Physical Activity Instructors of Older Adults* that form the basis of the content in this book. Special thanks are also given to Rosabel Koss, PhD, who was the first recognized leader in the United States to raise awareness of the need for specialized training for physical activity professionals working with older adults.

To the staff at Human Kinetics, we are indebted to you for your expertise and publishing skills and for your consistent support. You are all truly amazing, especially D.K. Bihler, the developmental editor; Amanda Ewing, the assistant editor; and Dalene Reeder, who served as the permissions manager for this book.

We extend our heartfelt gratitude to Dr. Rainer Martens, president of Human Kinetics, and Dr. Judy Wright, acquisitions editor, who believed in the importance of this groundbreaking book project, for their willingness to double the original length of the text to ensure that each of the nine training modules that comprise the *International Curriculum Guidelines for Preparing Physical Activity Instructors of Older Adults* was adequately covered.

Above all, to the thousands of older adults who have participated in our research and training programs over the course of the last 10 years at the Center for Successful Aging at California State University, Fullerton, thank you for your support—we have learned so much from each and every one of you!

Part I

Overview of Aging and Physical Activity

TRAINING MODULE 1:
Overview of Aging and Physical Activity

TRAINING MODULE 2:
Psychological, Sociocultural, and Physiological Aspects of Physical Activity and Older Adults

TRAINING MODULE 9:
Ethics and Professional Conduct

TRAINING MODULE 3:
Screening, Assessment, and Goal Setting

TRAINING MODULE 8:
Client Safety and First Aid

International Curriculum Guidelines for Preparing Physical Activity Instructors of Older Adults

TRAINING MODULE 4:
Program Design and Management

TRAINING MODULE 7:
Leadership, Communication, and Marketing Skills

TRAINING MODULE 5:
Program Design for Older Adults With Stable Medical Conditions

TRAINING MODULE 6:
Teaching Skills

Training to become a physical activity instructor of older adults begins with an introduction to the field of gerontology (the science of aging) and knowledge about the physiological and psychological dimensions of the aging process and the role of physical activity. Part I of this text addresses the first two training modules included in the *International Curriculum Guidelines for Preparing Physical Activity Instructors of Older Adults*. Module 1 recommends areas of study that include general background information about the aging process and the benefits of an active lifestyle. These are the topics of chapters 1 and 2. Module 2 recommends areas of study that include psychological, sociocultural, and physiological aspects of physical activity in order to develop safe and effective physical acitvity and exercise programs for older adults. Chapters 3 and 4 address areas of study contained in both modules 1 and 2.

- Chapter 1 provides an overview of the demographics of aging, compares various definitions of aging, and introduces the reader to a new field of study: gerokinesiology.
- Chapter 2 describes the predictors of successful aging. It discusses biological, psychological, and sociological theories of aging and how physical activity promotes successful aging. This information will help you communicate to your clients that successful aging depends on the interplay of many factors, especially staying physically active.

- Chapter 3 debunks common myths and misperceptions about the aging process. It then describes the psychological, cognitive, and social benefits of regular physical activity and ways to promote more physical activity among older adults at both a local and national level.

- Chapter 4 describes the major age-associated changes in physiological systems, the functional implications of these changes, and types of physical activity that have the potential to counteract or delay these age-related changes. With this knowledge base you will better understand the factors to consider when designing programs to meet the special needs of older adults. You will also be able to better articulate and promote the benefits of an active lifestyle to older adults once you have finished reviewing the chapters in part I and completing the questions and application activities at the end of each chapter.

1

The Field of Gerokinesiology

C. Jessie Jones
Debra J. Rose

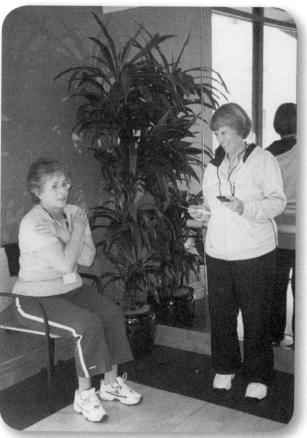

The academic disciplines of exercise science, kinesiology, and physical education have traditionally focused on children, youth, and younger adults. However, as the value of physical activity throughout the life span is recognized and supported by a growing body of research evidence, more attention is being directed to the training of instructors who specialize in leading physical activity programs for older adults. The purpose of this chapter is to describe the demographics of aging throughout the world, various definitions of aging, and the emerging field of gerokinesiology.

Demographics of Older Adults

Advancements in medical technology, health care, nutrition, and sanitation have resulted in lower birth and death rates throughout the world. People are living longer, and the population aged 65 years and older is rapidly increasing. Average life expectancy at birth in most developed countries now is approximately 80 years, an average increase of about 25 to 30 years since 1900, with women living between 6 and 8 years longer on the average than men. By the year 2020, the population over the age of 65 years will be greater than 20 percent in four countries. A national report by the U.S. Census Bureau, *An Aging World: 2001* (Kinsella & Velkoff, 2001), emphasized that global aging is occurring at an unprecedented rate. Whereas in 1950 there were only 131 million people over the age of 65 worldwide, in 1994 this number had risen to 357 million, and by 2000 it reached 420 million. The 65 and older population is projected to increase to nearly 1 billion by 2030. This equates to a growth rate of 800,000 older adults per month. International comparisons in the year 2000 showed that Italy was the nation with the highest percentage of total population aged 65 and over (18.1 percent), closely followed by Greece with 17.3 percent (see figure 1.1). The United States ranked 32nd on this list, with 13.3 percent of its population older than 65 years.

The rapid growth in the aging population, especially people over the age of 85, presents a number of health, social, and economic challenges for individuals, families, and governments throughout the world. Two of the greatest challenges will be the fiscal shortfall in health and social security programs for older adults and the rising medical costs associated with chronic disability. In response to these imminent challenges, a worldwide movement is under way to find effective ways to promote *active* life expectancy and reduce the number of years people live with chronic disabilities. Fries and Crapo (1981) defined **active life expectancy** as the number of years of life spent without significant disease or disability, while Katz and colleagues (1983) adopted a more positive tone by defining it as the number of expected years of physical, emotional, and intellectual vigor or functional well-being.

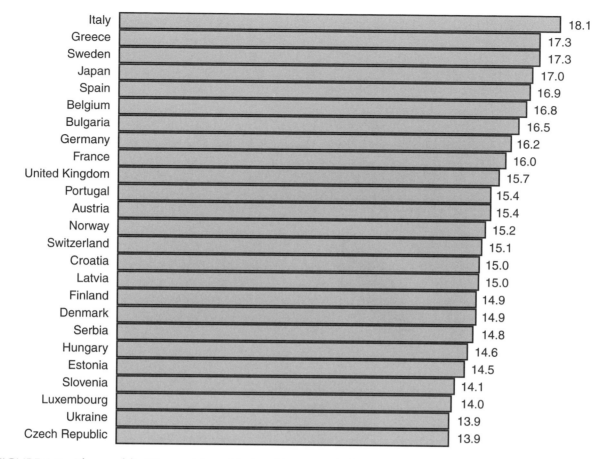

FIGURE 1.1   The world's 25 countries with the oldest populations: 2000.

From K. Kinsella and V.A. Velkoff, 2000, "The world's 25 oldest countries" U.S. Census Bureau, Series P95/01-1.

Benefits of Physical Activity

Professionals who have worked in the health and fitness field for many years are well aware of the importance of integrating physical activity into every individual's daily life. Numerous research studies have also reported many health- and performance-related benefits of engaging in regular physical activity, particularly for older adults. It has been shown that a certain level of fitness not only protects the individual from a number of chronic diseases (e.g., heart disease, diabetes, cancer) but also makes performing the many tasks of daily life, as well as participation in a variety of sports and recreational activities, considerably easier. A number of psychological benefits can also be derived from regular participation in physical activity, including emotional well-being, enhanced cognitive function, and a higher perceived quality of life.

Despite this large body of research evidence, statistics in the United States indicate that few older adults engage in physical activity on a regular basis. The U.S. Department of Health and Human Services (USDHHS, 2000) estimates that only 31 percent of people aged 65 to 74 years participate in 20 minutes of moderate physical activity three or more times a week, and an even smaller percentage (16 percent) report engaging in 30 minutes of moderate activity five or more days per week. Moreover, adults aged 75 and older are even less physically active: Only 23 percent report that they engage in moderate physical activity three or more days per week, and 12 percent engage in moderate physical activity five or more days per week. Unless the current trend is reversed, the costs of physical inactivity among the older adult population will place increasing demands on medical and social services and the public health system in general. It is already the case that approximately one third of total health care expenditures in the United States are for older adults (over 65 years), a proportion that is expected to rise substantially in the next 25 years. This alarming trend could be reversed if older adults were to become more physically active. The Centers for Disease Control and Prevention (2002) recently reported that the annual direct medical costs of physically inactive older adults (with no physical limitations) are significantly higher than those of their physically active peers (see figure 1.2).

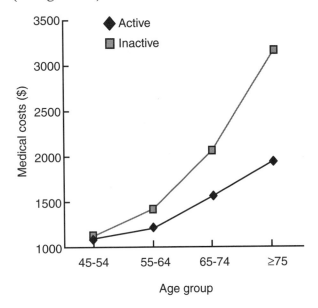

FIGURE 1.2   Annual medical costs of active and inactive women.

Promoting active lifestyle among older adults. U.S. Surgeon General, 1996. Http://www/cdc/gov/nccdphp/dnpa/physical/lifestyles.htm

Defining Old Age

Defining the term *old age* sounds simple, but it is actually very complex. For example, with the increase in anti-aging treatments (e.g., anti-aging products and cosmetic surgical procedures) available today, individuals may look and feel much younger than their chronological age. To help you understand the complexity of defining *old age,* the following is a brief description of three main definitions: chronological, biological, and functional aging.

Unfortunately, the most common indicator used to define *old age* is **chronological age,** that is, the passage of time from birth in years. People can be lumped together in a particular age category by chronological age and then provided a label such as "young-old" (aged 65-74 years), "middle-old"

(aged 75-84 years), "old-old" (aged 85-99 years), and "oldest-old" (aged 100 or more years). At the turn of the 21st century there were over 1 million centenarians (100 or more years old) worldwide, approximately 100,000 of them living in the United States.

Biological aging, also known as primary aging, refers to a group of processes within the body that eventually lead to loss of adaptability, disease, physical impairments, functional limitations, disability, and eventual death. There are several biological theories of aging, and a number of factors have been proposed that affect the rate of biological aging. The major theories of biological aging are discussed in chapter 2.

Functional age has to do with one's functional fitness in comparison with others the same age and gender. For example, an 80-year-old woman may have the aerobic endurance of a woman in the 60-64 age category (as measured by the six-minute walk; see chapter 6 for Senior Fitness Test items and national performance norms). Therefore her functional age relative to aerobic endurance is between 60-64 years of age. Impairments in physical fitness parameters (e.g., aerobic endurance, musculoskeletal integrity, flexibility, body composition, and the sensorimotor system) have a direct impact on a person's functional abilities (e.g., walking, stair climbing, rising from a chair), and functional limitations eventually lead to physical disabilities (refer to the Functional Fitness Framework in chapter 6). Spirduso (1995) hierarchically divided physical function into five levels: physically elite, physically fit, physically independent, physically frail, and physically dependent (see figure 1.3). This hierarchy of physical function in later life may be an effective way to categorize your clients once you have completed the preexercise screening and assessment described in chapters 5 and 6, respectively.

It is extremely important to recognize that as people age, they become increasingly more diverse in their medical, psychological, and physical status. Differentiating between usual (or normal), pathological (or abnormal), and successful aging is another way of categorizing the way people age. **Usual aging** refers to the way most people age and is characterized by a gradual decline in body function, leading to physical impairments, disease, functional limitations, and eventually the onset of disability and death. **Pathological aging** generally refers to the way individuals age who are genetically

Physically elite
- Sports competition, Senior Olympics
- High-risk and power sports (e.g., hang-gliding, weight lifting)

Physically fit
- Moderate physical work
- All endurance sports and games
- Most hobbies

Physically independent
- Very light physical work
- Hobbies (e.g., walking, gardening)
- Low physical demand activities (e.g., golf, social dance, hand crafts, traveling, automobile driving)
- Can pass all IADLs

Physically frail
- Light housekeeping
- Food preparation
- Grocery shopping
- Can pass some IADLs, all BADLs
- May be homebound

Physically dependent
- Cannot pass some or all BADLs
  - Walking
  - Bathing
  - Dressing
  - Eating
  - Transferring
- Needs home or institutional care

Disability

Physical function (y-axis label)

FIGURE 1.3 Hierarchy of physical function. BADL = basic activity of daily living. IADL = instrumental activity of daily living.

Reprinted, by permission, from W. Spirduso, 1995, *Physical dimensions of aging* (Champaign, IL: Human Kinetics), 339.

predisposed to certain diseases or have high-risk negative lifestyles (e.g., poor eating habits, smoking, excessive alcohol use) that lead to premature disability and death. **Successful aging,** on the other hand, is more difficult to define because the term *success* itself is quite ambiguous. Successful aging is a qualitative description of aging rather than one that refers to longevity or survival. Rowe and Kahn (1987) referred to successful agers as people with better than average physiological and psychosocial characteristics in late life and healthy genes. Successful agers are also more satisfied with life in general. Chapter 2 provides a more in-depth discussion of the major theories and predictors of successful aging.

Physical activity has great value in preserving functional capacity and reducing disease and physical frailty in later years, making physical activity programs for older adults especially important. However, most experts agree that specialized training is needed for activity professionals who develop and implement physical activity programs for older adults.

Gerokinesiology: A New Field of Study

Recognition of the importance of physical activity for older adults and the support of the medical community (Nied & Franklin, 2002) have resulted in more facilities and organizations (e.g., senior centers, hospitals, recreation departments, fitness clubs, churches, YMCAs, retirement communities) offering physical activity programs for this segment of the population. Shephard (1997), however, argued that because of the large range of medical conditions and functional abilities in the 65+ population, preparing to be a physical activity instructor for older adults requires more knowledge, skills, and experience than to be an instructor of younger adults. Because of the more numerous job opportunities for physical activity instructors of older adults and the recognized need for specialized training, universities have started developing advisement tracks, focus areas, and specializations in the area of fitness and aging.

In an effort to promote curriculum development and elevate the quality of professional training programs offered in this area, several experts representing numerous organizations throughout the world convened and developed International Curriculum Guidelines for preparing physical activity instructors of older adults. The guidelines are comprised of nine curriculum training modules. This text uses the term **gerokinesiology** to describe this rapidly growing field of study, a term based on the input of several expert physical activity instructors of older adults and many university professors who throughout the world currently prepare undergraduate and graduate students to work with older adults in a variety of physical activity settings.

Historically, the academic discipline of kinesiology and physical education focused on preparing students for careers in the areas of teaching and coaching children and young adults. In more recent years, however, the discipline has expanded to include specialized areas of study designed to prepare students for careers in such areas as fitness and health promotion, athletic training, and

> **Gerokinesiology** is a specialized area of study within the larger discipline of kinesiology that focuses on understanding how physical activity influences all aspects of health and well-being in the older adult population and the aging process in general.

cardiac rehabilitation (Jones & Rikli, 1993). As with a number of other subdisciplines in kinesiology—such as motor control and learning, biomechanics, exercise physiology, sport psychology, and pedagogy—the emerging new subdiscipline of gerokinesiology was preceded by scientific research and the development of unique curriculum offerings.

Gero- is the root of the word *gerontology.* As a field of study, gerontology adopts a multidisciplinary approach to examining the biological, economic, psychological, social, and health and fitness aspects of the aging process. The American Academy of Kinesiology and Physical Education uses the term *kinesiology* to describe a multifaceted field of study in which movement or physical activity is the intellectual focus. According to this definition, physical activity encompasses exercise performed for the improvement of health and fitness, activities of daily living, sport, dance, work, and play. Moreover, a variety of special populations are studied, including people with injuries, diseases, or disabilities; athletes; children; and the elderly. Elements of the two terms *gerontology* and *kinesiology* have been combined to describe a specialized area of study within the larger discipline of kinesiology that focuses on understanding how physical activity influences all aspects of health and well-being in the older adult population and the aging process in general.

Curriculum Development

Curriculum development to prepare physical activity instructors of older adults was minimal prior to the 1990s (Jones & Rikli, 1994). Until recently, instructors and personal trainers who led physical activity programs for older adults reported that they had to rely primarily on self-study, on-the-job training, or workshops and conferences to develop the specific knowledge and skills needed to work with older adults (Jones & Rikli, 1993). The slow response by academic institutions to develop curricula aimed at prepar-

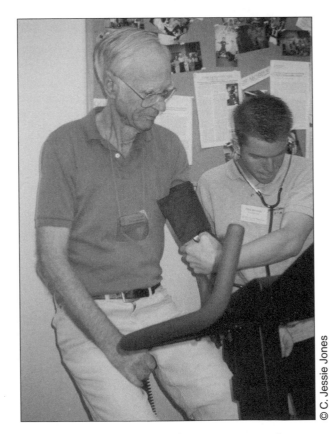

The gerokinesiology curriculum prepares undergraduate and graduate students to work with older adults in a variety of physical activity settings.

© C. Jessie Jones

ing physical activity instructors for older adults has resulted in a number of professional organizations and individual entrepreneurs offering training that culminates in some type of certification. Unfortunately, lacking curriculum guidelines to assist their development, some of these training programs failed to provide the essential knowledge and skills that are essential for safe and effective physical activity programs for older adults (Jones & Clark, 1998).

The International Curriculum Guidelines for Preparing Physical Activity Instructors of Older Adults, published by Ecclestone and Jones (2004) in the *Journal of Aging and Physical Activity,* recommend that the following nine curriculum training modules form the basis of any professional training program or academic curriculum subsequently developed:

1. Overview of Aging and Physical Activity
2. Psychological, Sociocultural, and Physiological Aspects of Physical Activity and Older Adults
3. Screening, Assessment, and Goal Setting
4. Program Design and Management
5. Program Design for Older Adults With Stable Medical Conditions
6. Teaching Skills
7. Leadership, Communication, and Marketing Skills
8. Client Safety and First Aid
9. Ethics and Professional Conduct

The content presented in this text is based on these training modules recommended by the international guidelines. Refer to appendix A for a detailed description of the training modules.

Summary

The increase in the number of people living beyond the age of 65 and the recognized value of physical activity for preventive medicine and health promotion have caused the proliferation of physical activity programs especially designed for older adults. Gerokinesiology is a new and specialized area of study that focuses on professional training in and research on physical activity and aging.

Key Terms

Recommended Readings

Howley, E., & Franks, B.D. (2003). *Health fitness instructor's handbook* (4th ed.). Champaign, IL: Human Kinetics.

Jones, C.J., & Clark, J. (1998). National standards for preparing senior fitness instructors. *Journal of Aging and Physical Activity, 6,* 207-221.

Study Questions

1. The average life expectancy at birth in most developed countries now is approximately
   a. 68 years
   b. 72 years
   c. 75 years
   d. 80 years

2. The country with the greatest percentage of its total population aged 65 and over in the year 2000 was
   a. Japan
   b. Germany

(continued)

      c. France
      d. Italy

3. What percentage of people in the United States between the ages of 65 and 74 years are estimated to participate in 30 minutes of moderate physical activity five or more days per week?
      a. less than 10 percent
      b. 16 percent
      c. 25 percent
      d. 35 percent

4. Gerokinesiology is defined as
      a. a specialized area of study within the larger discipline of kinesiology that focuses on understanding how physical activity influences all aspects of health and well-being in the older adult population and the aging process in general
      b. a subdiscipline within gerontology that focuses on understanding how physical activity influences all aspects of health and well-being across the life span.
      c. a new discipline that focuses on understanding how physical activity influences all aspects of health and well-being in the older adult population and the aging process in general
      d. a specialized area of study within kinesiology that focuses on physical activity across the life span.

Application Activities

1. Interview two or three physical activity instructors of older adults and ask them to describe what they consider to be the important knowledge and skills needed for their job.

2. Surf the Web and review the certification programs offered by different professional organizations (e.g., World Instructor Training School, American Senior Fitness Association, National Strength and Conditioning Association) for physical activity instructors of older adults. Which one would you recommend and why?

2

Predictors of Successful Aging

C. Jessie Jones

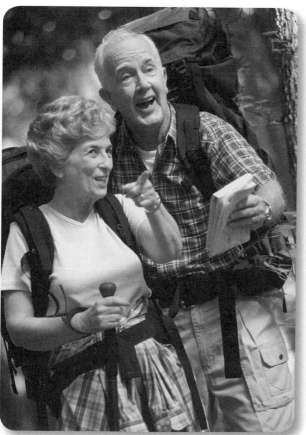

Because of advances in sanitation, public health, medical and pharmaceutical technology, and food science, most of us will live a long life. However, what is important to most people is the quality of that life. As stated in chapter 1, it is difficult to define successful aging because the term *success* itself is quite ambiguous. The concept of successful aging dates back several decades (Baltes & Baltes, 1980; Havighurst, 1961; Palmore, 1979; Rowe & Kahn, 1987; Ryff, 1989). Havighurst (1961) coined the term *successful aging,* referring to it as "adding life to the years" and "getting satisfaction from life." Palmore (1979) defined successful aging as including longevity, lack of disability, and life satisfaction. Rowe and Kahn (1987) further defined successful agers as people with better than average physiological and psychosocial characteristics in late life and healthy genes. Furthermore, they considered successful agers as having two additional traits: low risk for physical and cognitive diseases and disabilities until the age of 80 or more, and life satisfaction with their physical, mental, social, emotional, and spiritual well-being. Other experts in the field have added the following indicators of successful aging: autonomy (independence), financial and social status, sense of meaningful purpose in life, and self-actualization.

Successful aging should not be limited to one-dimensional stories about older adults who exhibit above average performance speed, intellectual function, and physical health. Gerokinesiologists also need to be careful not to make people feel that they have aged unsuccessfully because they have a disease or are unable to walk. However a person defines successful aging, it is certainly not determined by longevity (survival) alone but also by the quality of those years. It is important to remember that quality of life is defined by much more than physical health—it is also a state of mind. Reduced physiological reserve and increased vulnerability to illness constitute only a small part of the aging process. Later life is also a time for personal growth, discovery, and opportunities.

Although physiological aging is inevitable, the way in which a person ages depends for the most part on his or her lifestyle. Successful aging is not something that begins in later life; rather, it is an accumulation of where and how we have lived our lives, experiences we have encountered, people in our lives, how we feel about ourselves, and choices we make regarding how we care for ourselves and manage our lives (see figure 2.1). This chapter discusses various predictors (determinants) of successful aging addressed by biological, psychological, and sociological theories of aging. Why study theories of aging? Theories provide the basis for addressing basic and applied research questions, developing effective intervention strategies, and creating or changing public policies. At a practical level, this knowledge can help you as a physical activity instructor to create effective exercise programs and physical activity environments that help to promote the successful aging of your clients. The second part of this chapter discusses physical activity as a determinant of successful aging.

Biological Theories of Aging

The maximum life span (110-120 years) has not changed since prehistoric times, yet very few people live that long. Why? What are the underlying mechanisms that alter our physiology and determine our deterioration and eventual death? Why do people age at different rates? Several biological theories of aging attempt to answer these

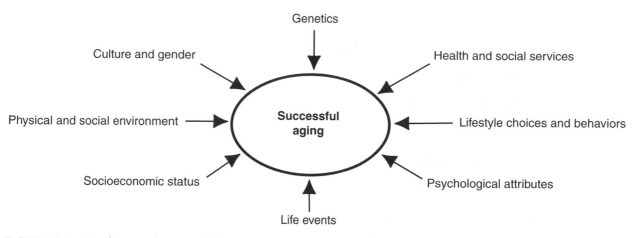

FIGURE 2.1   Predictors of successful aging.

Reprinted, by permission, from the World Health Organizations, 2002, "Growing older - Staying well." (Geneva, Switzerland: WHO).

questions. However, one of the major problems in developing a coherent aging theory is separating causes from effects. Many theories have been and are still being tested. It is important to remember that theories should not be considered fact and that no single theory can explain the phenomenon of **senescence,** which is defined as the aging of the body, the gradual decline in cell and body functions that eventually leads to death. Although many individual biological theories of aging have been developed over the years, for the purpose of this discussion, they are divided into three main categories: genetic theories, damage theories, and gradual imbalance theories.

Genetic Theories

Genetic theories focus on the role of heredity in determining the rate of aging within the body. Few genes actually control the rate of aging; however, thousands of genes have a significant role in development of pathologies (diseases). According to Medvedev (1981), aging of the body occurs as a result of the gradual breakdown of **deoxyribonucleic acid (DNA,** the chemical makeup of genes) sequences within the cells, causing incomplete cell reproduction. Genetic theories also suggest that the aging process is controlled by a biological clock that is programmed into each cell of the body. This process prevents human cells from growing and dividing forever. One of the oldest and most prominent theories of aging is the Hayflick limit, which states that a human cell can only divide a

limited number of times, approximately 50, and then it suddenly stops dividing and dies (Hayflick, 1961). Hayflick's theory has recently been challenged because it is now known that not all cells age or divide at the same rate. For example, cells of the immune and endocrine systems divide very few times, while neurons and muscle cells do not divide at all. Even Hayflick conceded that most people die of diseases before they reach the limit of possible cell life.

Damage Theories

The damage theories emphasize the accumulation of cell damage as a key determinant of cellular dysfunction and death. According to these theories, the cells are damaged by an accumulation of DNA errors or cross-linkages, waste products, glucose, or free radicals within the cells. One of the most accepted theories of cell damage is the free-radical theory (Harman, 1956). **Free radicals** are atoms or groups of atoms that have at least one unpaired electron, making them highly reactive. Although free-radical production provides the energy needed for daily living and kills bacterial invaders, excessive free radicals cause harmful oxidation that damages cell membranes, cell components of DNA and **ribonucleic acid (RNA)** synthesis, and enzymes needed for cell metabolism and correct cell division. Free radicals are especially damaging to the cardiovascular, neuromuscular, immune, and endocrine systems. Eventually the accumulation of cellular damage increases a person's risk for a host of dis-

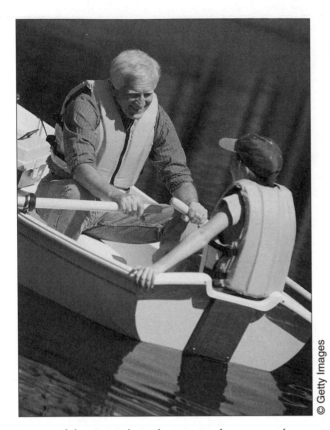

Successful aging is based on many factors, such as biology, genetics, and environment. Successful aging determines how active an older adult will be.

eases, such as cardiovascular disease, diabetes mellitus, neurodegenerative diseases, cancer, and macular degeneration. In addition to the body producing free radicals during metabolism (breakdown of food to make energy), cells are exposed to free radicals from environmental chemicals (especially tobacco smoke), the ultraviolet rays of the sun, and radiation.

Another highly supported damage theory relates to **cross-linkage.** As we age, important large molecules (called macromolecules) of connective tissue (elastin and protein collagen) become intertwined or cross-linked, decreasing the elasticity of tissue within the lungs, kidneys, vasculature, gastrointestinal system, muscles, ligaments, and tendons (Warner, Butler, Sprott, & Schneider, 1987). Cross-linkage of molecules also causes large tangles that interfere with intracellular transport of nutrients and chemical messengers. The cross-linkage of fibers is thought to be caused by increases in free-radical oxidation. Interestingly, leading a more active lifestyle and consuming a healthy diet seem to inhibit or delay cross-linking.

> An understanding of the genetic, damage, and gradual imbalance theories of aging will enable you to confidently convey to your clients that much of their aging process is within their control.

Gradual Imbalance Theories

Collectively, the gradual imbalance theories hypothesize that body systems age at different rates, causing imbalances in biological functions, especially within the central nervous system (brain and spinal cord) and the endocrine system (Frolkis, 1968; Finch, 1976). The central nervous system and the endocrine system, often together referred to as the neuroendocrine system, involve a complicated network of biochemicals that regulate the release of hormones to help the body adapt to real or perceived stress or environmental challenges. Malfunctions of these systems result in hormonal imbalances and deficiencies, causing other physiological and metabolic imbalances that negatively affect a number of body functions.

Each of the biological theories described in this section attempts to explain the deterioration of body systems (senescence) and eventual death. Although there is a lack of agreement on just how much genetics determine the aging process, it is generally believed to be somewhere between 30 and 40 percent (Rowe & Kahn, 1998). With some understanding of the biological theories of aging, you can confidently convey to your clients that much of how they age is within their control. The next section discusses various psychological theories of aging.

Psychological Theories of Aging

Psychological theories of aging attempt to explain the psychological development of a person and the psychological traits associated with successful aging. Three prominent psychosocial theories discussed here are Maslow's (1943) hierarchy of needs, Erikson's psychosocial stages of development (Erikson, Erikson, & Kivnick, 1986), and the theory of selective optimization with compensation developed by Baltes and Baltes (1990).

One of the most popular theories of successful aging is Maslow's (1943) hierarchy of needs. Maslow described a hierarchy of human needs in which lower-level needs must be satisfied before addressing needs at the next higher level (Maslow & Lowery, 1998). According to Maslow, the more self-actualized and transcendent an individual becomes, the wiser he or she also becomes. **Self-actualization** is defined as finding self-fulfillment and realizing one's potential. **Transcendence** is defined as helping others find self-fulfillment and realize their potential. Although there is little agreement about the order of basic human needs, or wording used to describe basic needs, it is at least generally accepted that people age in a more successful way when their basic needs are fulfilled (Deci & Ryan, 2002; Ryan, 1991).

One of the early theories of personality development is Erikson's psychosocial stages of development (Erikson et al., 1986). According to Eric Erikson, personality development proceeds through eight stages, each characterized by some type of psychosocial crisis, which must be resolved for successful aging to occur (see table 2.1). The last three stages (between young and late adulthood) describe positive personality development leading to successful aging as the ability to (1) form close relationships with friends and lovers, (2) be productive by raising a family or through some form of work, and (3) look back on one's life with pride and satisfaction.

TABLE 2.1 Erikson's Psychosocial Stages

Stages	Approximate age	Positive outcome	Negative outcome
Trust vs. mistrust	0-1 year	Child develops faith in people, believes that his or her needs will be taken care of.	Child comes to believe that other people cannot be counted on, believes that his or her needs will not be met.
Autonomy vs. shame and doubt	1-3 years	Child develops confidence in his or her ability to do basic tasks independently.	Child lacks self-confidence.
Initiative vs. guilt	3-5 years	Child feels OK about trying new things.	Child is afraid to try new things, afraid of failure or disapproval if he or she does try new things.
Competence vs. inferiority	6-12 years	Child takes pride in being able to accomplish normally expected tasks.	Child feels inferior because he or she cannot do things that other children appear to do with ease.
Identity vs. role confusion	13-18 years	Child develops a sense of who he or she is and how he or she wants to live life.	Child may be unable to settle on an identity (role confusion) or may adopt a negative identity.
Intimacy vs. isolation	Young adulthood	Person is able to form close relationships with friends and lovers.	Person has difficulty forming or sustaining close relationships.
Generativity vs. stagnation	Middle adulthood	Person is productive through raising a family or through some form of work.	Person is unable to be productive.
Ego integrity vs. despair	Late adulthood	Person is able to look back on his or her life with pride and satisfaction and approach death with dignity and acceptance.	Person feels that he or she has not accomplished what he or she set out to accomplish in life and is frustrated by the approaching end of life.

From Erik H. Erikson, 1963, *Childhood and society*, 2nd ed. (New York, NY: W.W. Norton and Company), 272-273.

Baltes and Baltes (1990) provided yet another perspective on the determinants of successful aging in their theory of selective optimization with compensation. According to this theory, successful aging has much to do with the ability of an older adult to adapt to physical, mental, and social losses in later life. This theory focuses on three behavioral life-management strategies for maintaining functional independence in later life: (1) focusing on high-priority areas of life, areas that result in feelings of satisfaction and personal control, (2) optimizing remaining personal skills and talents that enrich and enhance life, and (3) compensating for losses of physical and mental function by using various personal strategies and technological resources, either one's own or others', to achieve objectives. For example, one strategy, for a person with limited mobility, might be to use a cane or walker so that he or she can continue to participate in various occupational, social, and recreational activities. You can help your clients compensate for losses in later life by improving their **functional competence,** which not only affects their ability to perform daily activities but also the quality of their lives. Functional competence is defined as the degree of ease with which individuals think, feel, act, or behave in congruence with their environment. To a large extent, functional competence determines a person's social life, such as the ability to visit friends, participate in active vacations, and make use of public services and facilities, all of which promote successful aging.

Although various studies investigating psychological theories of aging have been published in numerous scientific journals, two easy-to-read books—*Sound Mind, Sound Body* (Pelletier, 1994) and *Successful Aging* (Rowe & Kahn, 1998)—summarize the research findings and also identify the key predictors of successful aging. According to these authors, people who age the most gracefully seem to indulge in many small, daily pleasures that cultivate positive attitudes and optimistic outlooks toward aging and life; they have a spirit that creates aliveness in everything they do; they have a passion for living life to the fullest; they have a drive toward a deeper purpose and meaning in life beyond themselves.

More specifically, factors identified as determinants of how we age include **intelligence** (e.g., the ability to learn and adapt to new environments, the ability to think nonverbally, knowledge of important facts in one's culture), **cognitive capacity** (e.g., mental processing speed, the ability to solve problems, memory), **self-efficacy** (i.e., a belief in one's capabilities to handle situations and tasks in life), **self-esteem** (i.e., feelings about oneself), **personal control** (i.e., belief in one's ability to exert control in life), **coping style** (e.g., how one adapts to transitions and handles daily hassles and crises), **resilience** (i.e., the ability to overcome adversity), and mental and physical stimulation.

According to Bandura (1997), a person's self-efficacy is critical for successful aging because it influences a person's thought patterns and emotional reactions, lifestyle choices and behaviors, effort put forth on a task or activity, and perseverance when confronting obstacles throughout life. Helping your clients set attainable goals and communicating your respect and support can help to build the self-esteem and the self-efficacy of your clients.

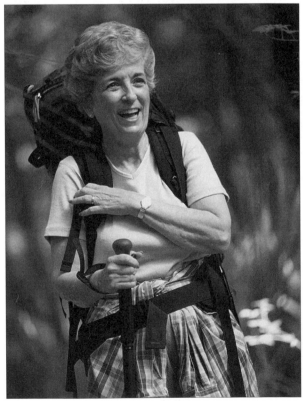

© Getty Images

This older woman's goal was to be able to hike again. Being able to do so has improved her self-esteem and self-efficacy.

Sociological Theories of Aging

The most widely accepted sociological theory of aging currently is activity theory. This theory simply states that people who stay engaged in mental and physical activities of daily living throughout life tend to age in a healthier and happier way (Fisher, 1995; Lemon, Bengtson, & Peterson, 1972). Another theory that has gained considerable support in the last several years is continuity theory (Atchley, 1972). This theory states that the people who age most successfully carry forward positive health habits, preferences, lifestyles, and relationships from midlife into later life.

A large body of literature provides consistent evidence that a person's social and physical environments influence the aging process (Lemon et al., 1972; Sugtswawa, Liang, & Liu, 1994; World Health Organization, 1998). Conversely, inadequate social and physical environments have been found to be associated with an increase in mortality and morbidity and a decrease in overall health and well-being (House, Landis, & Umberson, 1988; Seeman & Crimmins, 2001; Seeman et al., 2002). Evidence from a recent study indicated that positive cumulative social experiences and emotional supports are also associated with lower biological risk for morbidity and mortality (Seeman et al., 2002). As an instructor, you can do a lot to promote the successful aging of your clients by creating fun and social physical activity environments.

Physical Activity As a Determinant of Successful Aging

Many scholars believe that the single most important factor related to successful aging is remaining healthy. A strong body of scientific evidence that physical activity is a key ingredient for healthy aging of body, mind, and spirit has resulted in several national reports and position stands in the United States that endorse this premise (American College of Sports Medicine, 1998; Robert Wood Johnson Foundation, 2001; U.S. Department of Health and Human Services, 1996, 2000; World Health

> Creating a fun and social physical activity environment can do much to promote the successful aging of your clients.

Organization, 1998). Regarding longevity, a landmark study by Blair and colleagues (1996) found that among major risk factors for all-cause mortality, fitness level was the best predictor of premature death. Men and women with low fitness levels were twice as likely to die during an eight-year follow-up period than their more fit counterparts. The following discussion summarizes why physical activity is considered to be one of the main determinants of successful aging.

The Body

Two of the main indicators of successful aging defined in the literature are longevity and low risk for disease and disability (Rowe & Kahn, 1987). There is abundant research indicating that people who participate in regular physical activity have lower morbidity and mortality rates than their more sedentary counterparts. A consensus document published in the United States (Robert Wood Johnson Foundation, 2001) and an international proceedings and consensus document (Bouchard, Shephard, & Stephens, 1994) state that physical activity reduces the risk of developing various chronic diseases and disabilities, especially cardiovascular disease, diabetes, osteoporosis, sarcopenia (loss of muscle mass), certain forms of cancer (colon and breast), and mobility problems. Specific benefits are listed in figure 2.2. More in-depth discussion of the benefits of physical activity is provided in several chapters in this book.

The Mind

One of the key predictors of successful aging that has emerged from the psychological theories of aging is cognitive integrity. Although thousands of studies have investigated the effects of physical activity on reducing the risk of disease and improving physical fitness and mobility among older adults, far less research has been conducted on the impact of physical activity on cognition and state of mind. First, how is **mind** defined? The mind can be defined as a collection of conscious

Cardiovascular health

Improves myocardial performance
Increases peak diastolic filling
Increases heart muscle contractility
Reduces premature ventricular contractions
Improves blood lipid profile
Increases aerobic capacity
Reduces systolic blood pressure
Improves diastolic blood pressure
Improves endurance

Obesity

Decreases abdominal adipose tissue
Increases lean muscle mass
Reduces percentage of body fat

Lipoproteins, glucose

Reduces low-density lipoproteins
Reduces cholesterol and very-low-density lipoproteins
Reduces triglycerides
Increases high-density lipoproteins
Increases glucose tolerance

Osteoporosis

Slows decline in bone mineral density
Increases bone density

Psychological state

Improves perceived well-being and happiness
Increases levels of catecholamines and serotonin

Functional capacity

Reduces risk of musculoskeletal disability
Improves strength and flexibility
Reduces risk of falls by increasing strength
Reduces risk of fractures
Increases reaction time
Sustains cerebral perfusion and cognition

FIGURE 2.2   Benefits of physical activity.

Adapted, by permission, from W.J. Chodzko-Zaijko, 2001, "National blueprint for increasing physical activity among adults age 50 and older: Creating a strategic framework and enhancing organizational capacity for change," *Journal of Aging and Physical Activity* 9: S10.

and unconscious processes that direct and influence our mental and physical behavior. The mind perceives, thinks, reasons, feels, wills, imagines, and desires. According to Candace Pert (1993), a molecular biologist, the mind is not only in the brain but also in every cell of the body. In other words, there is no separation between mind and body. For example, when you experience a "gut" reaction, it is the wisdom of the body/mind speaking to you. Chapter 3 provides detailed information regarding the relationship between physical activity and psychological processes, including cognition and brain function. Here is a simple list of evidence-based benefits of physical activity on the mind (Chopra, 1993; Pelletier, 1994; Stathi, Fox, & McKenna, 2002):

- Better brain function: mental alertness, memory, concentration, abstract reasoning, verbal fluency, fluid intelligence (decision-making skills)
- Improved sensorimotor performance
- Improved attitude toward life
- Increased self-reliance and control over one's life
- Improved confidence
- Healthier self-image and self-esteem
- Increased energy

The Spirit

Very little research has investigated the impact of physical activity on spiritual health, yet studies indicate spiritual health is a major determinant of successful aging (Crowther, Parker, Achenbaum, Larimore, & Koenig, 2002; Pelletier, 1994; Leder, 1997; World Health Organization, 1998). After interviewing 51 prominent people, Pelletier (1994) reported that all the participants in his study emphasized the importance of inner balance and spirituality as a guiding force in their personal strategies for optimal health.

Among people who study the topic of human spirituality, there is a consensus that it is very difficult to define **spirituality** in words. Brian Seaward's *Health of the Human Spirit* (2001) is an excellent resource for understanding human spirituality and strategies to nurture spiritual health. For an understanding of how physical activity can be a vehicle to enhance spiritual health, a brief definition is in order. First, many people have a difficult time understanding the difference between spirituality and religion. Religion, according to Seaward (2001), is an organized system of worship that is defined by its institutional leaders and that has as its main goal the fostering of spirituality, a divine higher power. Regardless of one's ethnic and cultural background and personal beliefs, there is an implicit understanding that human spirituality refers to a feeling of connection to a higher power, often referred to by such names as God, Allah, Tao, the Creator, the Absolute, the Divine Source, the Universe, the Big Kahuna, Buddha, just to name a few. Connecting with this higher power is said to provide people with a special type of life force, characterized by such words as *energy, spirit,* and *chi.* The important point here is that a person can be very spiritual without attending a religious institution (e.g., temple, church, or mosque). With this very sketchy definition of spirituality, Seaward (2001) and others define **spiritual health** as involving (1) an insightful and nurturing relationship with oneself and others, (2) a strong personal value system, and (3) a sense of meaningful purpose in life.

Many scholars who study the impact of spirituality on health believe that the spirit illuminates our higher consciousness. Spirituality is the seat of emotional beauty and the manifestation of the heart and soul, it helps to set the analytical mind and ego free so that we can experience the beauties of inner peace and bliss. Research summarized by Pelletier (1994) indicates that spiritual health provides people with the courage and determination needed to face adversity and heightens enthusiasm and sense of purpose in life.

Physical activity can be a vehicle for people to connect with this higher power and enhance their spiritual growth. For example, mind–body physical activities such as tai chi and yoga provide older adults an opportunity both to be physically active and to quiet the mind and focus on the supreme spiritual center of the body. Chapter 15 discusses this topic at greater length.

Physical activity can also awaken the spirit or life force within that ignites the soul. This type of experience is often referred to in the literature as an aesthetic (beautiful) experience, which often defies verbal explanation. Imagine the rush of emotions a person feels who is able to stand or walk for the first time following rehabilitation after a stroke or injury, or who successfully reaches the top of a mountain after a long hike. The aesthetic experience is a feeling of the movement or of being in the moment. Perhaps you have felt this when dancing to music or standing on the top of a mountain. By making physical activity enjoyable, meaningful, and challenging, you can help your clients meet the soul of movement where the spirit dances.

Summary

Successful aging is a difficult concept to define because it is multifaceted. The indicators of successful aging include such factors as length of life, physical and mental health, social competence and productivity, personal control, and life satisfaction. Biological theories of aging—including genetic, damage, and gradual imbalance theories—focus on the factors that cause senescence of the body and increase the risk of morbidity and mortality with age.

Psychosocial theories of aging emphasize how much control people have over how they age. Psychological theories (e.g., Maslow's hierarchy of needs, Erikson's psychosocial stages of development, and the Baltes' theory of selective optimization with compensation) focus on the influence of psychological processes and personality characteristics on the aging process. Research has identified the following psychological factors as being important determinants of successful aging: intelligence, cognitive capacity, self-efficacy, self-esteem, personal control, coping style, and resilience.

Sociological theories focus on the influence of the social and physical environments on aging. Such theories include the activity theory and the continuity theory. Theories of aging are the basis for research, program development, and public policies. This theoretical knowledge can also help you as a physical activity instructor to create effective exercise programs and physical activity environments that promote the successful aging of your clients.

The final section of the chapter discussed the influence of physical activity on successful aging, including its impact on body, mind, and spirit. Successful aging depends on the interplay of such factors as genetics, personal and social environment, lifestyle behaviors, attitudes, adaptability, social supports, and certain personality characteristics. The key to successful aging, then, is to integrate positive physical, social, mental, emotional, and spiritual activities into our daily lives. Interactions with thousands of older adults in various environments support Pelletier's (1994) view that perhaps the most important determinant of successful aging is the wisdom to cultivate moral virtue, self-discipline, compassion, and a deep commitment to a spiritual purpose beyond ourselves.

The task of creating a physical activity environment that promotes the successful aging of your clients is not an easy one. Several chapters in this book are designed to prepare you with the knowledge and skills necessary to accomplish this task in a way that meets the needs, desires, and interests of your clients. The quality of life of every older adult you work with will be enhanced through your efforts.

Key Terms

Recommended Readings

Pelletier, K.R. (1994). *Sound mind, sound body: A new model for lifelong health.* New York: Simon & Schuster.

Rowe, J.W., & Kahn, R.L. (1998). *Successful aging.* New York: Pantheon Books.

Study Questions

1. The role of heredity in determining the rate of aging within the body is addressed by a
   a. damage theory of aging
   b. genetic theory of aging
   c. free-radical theory of aging
   d. gradual imbalance theory of aging

2. Maslow's hierarchy-of-needs theory is an example of a
   a. psychological theory of aging
   b. genetic theory of aging
   c. sociological theory of aging
   d. theory of selective optimization with compensation

3. The final stage of Erikson's psychosocial stages of personality development is
   a. generativity versus stagnation
   b. ego integrity versus despair
   c. competence versus inferiority
   d. autonomy versus shame and doubt

4. The theory of selective optimization with compensation states that successful aging has a lot to do with the ability of the older adult to
   a. focus on high-priority areas of life
   b. optimize personal skills and talents
   c. compensate for losses of physical function
   d. all of the above

5. A belief in one's capabilities to handle situations and tasks in life is referred to as
   a. self-actualization
   b. self-efficacy

    c. self-esteem

    d. resiliency

6. A person with strong spiritual health

    a. has a sense of meaningful purpose in life

    b. has a nurturing relationship with self and others

    c. attends church on a regular basis

    d. both a and b

Application Activities

1. Based on the psychological and sociological theories of aging discussed in this chapter, describe three ways you can promote the successful aging of your clients.

2. Describe three ways you can promote spiritual health through physical activity for your older clients.

3

Psychological and Sociocultural Aspects of Physical Activity for Older Adults

Wojtek J. Chodzko-Zajko

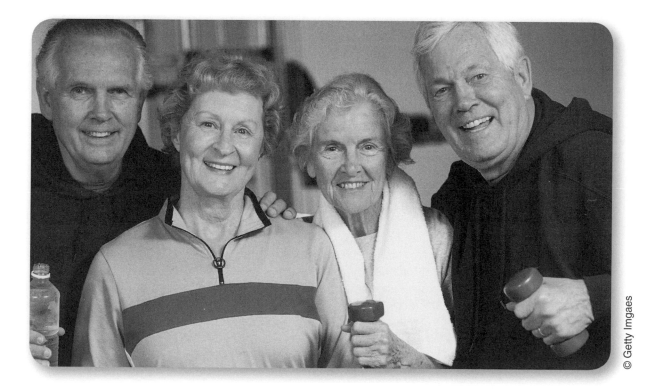

There is wide acceptance throughout the industrialized world of the importance of regular physical activity for successful aging. Major reports from the U.S. Surgeon General (1996), World Health Organization (1997), and the Robert Wood Johnson Foundation (2001) have concluded that participation in moderate levels of physical activity is associated with a reduction in risk factors for many chronic diseases and with the preservation of numerous aspects of physiological functioning, including cardiovascular function, muscle strength and endurance, balance, and flexibility. While the physical benefits are perhaps the most obvious outcome of regular physical activity, there are also significant psychological and sociocultural benefits, not only for older people themselves but also for society as a whole. Furthermore, there is increasing evidence that regular physical activity helps older adults maintain a high quality of life and independence in their later years. (Chodzko-Zajko, 2000).

This chapter begins with a discussion of attitudes toward old age and the aging process. Although aging is often portrayed in a stereotypical and negative manner, growing older is an extraordinarily heterogeneous process, with huge differences among older individuals. An explanation of what it means to grow older and some common myths and realities associated with aging are presented, followed by recommendations for dispelling common myths about physical activity and aging. Next comes an overview of the key social and psychological benefits of physical activity for older adults and the relationship between physical activity and cognitive function. The final section of the chapter discusses some of the broader social issues involved in the promotion of physical activity and strategies currently being implemented at the national level in the United States to help older adults increase their physical activity level.

Aging Stereotypes

One of the most persistent fallacies about aging is the widespread perception that aging is associated with nothing but losses and decline, doom and gloom (Chodzko-Zajko, 1995, 2000). The tendency to perceive aging as a negative condition or a social problem is inconsistent with current experimental evidence on the functional capacities of older individuals. It is also inconsistent with the self-perceptions of most older adults, who do not generally view themselves as disadvantaged or in decline (Bengtson & Schaie, 1999).

Robert Butler, the first director of the National Institute on Aging, suggested that there is a widespread tendency throughout society to focus disproportionately on the negative consequences of aging (Butler & Lewis, 1982). Butler referred to this tendency as **ageism,** which he defined as the practice of discriminating against an individual or group of individuals on the basis of their chronological age. He suggested that ageism has three constituent elements:

- Prejudicial attitudes toward the aged, toward old age, and toward the aging process
- Discriminatory practices against the elderly, particularly in employment, but in other social roles as well
- Institutional policies and procedures that perpetuate stereotypical beliefs about the elderly, reduce their opportunities for a satisfactory life, and undermine their personal dignity

Butler further concluded that these prejudicial attitudes, discriminatory behaviors, and unjust institutional policies have contributed to the transformation of aging from a natural process into a social problem.

Stereotypic attitudes about aging emerge as a result of widely held, false beliefs about aging. Physical activity and health professionals can do a great deal to correct these false beliefs by providing more accurate information about the aging process and what it means to grow old.

A common myth about growing older is that all aspects of health and physical function deteriorate with advancing age. There is now strong evidence to suggest that regular physical activity can alter the rate of decline of many physical and psychological variables. For example, numerous studies have shown that people who adopt lifelong patterns of physical activity often exhibit little or no decline in cardiovascular function for a long time, sometimes

> There is now strong evidence to suggest that regular physical activity can alter the rate of decline of many physical and psychological variables

for as long as several decades or more (Heath, Hagberg, Ehasani, & Holloszy, 1981; Pollock, Foster, Knapp, Rod, & Schmidt, 1987; Rogers, Hagberg, Martin, & Holloszy, 1990).

Physical activity and health professionals who work closely with older adults should emphasize that aging must not be viewed as a solely negative process. There is much that an individual can do to positively influence the aging process. By making healthy and active lifestyle choices, older adults can maximize their quality of life as they grow older. Regular physical activity is an excellent mechanism by which older adults can improve their physiological health, psychological well-being, and social opportunities.

Another common misconception about aging is that all changes in the health and functional abilities of older people are natural consequences of growing older. This is not necessarily true. For example, if you study large numbers of people, you will almost always find that muscular strength declines with advancing age. However, it is incorrect to conclude

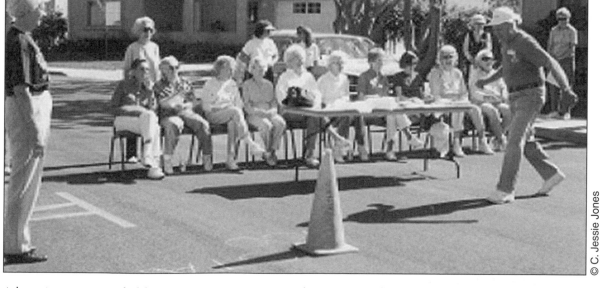

A large percentage of older Americans engage in no leisure-time physical activity, despite the wealth of research evidence proving its benefits.

that these changes are caused simply by the process of growing older. On the contrary, we now know that a substantial portion of the decline in muscle strength that usually accompanies advancing age is due to disuse atrophy resulting from extended periods of physical inactivity (Tzankoff & Norris, 1978).

For many years, exercise scientists, physicians, and other health professionals believed that loss of strength was a natural and inescapable consequence of normal human aging. As a consequence of this erroneous belief, older adults were actively discouraged from joining strength-training programs. Guidelines and position statements from the major professional organizations also actively discouraged strenuous resistance training for those over 60 years of age. We now know, however, that strength training has many beneficial outcomes for older adults, and a number of professional groups have reversed their positions and now actively endorse resistance training for older adults (American College of Sports Medicine, 1998).

There are numerous other examples in gerontology where causation is incorrectly attributed to chronological age. For example, it was once believed that clinical depression was a natural and unavoidable consequence of growing older. As a result of this false belief, clinicians were significantly less likely to treat depressive symptoms in older adults as aggressively as they would if the same symptoms were evident in younger patients. Although many studies do show that older adults are slightly more likely to suffer from depression than younger individuals, it is clear that aging itself does not cause this increase. Rather, older adults are more likely to be depressed due to a host of ancillary economic, social, and health-related factors that accompany but are not caused by advancing age (Chodzko-Zajko, 1990).

You can help dispel myths about aging by providing your older adult clients with numerous active role models in the community who are aging successfully. Following are some ideas to promote positive images of aging:

- Post biographical sketches and photos of physically active individuals who deviate from usual patterns of aging on a bulletin board in the facility where you teach.

- Contact the media to publish testimonials from your clients on how physical activity has improved their lives.

- Ask some of your model participants to be ambassadors in the promotion of physical activity to other older adults in the community.

If you observe a change in health status, a decline in physical performance, or a shift in mood state in an older client, never assume that such changes are a normal and expected aspect of aging. On the contrary, every effort should be made to ascertain the underlying cause of the change so that appropriate corrective measures can be initiated as soon as possible.

To summarize, negative stereotypes about older adults and the aging process often emerge as a result of inappropriate generalizations about aging. It is apparent that social stereotypes can play an important role in the lifestyle choices of older people (McPherson, 1994). For example, physical activity choices in later life often depend on an individual's perception of what is or is not age-appropriate behavior (Cousins, 1997; Cousins & Vertinsky, 1995). Many clinicians have encountered older people who consider it inappropriate to exert themselves in public. In "The Heidelberg Guidelines for Promoting Physical Activity Among Older Persons" (World Health Organization, 1997), the World Health Organization (WHO) actively encourages clinicians, health professionals, and older people themselves to break away from stereotypical perspectives on aging. Instead of encouraging older adults to follow expected patterns of behavior and "take it easy," the WHO urges practitioners to promote a more vigorous and healthful model of aging in which older people are invited to play a more active role (Chodzko-Zajko, 1997).

It is important for physical activity instructors to appreciate that it is not enough to simply inform clients that physical activity is good for them. Knowledge about the health benefits of physical activity is important, but it may not be sufficient to convince sedentary individuals to change their behavior (Dunn, Andersen, & Jakicic, 1998). Many older adults have developed long-term and deep-seated negative attitudes and values about growing older. These negative perceptions adversely influence their desire to participate in physical activity programs and are difficult to overcome (McPherson, 1990). Personal trainers and physical activity instructors can help to counter this learned helplessness by assisting older people to gradually begin to view themselves as legitimate participants in physical activity.

In recent years a variety of motivational strategies have been developed to assist older adults pass from sedentary living to habitual physical activity. For example, Dunn, Garcia, and colleagues (1998) have developed a behaviorally based counseling program known as Project Active. Project Active is designed to help sedentary people begin to view themselves as potential exercisers and gradually build more physical activity into their everyday lives. The program includes a wide variety of activities that can assist sedentary older adults to abandon stereotypical views of aging and retirement as a time for disengagement and decreased activity.

Physical activity instructors can further help older adults to develop more positive attitudes toward physical activity by actively discussing some of the common myths about physical activ-

ity with clients and potential clients (figure 3.1). Many professional groups provide books and brochures that are written for older adults and can help them view physical activity in a more positive light. For example, the *National Blueprint* initiative (www.agingblueprint.org) coordinates a public information campaign designed to dispel common myths and misunderstandings about physical activity.

Physical Activity, Psychological Well-Being, and Quality of Life

One way to help older adults make the transition from a sedentary to a physically active lifestyle is to educate them about the impact that regular

---

Myth 1: You have to be healthy to exercise.

Many older people resist exercising because they incorrectly believe that they have to be healthy to exercise. Physical activity can improve quality of life for the vast majority of older adults and may be most effective for people with chronic health conditions and diseases. Instructors can help dispel this myth by pointing out role models in the community who are regularly active despite having health concerns.

Myth 2: I'm too old to start exercising.

Many older people do not realize that physical activity has been shown to benefit individuals of all ages, including people as old as 90 or 100 years of age. Instructors can strategically display images of active older adults to help reinforce the notion that age need not be a barrier to activity.

Myth 3: You need special clothing and equipment.

No special clothing or equipment is needed. Safe and effective exercise can be performed while wearing comfortable street shoes and loose-fitting everyday clothes. Effective strength training can be achieved with inexpensive equipment such as elastic bands and water-filled jugs. For many older adults, cultural factors influence clothing and exercise choices. Instructors should be sure to take cultural and generational factors into consideration when choosing physical activity offerings.

Myth 4: No pain, no gain.

Many older adults learned about physical activity at a time when it was thought that exercise had to be of high intensity to be beneficial. It is now recognized that physical activity does not need to be strenuous or exhausting to provide significant health benefits. Exercise leaders may need to reinforce the notion that light to moderate physical activities, such as social dancing, walking, or gardening, are appropriate and effective ways to build more physical activity into daily life.

Myth 5: I'm too busy to exercise.

Few older adults realize that physical activity does not have to occur at a particular time and place but often can be built into daily activities such as shopping, gardening, and household chores. Physical activity professionals can help older adults review their busy schedules and identify opportunities for increasing physical activity.

FIGURE 3.1　Common myths and stereotypes about physical activity and aging.

physical activity can have on overall quality of life. Many people associate exercise only with changes in physical fitness. They fail to realize that there are many psychosocial benefits to be gained from regular physical activity. Over the past 20 years, numerous research studies with older adults have focused on the relationship of physical activity and psychological health and well-being, overall life satisfaction, quality of life, and cognitive function. The following sections provide an overview of research in these areas.

Physical Activity and Psychological Well-Being

Most of the early studies examining the relationship between physical activity and psychological function in older adults focused on the impact of physical activity on two specific psychological conditions: depression and anxiety neuroses. However, in recent years there has been less of this type of research. McAuley and Rudolph (1995) noted that only a relatively small proportion of the older adult population suffers from clinical levels of depression and anxiety and that it may be more appropriate to focus our attention on the effect of physical activity on **psychological well-being** (aspects of psychological good health such as self-esteem, self-efficacy, and general well-being) rather than mental illness. Accordingly, the last decade has witnessed a dramatic increase in the number of research studies examining the impact of physical activity on psychological well-being.

Although there is considerable evidence in support of the hypothesis that regular physical activity is associated with significant improvements in psychological health, the current research findings must be carefully interpreted (McAuley & Katula, 1998; Scully, Kremer, Meade, Graham, & Dudgeon, 1998). Relationship studies examine only whether two or more variables (characteristics) are related; they do not indicate that one variable actually causes a change in the other variable, in this case, that physical activity causes improvements in psychological health. Many other factors related to the physical activity environment must be considered, including the characteristics of the instructor, the cognitive and emotional state of the participant, and the dose of exercise (activity type, frequency, intensity, and duration). Early studies examined the relationship between physical activity and relatively general psychological constructs such as **self-concept** (one's perceptions, attitudes, and

> The evidence in support of the hypothesis that regular physical activity is associated with significant improvements in psychological health is considerable but must be carefully interpreted.

values about oneself as a person and one's role in society) and self-esteem (Folkins & Sime, 1981). The association between self-esteem and exercise appears to be strongest in cross-sectional studies; it is less clear whether short-term exercise training consistently *causes* changes in global aspects of self-esteem (McAuley & Rudolph, 1995; McAuley & Katula, 1998).

For many older adults, aging is associated with a loss of perceived control (Bandura, 1997). Since perceptions of control over one's own life are known to be related to psychological health and well-being (Rodin, 1986), exercise scientists have begun to focus more on the relationship between physical activity and various indices of psychosocial control, self-efficacy, and perceived competency (McAuley & Rudolph, 1995). McAuley and Katula (1998) reviewed the literature that examined the relationship between physical activity and **self-efficacy** (an individual's sense of control over his or her environment and ability to function effectively) in older adults. They concluded that most well-controlled exercise-training studies resulted in significant improvements in both the physical fitness and self-efficacy of older adults. Several studies further suggested that moderate-intensity physical activity may be more effective than either low- or high-intensity training regimens (King, Taylor, & Haskell, 1993; McAuley et al., 2000). Training programs of greater than 10 weeks' duration appear to have an appreciably greater effect on psychological well-being than programs less than 10 weeks in duration (McAuley & Rudolph, 1995).

In addition to the effect of physical activity on self-efficacy, there is growing interest in self-efficacy's effect on the ability of older adults to make the transition from a sedentary to an active

> Well-controlled exercise-training studies indicate that moderate exercise results in significant improvements in both the physical fitness and self-efficacy of older adults.

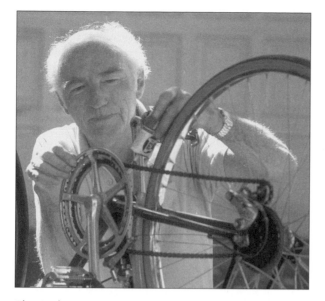

Physical activity can improve self-efficacy, the sense of control over one's environment and ability to function effectively.

Source: *Health Canada website and Media Photo Gallery,* Health Canada, http://www.hc-sc.gc.ca. Reproduced with the permission of the Minister of Public Works and Government Services Canada, 2004.

lifestyle. Dunn, Garcia, and colleagues (1998) demonstrated that physical activity promotion programs that are designed to increase self-efficacy among older adults can help sedentary individuals increase their daily levels of physical activity. There is growing recognition that self-efficacy is not only an important outcome of physical activity, it may also be an important predictor of sustained behavioral change in sedentary populations (Blair, Dunn, Marcus, Carpenter, & Jaret, 2001).

A number of unique stressors occur in later life, including retirement, fixed income, declining health, medical costs, caregiving, and the death of a significant other. Although much of the current research suggests that higher levels of physical fitness and physical activity are associated with a reduction in the physiological response to psychological stress, experimental studies investigating the effects of traditional exercises on reducing stress are rare (Scully et al., 1998).

Physical Activity and Cognitive Function

Maintaining cognitive function is vital to quality of life in later years. **Cognitive function** involves a combination of skills, including memory, attention, learning, goal setting, decision making, and problem solving. There is a long history of research into the impact of physical activity on the processing of information by the central nervous system. Because cognitive performance is known to decline significantly with advancing age, much of the literature on the relationship between physical activity and cognition (an umbrella term used to describe the function and efficiency of the central nervous system, particularly the processing of information) has involved older subjects. It is difficult, however, to separate the effects of aging, existing medical conditions, physical fitness levels, and lifestyle factors on cognitive function. The research on physical fitness, cognition, and aging has focused on two major questions:

- Do highly fit older adults exhibit cognitive performance superior to that of less-fit individuals of the same age?
- Can relatively short-term increases in physical activity bring about meaningful cognitive changes in previously sedentary older adults?

Studies investigating the relationship between physical fitness or health and cognitive decline in old age have also demonstrated that poor health and disease impair cognitive performance (Chodzko-Zajko & Moore, 1994). Furthermore, there is now a significant body of evidence to suggest that physically active and fit older adults often process cognitive information more efficiently than less-fit individuals of the same age (Etnier et al., 1997; Kramer et al., 2002). For example, DiPietro, Seeman, Merrill, and Berkman (1996) found that physically active older adults in the McArthur Study of Successful Aging significantly outperformed less-active older adults on a battery of five cognitive function tests. These differences were found to be independent of sex, self-rated health, and level of social activity.

Whether short-term training programs can bring about meaningful improvements in cognitive performance in previously sedentary older adults is less clear. Although several well-controlled studies discovered significant improvements in cognitive function in older adults after exercise training (Dustman et al., 1984; Hawkins, Kramer, & Capaldi, 1992; Kramer et al., 1999), others have not been able to replicate these training effects (Blumenthal & Madden, 1988; Panton, Graves, Pollock, Hagberg, & Chen, 1990; Hill, Storandt, & Malley, 1993).

In an attempt to clarify the confusion in the findings on exercise training and cognition, Kramer and his colleagues (1999) proposed that the benefits of exercise training may vary as a function of the cognitive demand imposed by the task. To test this hypothesis, Colcombe and Kramer (2003) recently conducted a meta-analysis of the 18 controlled research studies they were able to identify that examined the effect of exercise training on cognitive function. They organized the cognitive tasks employed in these studies into four categories:

- Speed tasks: Simple tasks requiring rapid responses that do not involve high-level cognition

- Visuospatial tasks: Tasks that require rotating real or imaginary objects in three-dimensional space

- Controlled processing tasks: Tasks that require the use of effortful processing strategies and that gradually become automatic with extended practice

- Executive control tasks: Tasks that require coordination, inhibition, and working memory and that also depend on effortful processing but do not become automatic over time

The results of the meta-analysis indicated that physical activity had the greatest impact on the performance of executive control tasks, followed by controlled processing tasks, visuospatial tasks, and then speed tasks.

Kramer and colleagues (2002) concluded that there is clear evidence that both aerobic exercise training and combined aerobic exercise and strength training are associated with improvements in cognitive function. However, they also noted that the effects of fitness are largest for tasks that require complex processing and executive control. Interestingly, combined aerobic exercise and strength training was found to be slightly more effective in improving cognitive performance than aerobic exercise training alone. Although the mechanisms responsible for these training-induced improvements in cognitive performance are not well understood, Kramer and his colleagues proposed that patterns of brain activation may vary between active and sedentary older adults. Future research using functional magnetic resonance imaging (fMRI) techniques may well be able to shed more light on this hypothesis (Kramer et al., 2002).

Although much remains to be learned about the exact nature of the relationship between exercise

> There is some evidence that regular physical activity improves the efficiency of cognitive processing on complex tasks; current research is examining whether these benefits extend to everyday life activities.

training and cognitive performance, the most recent evidence is promising in that it consistently identifies reliable effects for at least certain aspects of cognitive processing. The implications of the literature on exercise training and cognition for the physical activity practitioner are twofold. On the one hand, evidence suggests that aerobic exercise training alone and combined aerobic exercise and strength training positively affect a variety of laboratory tests of cognitive function. On the other hand, it is less clear to what extent these findings can be extrapolated to everyday cognitive tasks likely to be performed by the majority of older adults. For example, if your clients ask whether being physically active will improve their memory or other aspects of cognitive function, the responsible answer is that there is some evidence that regular physical activity improves the efficiency of cognitive processing on complex tasks and that research is currently examining whether these benefits extend to everyday life activities. A summary of the long- and short-term psychological and cognitive benefits of physical activity for older adults is presented in figure 3.2.

Physical Activity and Quality of Life

In the past decade there has been a dramatic increase in the number of research studies that have examined the relationship between physical activity and quality of life in old age (Rejeski & Mihalko, 2001). **Quality of life (QOL)** is a psychological construct that is most commonly defined as an individual's conscious judgment of satisfaction with his or her life (Pavot & Diener, 1991). In psychological research, QOL is most commonly measured using self-report inventories such as the Satisfaction With Life Scale (Diener, 1984) or the Life Satisfaction Inventory (Neugarten, Havighurst, & Tobin, 1961).

In medical research, quality of life is usually defined in more specific terms. For example, **health-related quality of life** is an umbrella term used to describe a constellation of characteristics related to overall physical and psychologi-

Immediate benefits

- Relaxation: Appropriate physical activity enhances relaxation. To promote relaxation, health professionals should encourage older adults to build physical activity breaks into their daily lives.

- Stress and anxiety reduction: There is evidence that regular physical activity can reduce stress and anxiety. Physical activity opportunities can be built into many social events, such as outings and shopping trips.

- Enhanced mood state: Numerous people report elevations in mood following appropriate physical activity. Physical activity can help counter some of the negative consequences of declining health and extended periods of isolation.

Long-term benefits

- General well-being: Improvements in almost all aspects of psychological functioning have been observed after periods of extended physical activity. Individuals who are regularly active have stronger self-esteem and self-efficacy. Active older adults have a greater sense of control over their own lives.

- Improved mental health: Regular exercise can make an important contribution in the treatment of several mental illnesses, including depression and anxiety neuroses. Physical activity is frequently recommended as an integral part of the treatment of many psychological conditions.

- Cognitive improvements: Regular physical activity may help postpone age-related declines in cognitive performance. There is a growing body of evidence that both aerobic exercise training and combined aerobic exercise and strength training improve cognitive function.

- Motor control and performance benefits: Regular activity helps prevent or postpone the age-associated decline in both fine and gross motor performance. Physical activity can help improve balance and reduce the risk of falling in old age.

- Skill acquisition: New skills can be learned and existing skills refined through physical activity by all individuals regardless of age. By being physically active, older adults can acquire new cognitive and motor skills that can help preserve cognitive functioning in old age.

FIGURE 3.2 Psychological and cognitive benefits of physical activity for older people.

Reprinted, by permission, from the World Health Organization, 1997, "The Heidelberg Guidelines for promoting physical activity among older persons," *Journal of Aging and Physical Activity* 5(1): 2-8.

cal health. The most common instrument for the assessment of health-related quality of life is the Medical Outcomes Study 36-item short-form survey (SF-36 Health Survey). This scale is used to evaluate 36 dimensions of health and well-being and generates an overall score for physical and psychological health (Ware, Kosinski, & Keller, 1994). For measuring QOL in older adult populations, Stewart, King, and Haskell (1993) recommended subdividing QOL into two domains: functioning and well-being. They operationally defined functioning to include physical ability and dexterity, cognition, and the ability to perform activities of daily living. In contrast, well-being is defined as physical symptoms and bodily states, emotional well-being, self-concept, and global perceptions of health and life satisfaction.

In a review of the literature that has examined the relationship between physical activity and QOL in old age, Rejeski and Mihalko (2001) reported that the majority of the evidence supports the conclusion that physical activity is positively associated

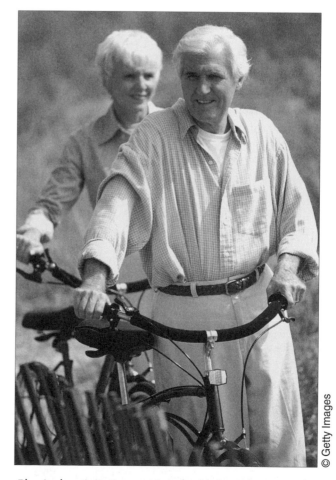

© Getty Images

Physical activity is associated with improvements in health-related quality of life.

with many but not all domains of QOL. Researchers have consistently shown that when physical activity is associated with significant increases in self-efficacy, improvements in health-related quality of life are most likely to occur (McAuley & Katula, 1998).

Social Implications of Regular Physical Activity

In addition to physiological and psychological benefits, physical activity also has significant benefits for the **social functioning** (such as the ability to adjust to changing roles and responsibilities associated with growing older) of older people (see figure 3.3). Among the social benefits of physical activity is the empowerment of older adults to play a more active role in society. Aging creates a need to adjust to changing roles. Because of factors such as the death of friends and loved ones, retirement, financial hardship, ill health, and isolation, many older adults are forced to systematically relinquish many of the roles that they consider a meaningful part of their identity. Physical activity can help older people better adjust to these changing roles

by providing opportunities to widen their social networks, stimulate new friendships, and acquire positive new roles in retirement.

In recent years, many new opportunities for lifelong learning, in which older adults participate in a wide variety of educational, social, and cultural activities, have been developed. There has been a tremendous growth in the number and variety of travel and learning experiences such as Elderhostel available to older adults. Institutes of Lifelong Learning and Universities of the Third Age are providing numerous opportunities for older adults to build ongoing learning experiences into their everyday lives. There is a growing appreciation of the importance of physical activity programs as an integral part of the curriculum for Elderhostels and other institutions of lifelong learning (Chodzko-Zajko, 2000). Health and physical activity professionals are encouraged to identify local commu-

> Physical activity can help older people adjust to their changing roles by providing opportunities to widen their social networks, stimulate new friendships, and acquire positive new roles.

Immediate benefits

- Empowerment: A large proportion of the older adult population voluntarily adopts a sedentary lifestyle, which eventually threatens to reduce independence and self-sufficiency. Appropriate physical activity can help empower older individuals and assist them in playing a more active role in society.
- Enhanced short-term social and cultural integration: Physical activity programs, particularly when carried out in small groups or other social environments, increase social and intercultural interactions for many older adults.

Long-term benefits

- Enhanced long-term social integration: Regularly active individuals are less likely to withdraw from society and more likely to actively contribute to the social milieu.
- New friendships: Physical activity, particularly in small groups or other social environments, stimulates new friendships and acquaintances.
- Widened social and cultural networks: Physical activity frequently provides individuals with an opportunity to widen available social networks.
- Role maintenance and new role acquisition: A physically active lifestyle helps foster the stimulating environments necessary for maintaining an active role in society and for acquiring positive new roles.
- Enhanced intergenerational activity: In many societies, physical activity is a shared activity that provides opportunities for intergenerational contact, thereby diminishing stereotypical perceptions about aging and the elderly.

FIGURE 3.3   Social benefits of physical activity for older people.

Reprinted, by permission, from the World Health Organization, 1997, "The Heidelberg Guidelines for promoting physical activity among older persons," *Journal of Aging and Physical Activity* 5(1): 2-8.

nity programs that provide continuing education opportunities to older adults. These programs are an excellent way to reach highly motivated older adults who may be excited about participating in physical activity programs.

Promoting Physical Activity

In addition to providing physical, psychological, and social benefits for older adults individually, physical activity is now recognized as an important factor in the public health and well-being of society as a whole. In May 2001 a major national planning document was released in the United States in an effort to develop a coordinated national strategy for promoting physical activity among older people.

The *National Blueprint: Increasing Physical Activity Among Adults Age 50 and Older* was developed with input from more than 60 individuals representing 46 organizations with expertise in health, medicine, social and behavioral sciences, epidemiology, gerontology and geriatrics, clinical science, public policy, marketing, medical systems, community organization, and environmental issues (Armstrong et al., 2001). The *National Blueprint* notes that despite a wealth of evidence about the benefits of physical activity for older people, there has been little success in convincing older Americans to adopt physically active lifestyles. For example, the U.S. Surgeon General's (1996) report estimates that between one third to one half of Americans over 50 years old engage in no leisure-time physical activity at all.

A major goal of the *National Blueprint* was to identify some of the societal barriers to physical activity by older adults and to outline specific strategies for overcoming these barriers. The blueprint identifies barriers in the areas of research application, home and community programs, workplace settings, medical systems, public policy and advocacy, and marketing and communications. Some of the barriers that have the greatest relevance for health professionals and physical activity instructors in local communities are summarized in figure 3.4.

In addition to identifying barriers to physical activity in society at large, the *National Blueprint* proposes a number of concrete strategies to overcome these barriers. While many of the strategies are complex and will require the combined efforts of many individuals and organizations before they

- Research findings are rarely translated into practical intervention strategies that can be widely incorporated into ongoing home and community programs.
- Many neighborhoods and communities are poorly planned, unsafe, and designed in a manner that discourages regular physical activity by older adults.
- Few models exist of integrated community approaches to promote physical activity.
- Community resources (senior centers, senior residences, community centers, neighborhoods and apartment units, schools, and places of worship) are often disconnected.
- Health organizations do not collaborate enough with professionals in urban and community planning, transportation, recreation, and design to develop strategies that can make communities more amenable to physical activity.
- Many older adults do not know how to start a safe and appropriate home-based physical activity program.
- Many older adults are isolated and lack transportation to community physical activity facilities and programs.
- Health care professionals do not have adequate, tested, and age-appropriate patient education materials on physical activity for older patients.
- Medical professionals do not have the information to make referrals to community resources. They often lack knowledge about quality programs, materials, and resources.
- Many of the messages and much of the information about physical activity and exercise have been unclear, at times inconsistent, and confusing to older people, as well as to the general population, health professionals, and policy makers.

FIGURE 3.4   Summary of the barriers to physical activity by the older adult population.

can be realized, several of the strategies can be implemented at the local level and have significant implications for physical activity instructors and health professionals. Figure 3.5 summarizes the key strategies for increasing physical activity by older adults.

The *National Blueprint* is a challenging document! It challenges organizations to rethink how they are addressing issues related to physical activ-

- Create a national clearinghouse to disseminate effective, tested public education, social marketing materials, and public policy information on physical activity and aging.
- Seek opportunities for nonprofit associations and agencies to work collaboratively with the for-profit sector to develop joint public education programs. Involve groups such as public health agencies, health care organizations, civic groups, religious institutions, schools, hospitals, and health clubs.
- Identify barriers to walking by adults, determine why these barriers exist, and develop specific recommendations for overcoming them.
- Establish and disseminate standards for fitness leaders who work with midlife and older populations.
- Locate examples of activity-friendly communities and home- or community-based programs, and devise a system to share best practices.
- Encourage more health, physical education, recreation, and dance professionals to become trained and certified to work with older adults.
- Identify professionals in the community who can share information and offer assistance.
- Obtain funding and implement physical activity programs for older adults through appropriate existing community facilities, such as YMCAs and YWCAs, community centers, senior centers, and places of worship.
- Provide community organizations with a template for good physical activity programs.
- Establish partnerships among health, aging, urban- and community-planning, transportation, environmental, recreation, social service, and private sector agencies. Encourage these groups to work together to define, create, promote, and sustain communities that support lifelong physical activity.
- Identify high-quality community sources of information on physical activity and older adults (YMCAs and YWCAs, certified trainers, fitness clubs, etc.), and provide this information to clients in health care settings.
- Develop a national scorecard that outlines what makes a community activity friendly for older adults, and publicize rankings.

FIGURE 3.5   Summary of strategies identified in the *National Blueprint: Increasing Physical Activity Among Adults Age 50 and Older*.

ity. It challenges them to develop partnerships to share resources and work collaboratively to begin to restructure society in such a way as to enable older adults to be more active. The blueprint also challenges each of us as individuals. It asks us to identify how we can best contribute to the redesign and restructuring of our local communities. We are challenged to become more active in creating environments that enable and promote physical activity. We are encouraged to join coalitions, form partnerships, and share our knowledge and expertise. Most importantly, we are challenged to think outside of the box.

There are many ways that physical activity and health professionals can begin to think outside the box and get more involved in local efforts to promote physical activity. For example, many senior centers and continuing-care retirement communities would greatly appreciate receiving expert advice and assistance on physical activity programming from local fitness experts such as personal trainers and kinesiology faculty and graduate students. Links can also be developed between local physicians' offices and community fitness clubs and sports centers. A number of cities have established community coalitions to promote active living, in which local industry representatives, health care organizations, service agencies for older adults, transportation specialists, health and fitness professionals, local government officials, and many others meet regularly to develop programs and projects designed to reduce barriers to active living in the community. Fitness professionals should make every effort to reach out to other professionals working in the area of healthy aging. A phone call to a local senior center or Area Agency on Aging is often an excellent way to start getting involved.

Summary

This chapter described the psychological, cognitive, and social benefits of physical activity for older adults. The dissemination of information on the health benefits of physical activity alone is not sufficient to motivate people to be more physically active. To achieve long-term changes in behavior, it is necessary also to address a variety of social, behavioral, and psychological barriers to physical activity both for the individual and for society at large. At the level of the individual, this requires applying theories of motivation and behavioral change. Physical activity instructors need to carefully assess their clients' readiness to adopt physical activity (see chapter 5) and provide advice, counseling, and supportive strategies as needed (see chapter 8). It is not sufficient to develop a generic exercise program and expect all older adults to fit in and participate enthusiastically.

Persistent myths and stereotypes that reinforce inactivity need to be challenged before many older adults can be expected to change their sedentary lifestyle. Physical activity instructors of older adults have a significant role in dispelling common myths and misconceptions. They can help their older adult clients realize that they do not have to be healthy to exercise, it is never too late to start, they do not need expensive clothing or equipment, and gains can be achieved without pain. Instructors also have an obligation to teach older adults that physical activity offers more than just physical benefits. Regular physical activity is also one of the most effective methods for increasing self-efficacy and self-esteem, reducing stress, and maintaining cognitive function. In addition, physical fitness is consistently associated with overall quality of life in old age.

At the societal level, much needs to be done to restructure our communities to promote physical activity. The *National Blueprint: Increasing Physical Activity Among Adults Age 50 and Older* has identified a number of societal impediments to the adoption of physical activity among older adults. The blueprint argues that in order to bring about significant changes, partnerships and coalitions need to be developed between individuals and organizations with an interest in active aging. There is little doubt that physical activity instructors of older adults will have many opportunities to participate in such coalitions and help to integrate opportunities for physical activity by older adults into the wider social, cultural, and economic context.

Key Terms

Recommended Readings

Robert Wood Johnson Foundation (2001). National blueprint: Increasing physical activity among adults age 50 and older. *Journal of Aging and Physical Activity, 9,* S5-S13.

U.S. Surgeon General. (1996). *Physical activity and health.* Washington, DC: U.S. Department of Health and Human Services.

World Health Organization. (1997). The Heidelberg guidelines for promoting physical activity among older persons. *Journal of Aging and Physical Activity, 5,* 2-8.

Study Questions

1. Why is it important for older adults to change stereotypic perspectives on aging?
   a. It is important that older people learn to act their age.
   b. Healthy aging can help promote international goodwill.
   c. Later-life physical activity choices often depend on an individual's perception of age-appropriate behavior.
   d. Stereotypes usually include an element of truth.

2. Recent research into the psychological benefits of physical activity for older people
   a. has focused mostly on the study of depression and anxiety
   b. has focused on psychological well-being rather than mental illness
   c. has ignored cognitive function and memory research
   d. demonstrates that physiological changes are more important than psychological adjustments

(continued)

3. Short-term exercise training should not be recommended as a means for improving cognitive function in older adults because
   a. exercise training is stressful
   b. there is no relationship between physical activity and cognitive function
   c. the effects of exercise training on cognitive function are relatively small
   d. cognitive function does not decline with advancing age

4. Which of the following is true of the *National Blueprint: Increasing Physical Activity Among Adults Age 50 and Over?*
   a. It was developed by the Office of the Surgeon General.
   b. It identifies societal barriers to physical activity.
   c. It proposes strategies to increase physical activity at national, regional, and local levels.
   d. b and c

5. Successful physical activity instructors of older adults should do which of the following?
   a. design physical activity programs that are adapted to meet the diverse needs of their older adult clients
   b. be prepared to negotiate with their clients
   c. get to know and understand their clients
   d. all of the above

Application Activities

1. Identify four or five organizations that could be recruited to form a coalition to promote physical activity in your community. Briefly describe how you would recruit them.

2. An 80-year-old woman wants to become involved in a physical activity program that you are teaching, but she has been led to believe that she will not derive any benefits from the program because she is too old. Briefly describe what you would say to this woman in response to her misperception.

4

Physiological Aspects of Aging

A. Paige Morgenthal
Roy J. Shephard

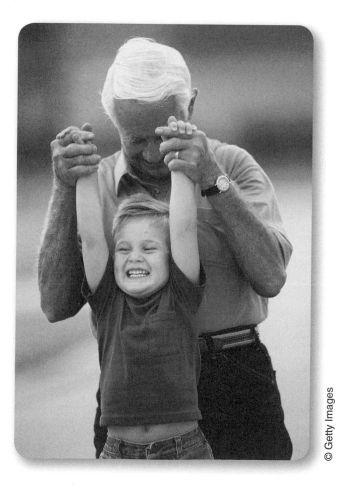

Objectives

After completing this chapter, you will be able to

1. recognize that the progressive decline in physiological systems is due more to chronic disease and sedentary lifestyle than to the aging process itself;
2. discuss how aging and physical inactivity lead to progressive declines in many body systems, including those related to cardiovascular and respiratory function, muscle integrity, joint mobility, bone mass, and neurological function;
3. explain how physiological declines in various body systems affect functional mobility and independence; and
4. identify types of regular physical activity that can improve the function of various body systems and thus help counteract age-related changes that progressively limit performance.

Although aging leads to a progressive decline in the function of most body systems (see figure 4.1), the good news is that much of the decline is preventable or reversible through participation in physical activity. Customary levels of physical activity decline at about age 30; as people typically become more sedentary and their repertoire of activities more limited, organs and tissues start to decline. This progressive decline occurs slowly at first, then proceeds more rapidly with prolonged inactivity. By age 60, many of the changes resulting from the interaction between advanced age and physical inactivity may be profound. Chronic diseases of the cardiovascular, metabolic, musculoskeletal, and neurological systems are also a major cause of physiological deterioration with age (Masoro, 2001). Moreover, declines in one system often have profound effects on other systems in the body, thereby compounding the decrease in functional mobility and performance and the risk of frailty and disability. These common chronic diseases, and their consequences, inevitably accompany aging and must be factored into any exercise or physical activity intervention.

- A decrease in peak oxygen transport of 5 ml $\cdot$ kg$^{-1}\cdot$ min^{-1} per decade between ages 25 and 65 years
- An increase in body fat content, with decreased glucose tolerance and a deterioration of blood lipid profile
- A 25% decrease in peak muscle force and lean tissue from age 40 to 65, with an accelerating loss thereafter; selective atrophy of fast-twitch muscle fibers; and less coordination of muscle contractions
- A 7% loss of flexibility per decade of adult life
- A progressive decrease in bone calcium and deterioration of bone matrix, beginning at age 25, and accelerating for 5 postmenopausal years in women
- Decrease in balance, slowing of reaction speed and movement time
- Deterioration of function in special senses (vision, hearing, smell, and taste), impaired memory, poor sleep patterns, and depression

FIGURE 4.1 Important functional changes associated with aging in sedentary older adults.

It is important that physical activity instructors of older adults understand that declines in body systems are affected by many factors besides genetic predisposition and that much of the aging process is within our control. Participating in regular physical activity can delay the normal aging process by 10 to 20 years (Shephard, 1997). Helping your clients understand how exercise can reduce problems associated with aging can motivate them to participate in your programs. Also, a working knowledge of the physiological aspects of aging is critical for leading safe and effective exercise classes for older adults with diverse functional capabilities. This chapter discusses age-related physiological changes in cardiovascular and respiratory function, muscle integrity, joint mobility, bone mass, and neurological function. In addition, the implications of these physiological changes for the design and implementation of exercise programs for older adults are addressed.

Cardiovascular and Respiratory Function

The age-related changes in the cardiovascular and respiratory systems are widespread and profound. However, they may be associated with the significant decrease in physical activity typical of older adults as much as the structural and functional changes in organs that stem from aging itself. These changes may initially limit both activities of daily living and physical activities. Although regular physical activity has the potential to reverse many of these changes, age-related changes in the heart, lungs, and vasculature must initially be factored into any activities prescribed for older adults.

Aerobic Capacity

Aerobic capacity is the ability of the cardiopulmonary system to deliver blood and oxygen to active muscles and the ability of those muscles to use oxygen and energy substrates to perform work during maximal physical stress. Aerobic capacity involves the interaction of four physiological functions carried out by various organs and tissues: pulmonary respiration (lungs), central circulation (the heart and the nerve conduction to it and to the blood vessels), peripheral circulation (arteries, veins, and capillaries), and aerobic respiration (in muscle cell mitochondria). Aerobic capacity is most accurately measured through gas analysis to determine the **maximal oxygen uptake ($\dot{V}O_2$max),** or the total amount of oxygen the body is able to utilize per minute of physical activity. Chapter 7 discusses different methods used to measure aerobic capacity.

The aging process causes a progressive decline in $\dot{V}O_2$max that stems from the functional deterioration in essentially all components of the cardiorespiratory system, from the lungs to the mitochondria in skeletal muscle (Hepple, 2000). Maximal aerobic capacity decreases with advancing age in both men and women, regardless of physical fitness level (Fitzgerald, Tanaka, Tran, & Seals, 1997). An average decline of about 10 percent per decade in $\dot{V}O_2$max occurs from age 25 to age 65 (Hawkins, Marcell, Jaque, & Wiswell, 2001), which then slows at age 80 and older (Paterson, Cunningham, Koval, & St. Croix, 1999). Because of this decline, less physically demanding tasks require more of the work capacity reserves of healthy older adults. The heart and lungs may function adequately at rest and during light physical activity but may be severely taxed as exercise intensity increases (Scheuermann, Bell, Paterson, Barstow, & Kowalchuk, 2002).

Many factors are responsible for reduced exercise capacity. Factors that determine both oxygen supply and its delivery from the heart and lungs to skeletal muscle play a role in determining $\dot{V}O_2$max, as does oxygen diffusion between the red blood cells and mitochondria (Richardson, Harms, Grassi, & Hepple, 2000). Some of the age-associated changes in these components are similar to those that accompany prolonged inactivity. Thus, regular exercise and physical activity of sufficient intensity may improve the cardiorespiratory components of fitness substantially, even in the oldest and frailest adults.

The changes in the central and peripheral circulation that accompany aging and inactivity are diverse (see figure 4.2). **Maximal cardiac output,** the maximal amount of blood leaving the heart per minute of peak exercise, is reduced with aging, and the fraction of the blood flow from the heart that is distributed to muscles is reduced (Ho, Beard, Farrell, Minson, & Kenney, 1997). Maximal cardiac output declines at roughly the same rate as $\dot{V}O_2$max, an average decrease of 1 percent per year between age 35 and age 65 (Holloszy, 2001), which may account for most of the decrease in $\dot{V}O_2$max associated with aging. Other cardiovascular changes associated with aging that affect maximal aerobic capacity include reduced **maximal heart rate (HRmax,** the heart rate attained in the final minute of a progressive exercise stress test carried to the point of exhaustion, which decreases 5 to 10 beats per decade; Wiebe, Gledhill, Jamnik, & Ferguson, 1999), reduced or unchanged **maximal stroke volume** (the volume of blood pumped with each heart beat; Proctor, Beck, et al., 1998), and decreased arteriovenous oxygen difference (the difference between the oxygen content of arterial and venous blood; Paterson et al., 1999). In many older adults, these changes place enormous strain on the heart and can lead to serious signs and symptoms (e.g., dizziness, muscle cramps, or

Central changes	Peripheral changes
• Decreased maximal cardiac output	• Decreased blood flow to working muscles
• Reduced maximal stroke volume	• Reduced arteriovenous oxygen difference
• Decreased maximal heart rate	• Decreased oxidative capacity of working muscles
• Prolonged myocardial contraction time	• Decreased muscle mitochondrial number and density
• Progressive increases in systemic blood pressure	
• Decreased heart muscle response to catecholamines released during exercise	

FIGURE 4.2   Age-associated cardiovascular changes.

chest pain) when exercise intensity overtaxes their aerobic capabilities.

In healthy older adults, muscle oxygen consumption may also be limited by inadequate muscle blood flow or oxygen delivery in working muscles, especially when exercise is begun without an adequate warm-up (Scheuermann et al., 2002). Three common cardiovascular diseases that result from atherosclerotic narrowing of the arteries limit oxygen delivery throughout the body: peripheral arterial disease (PAD) (Womack, Ivey, Gardner, & Macko, 2001), coronary artery disease (CAD), and cerebrovascular disease (CVD). These conditions may drastically limit the duration and intensity of physical activity that older people can perform safely. Reduced blood flow to the heart from CAD may result in **angina pectoris,** a crushing chest pain that occurs with exertion. Reduced blood flow to the legs from PAD leads to intermittent claudication, an intense cramping pain in the legs with physical activity. Reduced blood flow to the brain from CVD can lead to disorientation or light-headedness with exercise. Exercise should be stopped immediately if any of these symptoms occur. Refer to chapter 21 for a more in-depth discussion of exercise considerations for common medical conditions.

Another major contributor to the decline in $\dot{V}O_2$max in older adults is the reduction in the oxidative capacity of muscles, that is, the ability of the muscle cell to generate energy from oxygen and energy substrates within the mitochondria. Mitochondrial volume density, respiration capacity, and oxidative enzyme activity appear to be reduced in aging muscle (Short & Nair, 2001), which may greatly limit the amount of aerobic exercise an older client can perform before the onset

> Progressive declines in aerobic capacity in older adults may severely tax the heart and lungs during exercise and hasten the onset of fatigue. Regular exercise and physical activity may improve cardiorespiratory fitness substantially.

of fatigue. Regular participation in aerobic activity enables working muscles to extract more oxygen from the blood and increases the oxidative capacity of mitochondria, even for older adults (Holloszy, 2001; Short & Nair, 2001). This leads to improvements in $\dot{V}O_2$max and increased exercise capacity with less fatigue. This mechanism is especially important for postmenopausal women, because training-induced adaptations in skeletal muscle oxygen consumption and utilization (peripheral changes) are mostly responsible for their gains in $\dot{V}O_2$max (McCole et al., 1999).

Maximal oxygen intake is further affected by an individual's initial level of aerobic capacity and changes in activity levels (Pollock et al., 1997). Long-term aerobic exercise training has been shown to decrease the rate of decline of $\dot{V}O_2$max due to aging (about 6-7 percent per decade) but not the rate of decline in maximal heart rate (Kasch et al., 1999). Through endurance training, aerobic capacity can be maintained late in life at a level that is similar to sedentary younger adults (Bouvier, Saltin, Nejat, & Jensen-Urstad, 2001). Despite this, endurance-trained older athletes average 40 percent lower pulmonary oxygen uptake than young endurance athletes, demonstrating that the age-dependent decline in aerobic capacity may be slowed by endurance training but cannot be stoppped entirely. Although maintaining the same level of activity may slow the inevitable changes that accompany aging, those changes cannot be forestalled entirely. Nonetheless, both older men and women can increase their aerobic capacity with endurance training and, as a result, lead potentially more active and fulfilling lives.

Functional Implications of Reduced Aerobic Capacity

The age-related decrease in maximal aerobic capacity is associated with increased risks of disability and death from all causes, as well as reductions in cognitive function and quality of life. (Eskurza, Donato, Moreau, Seals, & Tanaka, 2002). Moreover, a minimal level of aerobic capacity is necessary for older adults to continue independent daily functioning. Healthy, sedentary individuals over 75 years of age generally have a $\dot{V}O_2$max of 7 to 14 milliliters per kilogram per minute (2 to 4 metabolic equivalents, or METs), and those under 75 years can attain a $\dot{V}O_2$max of 17.5 to 24.5 milliliters per kilogram per minute (5 to 7 METs; Daley & Spinks, 2000). Metabolic equivalents (METs) indicate the intensity of activities; 1 MET is equal to resting oxygen consumption, or approximately 3.5 milliliters of oxygen per kilogram of body mass per minute. However, the minimal level of aerobic capacity compatible with an independent life at age 85 appears to be approximately 18 milliliters per kilogram per minute (5 METs) for men and 15 milliliters per kilogram per minute (4.3 METs) for women (Paterson et al., 1999). Thus, by the age of 80 to 85 years, the maximal oxygen intake of many people has dropped to or below the threshold required for independent living. A short-term gain in aerobic capacity of 5 milliliters per kilogram per minute brought about through increased physical activity may be equivalent to a 10-year reduction in biological age (Shephard, 1997).

In addition, a person's ability to perform vigorous and prolonged exercise declines with age, as ventilatory and circulatory responses to exercise become attenuated (Ishida, Sato, Katayama, & Miyamura, 2000). A longer time is needed for ventilation, heart rate, blood pressure, and oxygen consumption to reach equilibrium at any given work rate. This can strain the cardiopulmonary systems of older adults, especially at the start of an exercise session, if the period of warm-up activity before beginning higher-intensity exercises is inadequate (Scheuer-

A sufficient warm-up before exercise and cooldown after exercise are absolutely essential for older adults to minimize the risk of many serious abnormal cardiac responses to sudden changes in cardiovascular demand.

mann et al., 2002). Older adults are also likely to fatigue if exercise is sustained for more than a few minutes at 70 to 75 percent of peak oxygen intake (an intensity perceived as hard or equivalent to a rating of perceived exertion [RPE] of 14 or 15). The 6-20 RPE scale is discussed in detail in chapter 7.

In addition, the aging heart is more vulnerable to rhythm disorders (Billman, 2001), particularly **ventricular fibrillation,** a dangerously rapid, erratic heart rhythm. An older exercise participant with heart disease may experience symptoms of chest pain, shortness of breath, or other signs of exertional intolerance because of insufficient cardiac blood supply during the critical period at the beginning of exercise. A sufficiently long warm-up period (10-20 minutes) of lower-intensity activity allows time for the cardiopulmonary adaptations necessary for safe exercise. Equally important is an adequate cool-down period that allows for the increased recovery time necessary for older adults (Franklin, 2000). Inadequate cool-down may result in venous pooling in the legs that leads to rapid drops in blood pressure and light-headedness or fainting after exercise. Inadequate cool-down also increases the likelihood of postexercise cardiac rhythm disturbances brought on by high levels of circulating exercise hormones (norepinephrine) after strenuous exercise (Billman, 2001). Refer to chapter 10 for more information on warm-up and cool-down.

Heart Rate

The autonomic nervous system exerts an enormous influence over homeostatic cardiovascular dynamics through the interplay of its two components, the parasympathetic and sympathetic nervous systems. Aging contributes to a reduction of autonomic regulation of the heart independent of physical fitness (Perini, Fisher, Veicsteinas, & Pendergast, 2002). Although resting heart rate largely remains unchanged with age (Franklin, 2000), the ability of the heart to increase contractions in response to both submaximal and maximal exercise is reduced as a result of changes in the cardiac conduction system or the dynamic regulation of the heart by the autonomic nervous system (Perini et al., 2002). Maximal heart rate (HRmax) decreases by as much as 10 beats per decade from its peak at age 20. Paterson and colleagues (1999) found, however, that HRmax is not well predicted by age. In fact, they question the use of age-predicted maximal heart rate in estimating aerobic fitness, because HRmax calculated from the common predictive equation (HRmax = 220 – age) underestimated the measured HRmax in both men (by 6-11 beats per minute) and women (7-9 beats per minute) in their study. Beta-blocker medication, commonly prescribed to older adults for high blood pressure and cardiac conditions, also has a profound impact on resting heart rate, lowering it by as much as 30 beats per minute. Thus, an RPE scale may be a much safer way to determine the appropriate exercise intensity for older clients than the use of exercise heart rate. Refer to chapter 13 for more information on aerobic endurance training and monitoring of RPE.

The age-related changes in both parasympathetic and sympathetic control of the heart may have other important clinical and exercise implications. Reductions in parasympathetic activity can lead to heart rate and arterial blood pressure variability, both of which may potentially (although very rarely) lead to lethally rapid heart rates and sudden cardiac death (Seals, Monahan, Bell, Tanaka, & Jones, 2001). These changes in heart rate and arterial blood pressure may lead to serious symptoms that should signal the immediate curtailment of exercise.

Blood Pressure

Resting and exercise blood pressures rise progressively with age (Franklin, 2000). Increased blood pressure elevates the heart's work rate and oxygen needs at any given intensity of exercise and may pose a threat to people with hypertension (blood pressure levels above 140/90 mmHg), especially when exercising at high intensity. Lifestyle factors that affect blood pressure include smoking, alcohol consumption, obesity, and sedentary living (Kasch et al., 1999). Dynamic aerobic training reduces blood pressure, although the mechanisms responsible for the reduction remain largely unknown (Moreau et al., 2001). The blood-pressure-lowering effect of exercise is more pronounced in people

with stage I hypertension (an approximately 7/6 mmHg decrease) than in people with normal blood pressure (an approximately 3/2 mmHg decrease). The blood pressure response to dynamic aerobic training does not appear to differ at training intensities between 40 percent and 70 percent of $\dot{V}O_2$max, equivalent to 55 to 80 percent of maximal heart rate or an RPE of 12 to 15 (moderate to hard intensity). It also appears to be similar at training frequencies between three and five sessions per week and for session durations between 30 and 60 minutes (Fagard, 2001).

Pulmonary Changes

Pulmonary efficiency also declines with age. The vital capacity of the lungs (the maximal volume of air that a person can exhale after maximal inspiration) decreases progressively, up to 40 or 50 percent by the age of 70. The efficiency of gas exchange within the lungs also declines steadily with age. Between the ages of 30 and 70, **maximal voluntary ventilation** (the maximal volume of air that can be breathed per minute by voluntary effort) diminishes up to 50 percent, while **residual lung volume** (the amount of air remaining in the lung at the end of a maximal expiration) increases 30 percent to 50 percent (Daley & Spinks, 2000).

Much of the steady, age-related functional decline stems from decreased respiratory muscle strength, increased chest wall stiffness, and small airway closure. Loss of elasticity in the pulmonary connective tissue results in reduced maximal alveolar ventilation (the maximal amount of air exchanged between the atmosphere and the alveoli in the lungs) during exercise in older adults. Reduced chest wall compliance increases the work of breathing for older people at any given ventilation level and leads to an increased demand for blood flow by the respiratory muscles. Greater competition for blood flow among respiratory muscles, locomotor muscles, and skin during exercise may lead to early onset of fatigue as exercise intensity increases (Proctor, Shen, et al., 1998). Moderate- to high-intensity physical training, however, may prevent the age-related decline in resting lung function until about age 60 (Pollock et al., 1997). Forms of exercise that focus on deep, diaphragmatic breathing and increasing elasticity in the thoracic cage, such as yoga, tai chi, qigong, and Pilates, have been shown to improve pulmonary function. Refer to chapter 15 for more information on the benefits of mind–body exercise, which

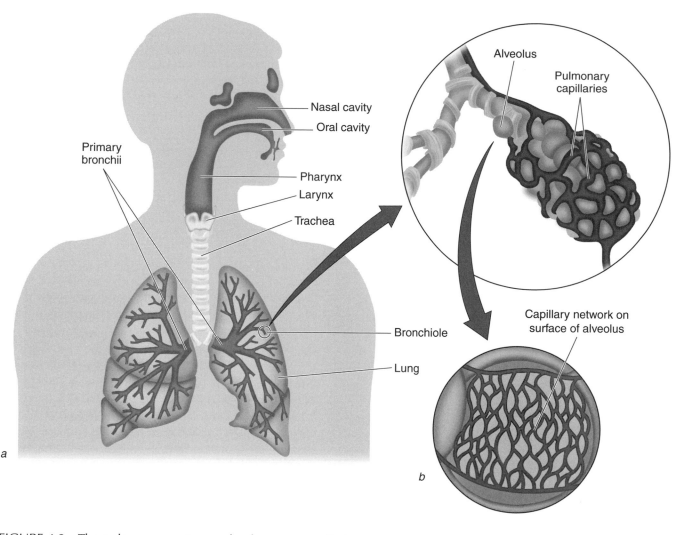

FIGURE 4.3   The pulmonary system and pulmonary ventilation.

Reprinted, by permission, from J.H. Wilmore and D.L. Costill, 2004, *Physiology of Sport and Exercise,* 3rd ed. (Champaign, IL: Human Kinetics), 245.

often focuses on breathing. Figure 4.3 illustrates pulmonary ventilation.

Pulmonary gas exchange does not usually limit exercise performance in older people unless they have some form of chronic cardiac or pulmonary disease. Shortness of breath, however, often causes older adults to voluntarily end exercise sessions when the volume of individual breaths reaches around 50 percent of vital capacity. This level of breathlessness appears to be less tolerated by older individuals who have not recently participated in moderate to strenuous physical activity. As physical activity becomes a regular habit, an older client will be able to use a larger fraction of the available vital capacity before stopping effort because of the sensation of breathlessness.

Muscle Function

Muscular weakness and **sarcopenia** (loss of muscle mass) are conspicuous age-associated deficits that lead to such consequences as reductions in aerobic capacity, bone density, insulin sensitivity, and metabolic rate and increases in body fat, blood pressure, and prevalence of cardiovascular disease and diabetes mellitus. Age-related strength reduction in the lower extremities has also been associated with balance and mobility problems leading to physical disability and loss of independence (Connelly, 2000). Age-related changes in muscle function are caused by a number of factors, including genetics, disease, diet, stress, and especially physical inactiv-

- Sarcopenia (decreased muscle mass)
- Decreased muscle strength
- Decreased muscle power
- Decreased muscle endurance
- Decreased aerobic enzyme activity in muscle mitochondria

FIGURE 4.4   Age-associated changes in muscle function.

ity. Figure 4.4 summarizes some of the age-related decreases in muscle function.

Muscle Mass

Skeletal muscle is composed of two principal types of contractile fibers. **Type I muscle fibers** are slow contracting and slow to fatigue, while **type II muscle fibers** are fast contracting and quick to fatigue. Researchers have found that type I fibers show little change with advancing age, with the exception of the antigravity muscles (Thompson, 2002). Type II fibers, on the other hand, have a 25 percent to 50 percent reduction in the number and size of muscle fibers. Because of the high concentration of type II fibers in the back and thighs (quadriceps and hamstrings), these muscles are the first to atrophy in older adults. Selective atrophy (shrinking) and loss of type II fibers, especially in the trunk and lower body, appear to be caused mainly by decreased use of these muscles and the lack of high-intensity physical activity needed to activate this fiber type (Landers, Hunter, Wetzstein, Bamman, & Wiensier, 2001).

One of the major consequences of sarcopenia and a reduction in the number of **motor units** (defined as a single motor neuron and all the muscle fibers it innervates) is loss of muscle strength (Fiatarone Singh, 2000). Muscle strength decreases approximately 30 percent on average between the ages of 50 and 70 years, with even more dramatic strength losses after age 80. As with muscle mass, there is a much greater loss of muscle strength in the lower extremities, which is highly associated with mobility problems. Therefore, exercise interventions designed for older adults should concentrate on maximizing recruitment of motor units and promoting hypertrophy of existing muscle fibers, especially type II fibers in the muscles of the back, buttocks, thighs, and calves.

Muscle Power

Power is defined as the rate at which work is performed and is calculated by dividing work by time. The ability of skeletal muscles to generate power is important for the performance of many daily activities, ranging from instrumental tasks (e.g., bathing, dressing, cooking, etc.) to recreational activities (Krivickas et al., 2001). However, the ability to develop muscle power diminishes with age to an even greater extent than muscle strength (Foldvari et al., 2000). The diminished ability of older muscles to produce power is caused by a combination of factors including decreased habitual physical activity, selective atrophy of type II muscle fibers, and a decrease in the number of motor units, particularly those of high-threshold, fast-twitch fibers. This combination results in decreased force production and decreased contraction speed, that is, loss of the ability to move quickly against force (Krivickas et al., 2001).

Age- and sex-related differences in muscle power may partially explain the impairments in muscle function that occur with aging and the greater muscle impairment observed in older women than in older men. Reduced leg power, for example, may impair performance more than reduced strength does in older adults because many basic daily activities, including fast walking, climbing stairs, quickly rising from a seated position, or recovering from tripping, require leg muscle power.

Effect of Endurance and Resistance Training on Muscle Function

Fortunately, many of the age- and disuse-associated changes in muscle physiology and function can be modified with exercise. Endurance training can improve the aerobic function of muscle. Resistance training can improve central nervous system recruitment, increase muscle mass (Short & Nair, 2001), and improve both aerobic and anaerobic function in older individuals (Slade, Miszko, Laity, Agrawal, & Cress, 2002; Vincent & Braith, 2002). Resistance training has been shown

> Aerobic endurance training and resistance training both can minimize, and even reverse, many of the age-associated losses in muscular integrity.

to reduce or prevent a number of functional declines associated with aging. It is considered an important intervention for reversing sarcopenia, muscle weakness, and loss of muscle power (Roth et al., 2000). Resistance training is also an effective way to improve bone health, improve postural stability, increase flexibility and range of motion, increase energy requirements, decrease body fat mass, and maintain metabolically active tissue in healthy older people (Hunter, Wetzstein, Fields, Brown, & Bamman, 2000; Fatouras et al., 2002). Additional information related to resistance training is presented in chapter 12.

Joint Mobility

Flexibility, the ability to move a joint through its full range of motion, is an important component of health that is related to bone, muscle, and connective tissue integrity. Limitation of joint movement and some degenerative change in the musculoskeletal system are the natural consequences of aging and prolonged physical inactivity. One of the major causes of joint stiffness, a common problem in older adults, is **joint contracture,** a stiffening or shortening of the ligaments, tendons, joint capsules, muscles, fascia, and skin around the joint that reduces joint mobility (Harada, 1995).

Flexibility has been found to decline 20 to 50 percent between the ages of 30 and 70 years, depending on the joint examined (Fatouras et al., 2002). Reductions in range of motion (ROM) often lead to problems performing such essential daily tasks as climbing stairs, dressing without assistance, and getting into and out of a bath or a car (Barbosa, Santarem, Filho, & Marucci, 2002). Loss of flexibility also increases the possibility of injury to the joint or muscles crossing the joint and the likelihood of falls from loss of balance and stability (Fatouras et al., 2002).

Fortunately, most musculoskeletal flexibility can be maintained in later years by using joints through their full ROM and by participating in physical activities that stretch the muscles that span joints. Active older adults are more flexible than inactive ones, particularly in the hips, spine, ankles, and knees (Daley & Spinks, 2000). Static and dynamic stretching, aerobic exercise, and resistance training have been shown to increase ROM in older adults, although the training effect is joint specific (Barbosa et al., 2002; Fatouras et al., 2002). In addition, regular activity may reduce the degree of pain or disability associated with degenerative joint disease (Ettinger et al., 1997). It is crucial that the joint be moved safely through its full ROM for the greatest improvements in flexibility. The topic of flexibility training is discussed in greater depth in chapter 11.

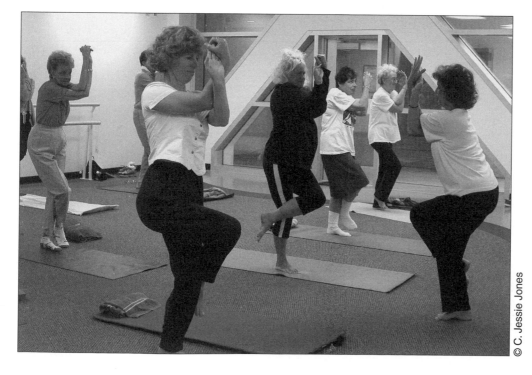

© C. Jessie Jones

Joint mobility can be maintained in later years by stretching the muscles that span joints.

Bone Mass

Both women and men lose bone mass as a normal part of skeletal aging (Bougie, 2001). At any given age, **bone mineral density (BMD),** the proportion of deposited mineral salts to organic bone matrix, is lower in women than in men. BMD is related to bone mass at maturity (peak bone mass) and subsequent bone loss. Peak BMD is usually reached by approximately 25 years of age (Marcus, 2001). BMD then remains fairly stable until about the age of 50, when progressive losses of calcium and deterioration of the organic matrix of bones occur in men and women. Women lose calcium particularly rapidly in the five years after menopause (Drinkwater, 1994). Bone density losses with aging parallel those of lean body mass, though most people lose muscle strength well before the onset of bone loss (Burr, 1997). However, these changes do not usually have a substantial effect until age 70. When a person's BMD measurement is 2.5 standard deviations below that of a young, normal adult, he or she is diagnosed with osteoporosis. BMD is typically measured at the hip and spine using dual-energy X-ray absorptiometry (DEXA; see figure

4.5). Although women are three times more likely to develop osteoporosis than men, statistics indicate that approximately 1.5 million American men over 65 years of age also have osteoporosis (Siddiqui, Shetty, & Duthie, 1999).

The major consequences of osteoporosis are spine, hip, and wrist fractures that often occur in response to minor stresses. Women have a 40 percent chance of sustaining a fracture during their lifetime (Metcalfe et al., 2001). Older adults with smaller bones (e.g., women and Asians) are more susceptible to fractures (Bougie, 2001). People suffering hip fractures often experience a loss of independence; less than one third of those who fracture their hips recover sufficiently to perform basic and instrumental activities of life. The mortality rate for hip fractures is also very high in frail, older adults. Vertebral fractures, which often are not diagnosed, can lead to loss of height, postural changes, increased thoracic kyphosis (humpback), and persistent pain when multiple fractures occur (Eagan & Sedlock, 2001). Unfortunately, many patients diagnosed with osteoporosis are told by their physicians to reduce physical activity to prevent fractures. Although exercises that involve spinal flexion (bending forward), twisting, and sudden

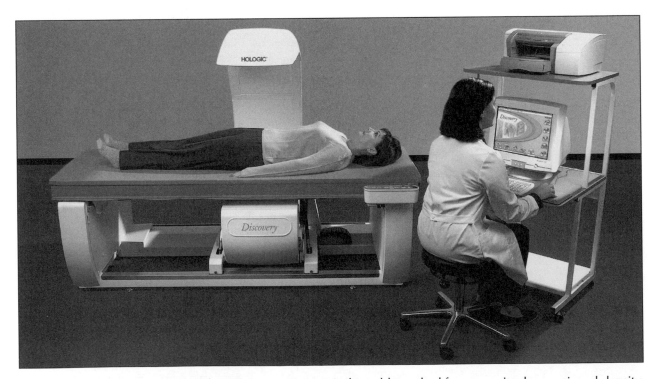

FIGURE 4.5   Dual-energy X-ray absorptiometry (DEXA) is the gold standard for measuring bone mineral density.
Centers for Disease Control and Prevention (2002). Promoting active lifestyles among older adults. National center for chronic disease prevention and health promotion. Nutrition and Physical activity. http://www.cdc.gov/nccdphp/dnpa/physical/lifestyles.htm.

movements should be avoided, physical activity is essential for preserving bone mass and functional mobility. Special exercise considerations for clients with osteoporosis are discussed in chapter 21.

Effective exercise-training programs may prevent or reverse bone loss at the lumbar spine and femoral neck (hip) of pre- and postmenopausal women by almost 1 percent per year (Blanchet et al., 2002). For bone modeling to result from exercise, however, the intensity of the stimulus appears to be more important than its frequency (Vincent & Braith, 2002). Greater loads and fewer repetitions result in greater gains in bone mass than lower loads repeated more times (Metcalfe et al., 2001). Weight-bearing endurance exercise and resistance exercise have both been found to increase bone mass at clinically relevant sites (hip, spine, wrist) in older men and women, but only when the exercise is quite vigorous (Kohrt, 2001). Activities of low to moderate intensity have had mixed results in elderly adults; appreciable gains in strength but variable changes in bone density have been documented (Humphries et al., 2000).

Exercises that introduce skeletal stress through ground-reaction forces (e.g., walking, jogging, and stair climbing) appear to be more effective for building bone in the femoral neck, a common fracture site, than those that introduce skeletal stress through joint-reaction forces (e.g., weightlifting and rowing). Both types of exercise, however, effectively increase bone density of the whole body, lumbar spine, and proximal femur (Kohrt, Ehsani, & Birge, 1997). Long-term training using weighted vests and jumping has also been found to maintain BMD and to prevent significant bone loss in older postmenopausal women (Snow, Shaw, Winters, & Witzke, 2000). Other investigations show that leg press, overhead press, and lumbar extension exercises have the greatest influence on both site-specific and total-body BMD (Vincent & Braith, 2002). In addition, a program of gradually progressive resistance training that strengthens the back extensor muscles can be safely done by patients with vertebral osteoporosis and results in reduced pain and improved ability to perform activities of daily living (Marcus, 2001). Though resistance training may produce small gains in bone strength after relatively short (three-month) training periods in bone-depleted older individuals, resistance training must be continued over the long term to preserve bone mass in all older individuals (Snow et al., 2000).

Neurological Function

Disorders of the nervous system are some of the most common causes of disability in people over age 65 (Silvestrone, 2001). Normal aging of the nervous system is characterized by slow, sometimes continuous changes in cognition, motor function, and the special senses (vision, hearing, smell, and taste). Although we accept these changes as inevitable, they may be greatly influenced by factors such as nutritional status and continued intellectual, sensory, and motor stimulation (Timiras, 1994). The most important areas of neurological change that accompany normal aging occur in cognitive abilities and memory, movement speed, posture, balance, and gait (Katzman & Terry, 1991). Age-associated changes in the special senses of vision and hearing may also have a profound impact on the lives of older adults.

Changes in Cognition

Aging is associated with a decline in cognitive functions, including memory, attention, intelligence, and speed of information processing (slowed reaction time is the outcome of this neurological change; see figure 4.6). These declines may eventually make it difficult, if not impossible, for an older adult to live independently (Van Boxtel et al., 1997). Aging does not affect all individuals in the same way, so the degree to which cognitive function declines varies considerably among older adults (Etnier & Landers, 1997). Most, though not all, older adults develop some degree of memory impairment as they age, especially after age 70. Moreover, women over age 85 are more likely to experience cognitive loss than are men (Gonzales McNeal et al., 2001). Although this sex-related effect is not fully understood, several explanations have been proposed. They include

---

- Short-term, or recent, memory loss
- Slower information-processing speed, especially at points of decision making
- Cognitive performance declines, especially when attention is divided
- Slower reaction time

FIGURE 4.6   Common age-associated changes in cognition.

sex differences in disease causation, stronger natural selection on men that ensures that only those men with the healthiest overall constitution live to advanced age, and social or environmental differences that give men an advantage.

The aging process does not affect all aspects of intelligence and memory equally, and it appears to affect motor performance differently based on the nature of the task (Silvestrone, 2001). General intelligence consists of two components: fluid and crystallized intelligence. **Fluid intelligence** is the ability to think on one's feet, that is, performance in abstractions and relations, reasoning, and problem solving. Conversely, **crystallized intelligence,** or what someone knows, involves verbal, numerical, spatial, and mechanical abilities. Age negatively affects performance on tests of fluid intelligence but appears to have no effect or even a positive effect on tests of crystallized intelligence (Etnier & Berry, 2001).

Memory changes with aging may be sporadic and scattered and are more related to changes in fluid intelligence. The most common complaints from older adults concern retention of names, misplacement of items, and impaired recall of daily events (Silvestrone, 2001). These complaints involve mostly short-term memory of events that are considered irrelevant or not associated with other ideas or memories. One explanation for this is an age-related limitation in physiological resources: Older adults in general may have insufficient oxygen transport to the brain, decreased neurotransmitter synthesis, and an overall decrease in cerebral metabolism that may explain declines in fluid intelligence (Etnier & Landers, 1997).

Some loss of cognitive processing speed is normal as we age; steady declines are evident from the third decade of life (Silvestrone, 2001). Dividing the attention tends to further slow the cognitive performance of older adults. Older individuals find it particularly difficult to simultaneously store and manipulate or reorganize material or to perform one task when a secondary concurrent task is added. During an exercise class, for example, when an older client is intently concentrating on a particular movement or exercise (e.g., cycling, stair climbing), she or he may stop that movement completely if someone asks her or him a question. Processing incoming information, especially when it is complex, is more problematic for older adults than is holding and rehearsing the information. The increase in central processing time with aging

underlies part of the difficulty older clients have in learning and remembering information presented to them. Your clients may also require more time to register and process new information, especially if it is abstract. They may also find it more difficult to recall information spoken faster.

Researchers have demonstrated that physical activity and resulting gains in physical fitness have many beneficial effects on memory and other aspects of cognition in elderly persons (Etnier & Berry, 2001; Laurin, Verreault, Lindsay, MacPherson, & Rockwood, 2001; Yaffe, Barnes, Nevitt, Lui, & Covinski, 2001). The cognitive tasks that demonstrate the closest correlation to physical fitness tend to be those that are novel and unpracticed and require considerable attentional demand for successful performance (Etnier & Landers, 1997; Van Boxtel et al., 1997). Moreover, greater gains in aerobic fitness may also confer bigger gains in cognitive function for both men and women (Yaffe et al., 2001).

Several physiological mechanisms may explain the potentially protective effects of physical activity on cognitive function (Laurin et al., 2001; Yaffe et al., 2001). Physical activity appears to sustain cerebral blood flow by decreasing blood pressure, lowering blood lipid (cholesterol and triglyceride) levels, inhibiting platelet aggregability (preventing blood clotting), and enhancing cerebral metabolic demands. There is also evidence that exercise may improve aerobic capacity and cerebral nutrient supply and stimulate neuronal growth and survival.

Functional Implications of Cognitive Decline

A minimal level of cognitive function is necessary for independent living. Cognitive abilities also have a clear relationship to risk of falls (Rappaport, Hanks, Millis, & Deshpande, 1998). The ability to think flexibly and to incorporate external feedback appears to be essential for safe mobility. Older adults with motor and sensory impairments whose judgment and cognitive abilities remain intact are aware of the difficulties imposed by their functional limitations and interact with their environment in an efficient, effective manner, particularly under novel circumstances. They are less likely to initiate behavior that jeopardizes their safety. In contrast, older adults with severe cognitive impairments engage in dangerous behaviors that place them at high risk of falls because of impulsiveness, difficulties in problem solving, and inability to benefit from feedback (Morgenthal, 2001).

Changes in Sensory and Motor Function

Age-related changes in the central and peripheral nervous systems result in slowed simple and choice reaction times and reduced nerve conduction velocities (by 10 to 15 percent), as well as changes in the ability to integrate incoming sensory information (Daley & Spinks, 2000; Morgenthal, 2001). Significant neurological changes include decreased **proprioception** (sense of limb position and movement) at the foot and ankle, decreased vibratory sensation in the feet, and reduced vestibular system function (Morgenthal, 2001). These changes are continuous and progressive with advancing age and affect the lower extremity more than the upper extremity.

The performance of motor tasks requiring central nervous system (CNS) processing is slowed with age, particularly those requiring sensory integration, organization, or response preparation (Alexander, 1994). Slower reaction times may be related to the loss of precise control over the speed at which responses can be made or to the loss of fine differentiation between fast and slow responses. Older adults may commit more serious motor performance errors when they are required to move faster than their ability to move accurately. Slowing the pace of activities performed by older clients may increase their motor performance success and their safety.

Somatosensory abnormalities, such as impaired position sense (knowledge of the position of body parts relative to each other and the orientation of the body in space) or touch sensitivity, are associated with increased incidence of falls and postural instability (Hughes, Duncan, Rose, Chandler, & Studenski, 1996). Age-associated changes in posi-

> Older adults may make more errors when they are required to move faster than their ability to move accurately. As with other types of movement, the compensatory movements that enable a person to adjust to a demand for increased speed come into play more slowly for older adults.

tion sense occur earlier in men than in women. Age-related changes in CNS processing also affect lower-extremity motions directly related to maintaining stance (Alexander, 1994). When multiple joints and multiple movement options are involved, age-related slowing in central processing may substantially influence responses to an unexpected loss of balance.

Foot position awareness also declines with age, and inappropriate footwear can significantly exacerbate this impairment (Robbins, Waked, & McClaran, 1995). Age and footwear affect position sense mainly through plantar (sole of the foot) tactile sensibility. Footwear with low heels and thin, hard soles should be recommended for use by unstable older persons to maximize proprioceptive input. More detailed information about age-associated changes in the sensory, cognitive, and motor systems, including the benefits of balance and mobility training, is given in chapter 14.

Changes in Vision and Hearing

Both optical and neurological elements of vision undergo age-related changes (Silvestrone, 2001). Anatomic changes in the cornea, lens, iris, vitreous humor, and visual cortex result in progressive visual changes, some of which may start early in life. Visual acuity decreases with age, with some impairment of near vision and focus, particularly after age 50. Changes in spatial frequency sensitivity, peripheral vision, glare sensitivity, dark adaptation, depth perception, and contrast sensitivity are also observed with aging (Morgenthal, 2001). Increased light is necessary to see an object because of decreased contrast sensitivity. A 12 to 14 percent loss of visual field in older adults, coupled with sensory and motor deficits, results in an increase in automobile accidents involving adults over 65 years old. Compromised dark adaptation and problems associated with glare may compound difficulties in driving at night, negotiating obstacles, and maintaining balance and mobility.

Hearing and vestibular function also diminish with age (Daley & Spinks, 2000). Normal hearing and interpretation of sounds depend on acuity, localization of sound, and the ability to mask extraneous sounds, all of which decline with age (Silvestrone, 2001). Older people commonly complain of hearing someone speak but not being able to make sense of the words. In addition, the ability to listen selectively to sounds or to mask

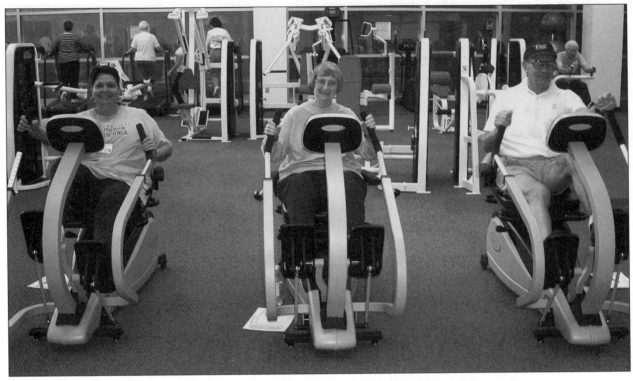

© C. Jessie Jones

An exercise environment that is well lighted and clutter free is safer for participants who have vision or hearing impairments.

> The most important neurological changes associated with aging are changes in cognitive ability and memory, decrements in vision and hearing, loss of motor speed, and balance and gait impairments.

background noise is required for interpreting conversation or other situations involving multiple auditory inputs, yet this ability is often impaired with age. Hearing impairment is complicated by reverberating or echoing noises, presentation that is too rapid, frequent interruptions, or tinnitus (ringing in the ears). Tinnitus may be a more common complaint in older adults because they cannot mask background noises.

Functional Implications of Vision and Hearing Impairments

An exercise area should be well lighted to compensate for age-associated visual deficits. Impairments

of vision or hearing may hamper the comprehension of instructions during activity sessions. Instructions should be written in large type or spoken clearly and slowly, and the instructor should observe clients' comprehension. The exercise area should be kept free of objects that might cause tripping or collisions. If a client has a history of frequent falls or postural instability, physical activity can still be performed in a seated or standing position if adequate external support is available (e.g., chair, wall bars). Impaired sight and hearing, poor balance, slower reaction times, slower movement times, impaired righting reflexes, and less-powerful muscles make older adults increasingly susceptible to falls during exercise (Overstall & Downton, 1998).

Summary

The functions of most body systems decline with age. These changes progressively limit the functional capacity of older adults and increase their risk for various diseases and injuries. The normal effects of aging are worsened by age-related decreases in habitual physical activity and the onset of chronic disease to the extent that functional declines are due mostly to the cumulative burden imposed by sedentary lifestyles and chronic diseases, not aging alone. Cardiovascular capacity, respiratory function, muscle integrity, joint mobility, bone mass, and neurological function all decline with age but much more so in physically inactive older adults and those afflicted with chronic conditions involving these systems. Furthermore, declines in these body systems contribute to and perpetuate functional mobility deficits and disability, as threshold levels of aerobic capacity, lung function, and muscle strength determine one's ability to live independently.

However, a well-designed exercise-training program for older adults can increase function by a similar percentage as in young adults. The optimal program should provide aerobic activities to enhance cardiorespiratory function, resistance exercises to strengthen the main muscle groups, weight-bearing exercises to strengthen the bones, range-of-motion exercises to increase flexibility in the major joints, and activities designed to enhance balance. Although the aging process is not reversed by physical activity, it is slowed, and at any given age, gains in functional capacity can counteract the adverse effects of 10 to 20 years of aging. Enhanced function extends independence and improves quality-adjusted life expectancy.

Key Terms

Recommended Readings

Bougie, J.D., & Morgenthal, A.P. (Eds.). (2001). *The aging body: Conservative management of common neuromusculoskeletal conditions.* New York: McGraw-Hill.

Shephard, R.J. (2001). *Gender, physical activity and aging.* Boca Raton, FL: CRC.

Study Questions

1. The maximal oxygen intake of a 50-year-old man has decreased by 20 percent over the past 10 years. How should this be interpreted?
   a. This is a fairly typical rate for the aging of oxygen transport.
   b. The rate is slower than normal; the client should be congratulated on a healthy lifestyle.
   c. This individual will be unable to participate in regular physical activity.
   d. The normal effects of aging have probably been exacerbated by a decrease in daily activity and an accumulation of body fat.

2. Which of the following does not contribute to the decrease in cardiac output in an older person?
   a. an increase in extraction of oxygen from the circulating blood
   b. a decrease in filling of the ventricles
   c. a decrease in maximal heart rate
   d. a decrease in responsiveness of the heart to catecholamines

(continued)

3. Why would a sedentary 60-year-old woman complain of severe breathlessness when exercising on a cycle ergometer, even at a light to moderate level of exercise intensity?
   a. She has reached maximal effort.
   b. Because of her sedentary lifestyle, she has no recent experience with sensations associated with vigorous effort.
   c. She has some form of acute respiratory disease.
   d. There is some technical error in the pulse counter.

4. A 60-year-old woman claims to have maintained a constant body weight over the past 10 years, although she engages in little physical activity. What would you think is the most likely explanation of this?
   a. She has managed to avoid an accumulation of fat by careful dieting.
   b. Her activities of daily living are sufficient to control her weight.
   c. There is little tendency for most people to accumulate fat over the second half of adult life.
   d. Fat accumulation has been masked by the loss of an equal mass of lean tissue.

5. Which of the following would be unlikely to contribute to maintenance of bone density in an older adult?
   a. weight-supported activities such as pool exercises
   b. a resistance-training program
   c. a high-calcium diet
   d. ingestion of vitamin D supplements

6. An 80-year-old man has a maximal oxygen intake of 15 milliliters per kilogram per minute. What comment would you make to him?
   a. This is an above-average value for your age. Keep up the good work!
   b. You have allowed your level of aerobic fitness to drop to a level where you will soon have difficulty living independently.
   c. Given the level of fitness that you have reached, you should have no difficulty completing a masters marathon this summer.
   d. Your aerobic fitness is good, but you should engage in more resistance exercises.

7. A 90-year-old woman has engaged in resistance exercises for 10 weeks. What changes would you expect to see?
   a. No changes in muscle strength can be achieved at this age.
   b. Strength can be enhanced, but no gains are likely to be seen in less than a year of steady activity.
   c. Strength will increase, but there will be little if any increase in lean tissue mass in such a period of time.
   d. Her muscle bulk will be restored to that of someone 10 to 20 years younger.

Application Activities

1. Now that you better understand the effects of age-related changes in various body systems, make a list of all the important things that you, as an instructor, must do to ensure that the exercise environment is safe for older adults. Which types of exercises are appropriate for older adults, and which might prove unsafe for them because of age-related physiological changes?

2. What elements of program design would you emphasize to improve the overall health and fitness of a recently retired, relatively sedentary 67-year-old man referred by his physician? In general, his health is good, although he is slightly overweight. His former career was very

stressful and time-consuming, and he has not participated in any regular physical activity for many years.

3. What elements of program design would you emphasize to improve the overall health and fitness of a frail 85-year-old woman who entered an assisted-living residence this year? She has been diagnosed with osteoporosis and has a history of wrist fracture. What special considerations or accommodations should you make because of her condition? Which types of exercise would be both safe and beneficial for her? Which types would be inappropriate?

Part II

Screening, Assessment, and Goal Setting

TRAINING MODULE 1:
Overview of Aging and Physical Activity

TRAINING MODULE 2:
Psychological, Sociocultural, and Physiological Aspects of Physical Activity and Older Adults

TRAINING MODULE 9:
Ethics and Professional Conduct

TRAINING MODULE 8:
Client Safety and First Aid

International Curriculum Guidelines for Preparing Physical Activity Instructors of Older Adults

TRAINING MODULE 3:
Screening, Assessment, and Goal Setting

TRAINING MODULE 4:
Program Design and Management

TRAINING MODULE 7:
Leadership, Communication, and Marketing Skills

TRAINING MODULE 6:
Teaching Skills

TRAINING MODULE 5:
Program Design for Older Adults With Stable Medical Conditions

Now that you have a basic understanding of the aging process, the psychological, sociocultural, and physiological aspects of physical activity, and have been introduced to the field of gerokinesiology, the next step is learning how to gather information that is specific to the needs and goals of your prospective clients. This second part of the book addresses training modules 3 and 4 of the *International Curriculum Guidelines for Preparing Physical Activity Instructors of Older Adults*. Module 3 recommends areas of study that include information on selection, administration, and interpretation of preexercise health and activity screening, and fitness and mobility assessments appropriate for older adults. Module 3 also recommends areas of study that include information on establishing, with client input, realistic and measurable short-, medium-, and long-term goals. This information will provide the basis for exercise program design and appropriate referrals to other health professionals. Module 4 recommends areas of study that include information about how to use the results obtained from screening, assessment, and client goal-setting activities to make appropriate decisions regarding individual and group physical activity and exercise program design and management. These topics are addressed in chapters 5 through 8.

• Chapter 5 presents guidelines for the choice and use of screening tools to determine the overall health, physical activity, and disability status of older adult participants. A screening tool to identify risk factors of coronary heart disease is also introduced in this chapter. How to share screening results with clients and how to maintain confidentiality is also discussed in this chapter.

• Chapter 6 introduces you to the functional fitness framework that can be used to guide the selection of sound field-based assessment tools.

These tools are used to assess physical impairments and functional limitations among older adults. This chapter describes several assessment tools that are appropriate for use in field settings as well as guidelines for the administration of the various assessments in group settings.

• Chapter 7 discusses various laboratory-based physiological assessments, including tests that objectively measure cardiorespiratory function, muscle strength and endurance, body composition, and balance. This chapter also addresses when these tools should be used in the assessment of older adults. Detailed instructions for administering and interpreting the results of key laboratory tests are also provided. The knowledge and skills gained from these chapters will serve as the basis for the development and implementation of exercise programs that are effective, safe, and target the specific needs of older adults at different functional levels. The screening and assessment tools described will also help the physical activity instructor monitor client progress and evaluate the training program.

• Chapter 8 describes the major personal, environmental, and program-related factors that influence the older adults' motivation to be physically active. Important theories of behavioral change that guide the planning, delivery, and evaluation of physical activity programs are also discussed. The cognitive and behavioral strategies presented for both group and individual settings will help you motivate older adults to make physical activity an integral part of their lives. Finally, you will learn how to develop an individualized behavior modification plan, including short- and long-term goal development, progress monitoring, problem-solving skills to help clients overcome obstacles to physical activity, and rewards and incentives to support behavioral change.

5

Preexercise and Health Screening

Michael E. Rogers

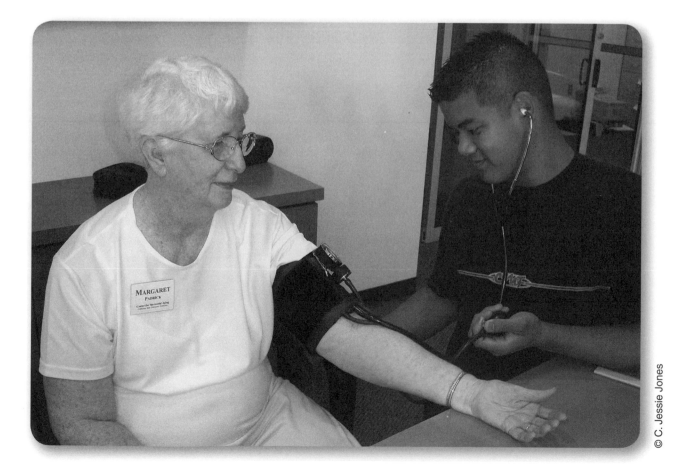

1. select, administer, and interpret the results of screening tools to determine the health, physical activity, and disability status of older adult participants;
2. evaluate the risk factors for coronary artery disease, which restricts blood flow to the heart;
3. identify medical conditions that require referral to a physician;
4. recognize the signs and symptoms of diseases that place an individual at risk during physical testing and exercise;
5. design and administer a health history and activity questionnaire;
6. design and administer an informed consent and a physician consent document; and
7. identify when screening should be repeated to determine changes in health status.

An important responsibility of physical activity instructors of older adults is to conduct a thorough screening of each client's health, physical activity, and disability status. The risk of injury during physical activity is present for all people but is particularly high for an older adult who has a serious medical condition, has been physically inactive for a prolonged period of time, or participates in an exercise program that exceeds his or her physical capacity. Given this risk, it is therefore important to conduct an initial screening of all older adults who are interested in joining your physical activity program. The screening will help you identify your client's (1) health and disability status, (2) signs and symptoms associated with certain diseases, and (3) risk factors that predispose him or her to certain diseases. A systematic approach to screening is essential in order to optimize the older adult's safety during performance testing and exercise and to develop effective exercise prescriptions (American College of Sports Medicine [ACSM], 2000).

Preexercise screening is a process whereby you obtain information from a new client before he or she undergoes performance testing or begins physical training. The primary goal of this process is to become familiar with the physical condition of each older adult who wishes to join your program. The screening process also helps you to determine a client's readiness for physical activity. The screening tools needed include an informed consent form (which explains the purpose, procedures, risks, and benefits of performance testing and your program in simple language and which must be signed by the client to indicate his or her written consent to participate in testing or exercise), a physician consent form, the **Physical Activity Readiness Questionnaire (PAR-Q,** a screening tool to determine a client's readiness to participate in a low- to moderate-intensity exercise program), a health history and physical activity questionnaire, and other tools to evaluate a client's coronary artery disease risk factors, body composition, and blood pressure. Also known as ischemic heart disease, **coronary artery disease** is caused by the narrowing of the coronary arteries (atherosclerosis), which decreases the supply of blood to the heart (myocardial ischemia). In certain moderate- to high-risk cases, a physical exam and additional laboratory tests may also be necessary. Laboratory-based tests are discussed in greater depth in chapter 7.

This chapter focuses on the procedures for conducting preexercise health screenings. It will help you recognize conditions that place an individual at risk during performance testing or exercise and conditions that require medical referral before the individual can participate in an exercise program. You will learn when it is appropriate to repeat the screening process to determine any changes in health status. Examples of each of the screening forms are also presented in this chapter.

Preexercise Screening

The screening process identifies clients who (1) have diseases, symptoms, or risk factors that require medical examination and clearance before starting an exercise program, (2) are at risk of a cardiac event while exercising, (3) should be excluded from participation in an exercise program, or (4) should participate in a medically supervised exercise program because their relative risk is too great or because they have clinically significant disease. In addition to identifying individuals at risk of a cardiac event during exercise, the screening process provides valuable information to address a variety of other important programming issues. Screening also helps you to identify clients who may need additional attention or accommodation in your program. For example, you may need to prescribe aquatic exercise rather than a walking program for someone with severe osteoarthritis.

A review of the client's medical history reveals the number, types, and dosages of medications the client takes. This can help you identify any medical conditions that are being supervised by a physician and any potential adverse effects from medication that may occur during exercise participation. For example, taking sedatives or narcotics can reduce alertness, and blood-pressure-lowering medication may lead to hypotension during exercise. (Refer to chapter 21 for additional information on this topic.)

Previous or current injuries that place the client at greater risk of an accident or reinjury during exercise can also be identified during screening. For example, you may find that a client has sustained a previous ankle fracture or a neck injury during a car accident. Screening helps you determine contraindicated exercises that place the client at risk of reinjury. In addition to the health and disability status of your client, determining his or her current physical activity level (frequency, duration, and intensity) and the types of activities your client enjoys helps you to choose appropriate fitness and functional testing and to develop an individualized exercise prescription that will increase compliance.

Contraindications to Performance Testing

By referring to figure 5.1, you can determine whether your clients have any diseases or conditions that are considered relative or absolute **contrain-**

Why Screen?

- Find out as much as you can about the person in order to provide a safe and effective exercise program.
- Identify relevant health problems, the amounts and types of medications used, and current level of physical activity.
- Identify risk level and determine the need for medical referral.
- Choose the correct type of follow-up fitness and mobility tests.
- Identify the client's goals, interests, barriers, motivators, quality of life, family support, and psychological state.

dications (conditions that make it inadvisable to prescribe exercise) to exercise testing or participation. Clients who have any of these conditions must visit their physicians for medical clearance before participating in any type of moderate- or high-intensity physical activity under your supervision. During the preactivity screening you should also identify whether your clients have any signs or symptoms of cardiovascular or pulmonary diseases. Clients who have one or more of the following signs or symptoms should be referred to their physicians for medical clearance before exercise testing or participation.

- Pain or discomfort in the chest. This may be a sign of obstructed blood flow to the heart, known as myocardial ischemia, and may be related to coronary artery disease or atherosclerosis.

- Shortness of breath at rest or with mild exertion. This may be a sign of obstructed blood flow to the lungs, lung disease, or heart disease.

- Dizziness or fainting. This may be a sign of insufficient blood flow to the brain.

- Swelling around the ankles. This may indicate a reduced ability of the heart to pump blood.

- Fast or irregular heartbeat. This may indicate a problem with the heart's electrical signals.

- Pain in the lower legs. This is called **intermittent claudication** and indicates blocked blood vessels in the legs. This is a sign of severe circulation problems (peripheral arterial disease). Brought on by exercise and relieved within 10 minutes of rest, the pain is caused by a lack of oxygen to the muscles as a result of narrowed or blocked arteries.

Relative contraindications to exercise

- Left main coronary stenosis (narrowing of coronary artery)
- Moderate stenotic valvular heart disease (narrowing of heart's mitral valve)
- Electrolyte abnormalities such as hypokalemia (decreased serum potassium levels) or hypomagnesemia (decreased serum magnesium levels)
- Severe arterial hypertension (resting systolic blood pressure over 200 mmHg or diastolic blood pressure over 110 mmHg)
- Tachyarrhythmia (rapid, irregular heartbeat) or bradyarrhythmia (slow, irregular heartbeat)
- Hypertrophic cardiomyopathy or other forms of outflow obstruction
- High-degree atrioventricular (AV) heart block (no conduction between the sinoatrial and atrioventricular nodes that serve as the heart's pacemaker; symptoms include slow heart rate and fainting)
- Ventricular aneurysm
- Neuromuscular, musculoskeletal, or rheumatoid disorders exacerbated by exercise
- Uncontrolled metabolic diseases such as diabetes, thyrotoxicosis (excessive thyroid hormone), or myxedema (hypothyroidism characterized by relatively hard edema of subcutaneous tissue)
- Chronic infectious diseases such as mononucleosis, hepatitis, or acquired immune deficiency syndrome (AIDS)

Absolute contraindications to exercise

- Recent significant change in resting ECG suggesting significant ischemia (restricted blood flow to the heart), recent (within two days) myocardial infarction (death of heart tissue caused by insufficient blood supply to the heart), or other acute cardiac events
- High-risk unstable angina (chest pain)
- Uncontrolled cardiac arrhythmia (irregular heartbeat) causing symptoms or compromised cardiac function
- Severe symptomatic aortic stenosis (narrowing of aortic valve opening)
- Uncontrolled symptomatic heart failure (right ventricular failure, decreased venous flow to lungs)
- Acute pulmonary embolus (occluded vessel caused by a detached clot, mass of bacteria, or foreign body)
- Acute myocarditis (inflammation of heart tissue) or pericarditis (inflammation of the membrane surrounding the heart and major blood vessels)
- Suspected or known dissecting aneurysm (splitting of an arterial wall by blood entering through a tear, commonly in the aorta, near the aortic valve)
- Acute infections

FIGURE 5.1   Relative and absolute contraindications to exercise. Testing of individuals with relative contraindications should be done only after careful evaluation of potential benefits and complications; testing of individuals with absolute contraindications should not be performed until conditions are stabilized or treated.

Gibbons RJ, Balady GJ, Bricker JT, Chaitman BR, Fletcher GF, Froelicher VF, Mark DB, McCallister BD, Mooss AN, O'Reilly MG, Winters WL Jr. ACC/AHA 2002 guideline update for exercise testing: a report of the American College of Cardiology/American Heart Association Task Force on Practice Guidelines (Committee on Exercise Testing). 2002. American College of Cardiology Web site. Available at: www.acc.org / clinical / guidelines / exercise / dirIndex.htm.

• Heart murmur. This suggests a heart problem in which the valves fail to close completely.

• Undue fatigue. This may be a sign of poor blood circulation or low oxygen levels in the blood.

Risk Factors for Coronary Artery Disease

The most serious risk associated with vigorous exercise is sudden cardiac death. Although the risk of sudden cardiac death is elevated during vigorous activity, the long-term benefits of physical activity on cardiac risk far outweigh the temporary elevation in risk during exercise. In fact, the incidence of death from coronary artery disease is much less among adults who are physically active than among those who are sedentary (Siscovick, Weiss, Fletcher, & Lasky, 1984). The cardiac risks are primarily associated with vigorous exercise when the individual has an existing medical condition that can precipitate a medical emergency during exercise. Therefore, one of the primary objectives of preexercise screening is to identify individuals with known cardiovascular disease, symptoms of cardiovascular disease, or risk factors associated with the disease before the client participates in any performance testing or physical activity.

During the screening you can determine the presence of risk factors for coronary artery disease. Based on this information, you can determine the participant's level of risk (see table 5.1). It is believed that individuals who have risk factors are more likely to develop coronary artery disease that may go undetected for some time. Individuals with undetected heart disease are at greater risk of sudden death while participating in performance testing or exercise. However, once these risk factors are identified, several of them can be reduced through behavioral and lifestyle modification. The risk factors to consider include the following:

• Age. Over 45 for men and over 55 for women.

• Family history of cardiovascular disease. A parent or sibling who has cardiovascular disease (e.g., heart attack) before age 55 for male relatives and before age 65 for female relatives.

• Smoking. Currently smoking cigarettes on a daily basis or having smoked on a regular basis during the past two years.

• Hypertension. High blood pressure, or **hypertension,** is defined as a systolic reading of 140 mmHg or greater or a diastolic reading of 90 mmHg or greater. **Systolic blood pressure** is the pressure in the arteries during the contraction phase of the heart cycle, and **diastolic blood pressure** is the pressure in the arteries during the resting phase.

• High cholesterol. Cholesterol is a fatty substance found in nerves and other tissues, and high levels are associated with elevated risk for heart disease. Total cholesterol of 200 milligrams per deciliter or higher is a risk factor.

• Low levels of **high-density lipoprotein (HDL).** This is the "good" cholesterol that carries "bad" cholesterol (**low-density lipoprotein, or LDL**) from the tissues to the liver for removal. Higher levels of HDL are associated with lower risk for heart disease. An HDL level less than 35 milligrams per deciliter is a risk factor. However, an HDL level greater than 60 milligrams per deciliter cancels out another risk factor.

• Diabetes. **Diabetes** is a metabolic disease that results in high blood sugar (glucose) levels. Insulin-dependent diabetes mellitus (also called juvenile-onset or type 1 diabetes) usually has a sudden onset at a young age, leads to insulin deficiency, and typically requires daily insulin injections. Non-insulin-dependent diabetes mellitus (also called adult-onset or type 2 diabetes) usually has a gradual onset and is caused by inadequate insulin production by the pancreas, inadequate insulin utilization, or excessive liver glucose release. Diabetes is a risk factor if an individual has type 1 diabetes and is over the age of 30 years, has had type 1 diabetes mellitus for more than 15 years, or has type 2 diabetes and is over the age of 35 years.

• Obesity. **Body mass index (BMI)** is a measure of body weight relative to body height (height in meters squared divided by weight in kilograms) that is used to evaluate body composition. A BMI of 30 or more with a waist girth greater than 102

TABLE 5.1   ACSM Initial Risk Stratification

Classification	Criteria
Low risk	Younger individuals (men under 45 years and women under 55 years) who are asymptomatic and have no more than one risk factor
Moderate risk	Older individuals (men 45 years or older and women 55 years or older) or individuals of any age having two or more risk factors
High risk	Individuals with one or more signs or symptoms of cardiovascular or pulmonary disease or individuals with known cardiovascular, pulmonary, or metabolic disease

Adapted from American College of Sports Medicine, 2000, *ACSM's Guidelines for exercise testing and prescription*, 6th edition (Philadelphia, PA: Lippincott, Williams, and Wilkins), 26.

centimeters for men and 88 cm for women is a risk factor.

• Sedentary lifestyle. This includes a combination of not participating in any regular exercise or recreational physical activity and having a job that does not involve physical activity.

Several tools are available to identify these risk factors. For example, a health history and activity questionnaire can be used to determine age, family history of heart disease, history of smoking, and sedentary lifestyle. Blood pressure can be measured to detect hypertension. A blood profile can identify those with high cholesterol or with high glucose (or blood sugar) levels associated with diabetes. Body mass index (BMI) and measures such as waist-to-hip ratio or waist circumference that indicate an individual's abdominal fat can be used to identify obesity. Each of these measurement tools are described later in this chapter.

Screening Steps

Many different approaches have been taken to preexercise screening procedures. As a physical activity instructor for older adults, you should become familiar with at least one approach to screening potential program participants. To keep the process simple, this discussion is limited to five essential steps and some sample screening forms. Some additional screening tools are discussed in the next section; you may want to consider incorporating them into your screening process.

Step 1: Informed Consent

Before you allow your clients to participate in any performance testing or your physical activity program, they need to complete an informed consent form. The purpose of **informed consent** is to ensure the participant's autonomy in deciding whether or not to take part in the performance testing or program activities. True informed consent involves an ongoing process of communication between the physical activity instructor and participants to ensure that all elements of a program or procedure are clearly understood. The consent document is not only part of that communication process but also a legal obligation to your exercise participants. The use of an informed consent document is mandated by federal law anytime an

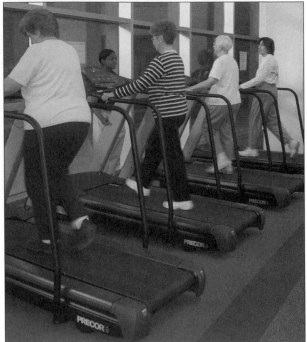

Staying physically active in later life reduces the incidence of coronary artery disease.

individual may be exposed to possible physical, psychological, or social injury as a result of participating in a physical activity program. Although an informed consent document won't protect you from legal action, it will improve your defense and increase the odds of a favorable outcome of any legal action if your program is supervised by qualified individuals and operated according to an established set of guidelines.

Typically informed consent documents are reviewed by the institutional review board (IRB) or a risk management unit that is responsible for reviewing an organization's protocols to ensure that appropriate laws and ethical standards are met. If your organization does not have a mechanism for reviewing these types of documents, you should consult with a lawyer to ensure that your informed consent document conforms to legal and ethical requirements. Many sample consent forms are available that can be tailored for use in exercise settings and that address performance testing as well as exercise program issues. Figure 5.2 provides an example of an informed consent form that addresses both performance testing and exercise program issues.

Informed consent is typically obtained by having the participant read and sign a document

Center for Physical Activity and Aging
Health Promotion Clinic of Healthy State University
Senior Fitness Program

Participant Consent Form

In response to the growth in the programs at the Health Promotion Clinic, Healthy State University has developed a new Center for Physical Activity and Aging. The director of the center is Kurt V. Trout, PhD. Through its educational, research, and service activities, the center has as its mission the promotion of health, vitality, and well-being in later years. The Senior Fitness Program is one of several programs under the direction of the center. The center provides a safe environment where people 50 years of age and over can improve their fitness. The center also provides a learning environment to train specialists in older adult fitness and to provide students with research experience necessary for graduate school.

Purpose: I understand that the purpose of this exercise program is to improve my physical and functional fitness. During this program I may perform exercises to improve the capacity of my heart and lungs, my muscle strength and endurance, my joint flexibility, my body composition (amount of fat and lean tissue), my mobility, and my balance.

Procedures: The fitness classes will meet for 12 weeks, three times per week for 60 minutes. Each class will be instructed by trained students and supervised by personnel with extensive education and experience in exercise science and aging. The class consists of a 10-minute warm-up followed by three 15-minute exercise stations, including aerobic, strength, and flexibility and mobility training. The class ends with a five-minute cool-down. Before starting the training program, I will be asked to obtain medical clearance and complete a medical and activity history questionnaire. I will also be asked to participate in a series of functional fitness tests to identify weaknesses in my physical ability to do activities of daily living and to allow the class supervisors to more effectively prescribe appropriate exercises. These tests will include a six-minute walk (walking as far as I can in six minutes), a two-minute step-in-place (stepping in place for two minutes), an eight-foot (2.4-meter) up-and-go (standing up from sitting in a chair, walking eight feet [2.4 meters], and returning to the chair as quickly as possible), walking speed (walking 50 feet, or 15.2 meters), a chair sit-and-reach (reaching toward my foot while seated in a chair with my leg straight), a back-scratch test (reaching over my shoulder and behind my back), a 30-second chair stand (standing from sitting in a chair as many times as I can in 30 seconds), and a 30-second arm curl (lifting a five-pound [2.3-kilogram] weight for women or an eight-pound [3.6-kilogram] weight for men as many times as I can in 30 seconds).

Risks: The risks associated with the classes are minimal, but the exercises performed during the testing and training sessions may cause me some immediate and delayed muscle soreness and physical fatigue. If I experience any physical discomfort (chest pain, leg pain, muscular discomfort, etc.) during the class or testing, I should immediately inform the class supervisor.
I understand that I am being asked to exercise within my own comfort level. During exercise my body may show signs that I should stop exercising. I understand that it is my responsibility to report any of these signs or symptoms to my instructor and doctor. These signs include:

- light-headedness or dizziness;
- chest heaviness, pain, or tightness, or angina;
- palpitations or irregular heartbeat;
- sudden shortness of breath not due to increased physical activity; or
- discomfort or stiffness in muscles and joints persisting for several days after exercise.

FIGURE 5.2   Sample informed consent form.

(continued)

Benefits: I understand that the results of these tests will help determine my fitness levels, which will be useful in developing my individualized exercise prescription.

All questions that I have about these procedures have been answered to my satisfaction. If I have additional questions, I can contact Dr. Kurt V. Trout at 316-555-9595. I understand that participation in the program is completely voluntary, and I am free to stop participation at any time. I understand that the center does not provide compensation for injuries that I may sustain. If I am accidentally injured during the classes, the program personnel will be unable to offer treatment, and I will be required to seek treatment with my own physician. I understand that any information obtained in this program will remain confidential and will not be disclosed to anyone other than my physician or those responsible for my exercise prescription without my written permission. I agree that results from these tests can be used for research purposes. My name will not be directly associated with any of the results in a published report.

My signature indicates that I have carefully read the information provided above and have voluntarily decided to participate. Furthermore, I, for myself and my heirs, fully release from liability and waive all legal claims against Healthy State University and all testing and training personnel for injury or damage that I might incur during participation in the Senior Fitness Program.

Signature of participant _____ Date_____

Signature of witness _____ Date_____

FIGURE 5.2 *(continued)*

that describes the performance tests and exercise program. Therefore, the informed consent document has two basic components: information and consent. The information provided is not meant simply to disclose information but also to educate participants. The informed consent document normally includes a description of the objectives of the screening procedures and performance tests, a description of the physical activity program, a summary of the risks and benefits, a statement that the participant is voluntarily choosing to participate and is free to withdraw from the program without prejudice at any time, a statement concerning confidentiality, a description of medical coverage (even if there is none) in case of injury, an offer to answer any questions, and the contact information of someone who can answer questions or address concerns (ACSM, 2000). It is important that you provide participants with sufficient time to read and complete this form and to ask any questions they might have about any aspect of the form, the program, or the performance tests to be conducted. You should also allow them time to consider their involvement in the context of their other daily commitments and to discuss their involvement with family and friends. Therefore, you may want to provide this document to your clients before the day when performance testing or the exercise program is to commence, thus allowing them time to consider their participation.

Comprehension is a key element of the informed consent document. The participant must be able to read and comprehend the document. First, the document should be as short as possible while still containing all the necessary elements. Second, although these documents have some legal merit, they are not to be written in "legalese." Rather, they are to be written at approximately an eighth-grade reading level. This helps to overcome many problems with literacy and understanding. Third, when preparing these (and other) documents for older adults, it is better to make the print size larger than normal to accommodate visual limitations. A font size of 14 or 16 points is often sufficient.

Step 2: The Physical Activity Readiness Questionnaire

The Physical Activity Readiness Questionnaire (PAR-Q; see figure 5.3) was developed by the Canadian Society for Exercise Physiology and is considered to be a minimal evaluation of individuals prior to the beginning of a *low- to moderate-intensity* exercise program. It was designed to identify the

PAR-Q & YOU

(A Questionnaire for People Aged 15 to 69)

Regular physical activity is fun and healthy, and increasingly more people are starting to become more active every day. Being more active is very safe for most people. However, some people should check with their doctor before they start becoming much more physically active.

If you are planning to become much more physically active than you are now, start by answering the seven questions in the box below. If you are between the ages of 15 and 69, the PAR-Q will tell you if you should check with your doctor before you start. If you are over 69 years of age, and you are not used to being very active, check with your doctor.

Common sense is your best guide when you answer these questions. Please read the questions carefully and answer each one honestly: check YES or NO.

YES	NO		
☐	☐	**1.**	**Has your doctor ever said that you have a heart condition <u>and</u> that you should only do physical activity recommended by a doctor?**
☐	☐	**2.**	**Do you feel pain in your chest when you do physical activity?**
☐	☐	**3.**	**In the past month, have you had chest pain when you were not doing physical activity?**
☐	☐	**4.**	**Do you lose your balance because of dizziness or do you ever lose consciousness?**
☐	☐	**5.**	**Do you have a bone or joint problem (for example, back, knee or hip) that could be made worse by a change in your physical activity?**
☐	☐	**6.**	**Is your doctor currently prescribing drugs (for example, water pills) for your blood pressure or heart condition?**
☐	☐	**7.**	**Do you know of <u>any other reason</u> why you should not do physical activity?**

If

you

answered

YES to one or more questions

Talk with your doctor by phone or in person BEFORE you start becoming much more physically active or BEFORE you have a fitness appraisal. Tell your doctor about the PAR-Q and which questions you answered YES.

- You may be able to do any activity you want — as long as you start slowly and build up gradually. Or, you may need to restrict your activities to those which are safe for you. Talk with your doctor about the kinds of activities you wish to participate in and follow his/her advice.
- Find out which community programs are safe and helpful for you.

NO to all questions

If you answered NO honestly to <u>all</u> PAR-Q questions, you can be reasonably sure that you can:
- start becoming much more physically active — begin slowly and build up gradually. This is the safest and easiest way to go.
- take part in a fitness appraisal — this is an excellent way to determine your basic fitness so that you can plan the best way for you to live actively. It is also highly recommended that you have your blood pressure evaluated. If your reading is over 144/94, talk with your doctor before you start becoming much more physically active.

DELAY BECOMING MUCH MORE ACTIVE:
- if you are not feeling well because of a temporary illness such as a cold or a fever — wait until you feel better; or
- if you are or may be pregnant — talk to your doctor before you start becoming more active.

PLEASE NOTE: If your health changes so that you then answer YES to any of the above questions, tell your fitness or health professional. Ask whether you should change your physical activity plan.

<u>Informed Use of the PAR-Q</u>: The Canadian Society for Exercise Physiology, Health Canada, and their agents assume no liability for persons who undertake physical activity, and if in doubt after completing this questionnaire, consult your doctor prior to physical activity.

No changes permitted. You are encouraged to photocopy the PAR-Q but only if you use the entire form.

NOTE: If the PAR-Q is being given to a person before he or she participates in a physical activity program or a fitness appraisal, this section may be used for legal or administrative purposes.

"I have read, understood and completed this questionnaire. Any questions I had were answered to my full satisfaction."

NAME _____

SIGNATURE _____   DATE _____

SIGNATURE OF PARENT _____   WITNESS _____
or GUARDIAN (for participants under the age of majority)

Note: This physical activity clearance is valid for a maximum of 12 months from the date it is completed and becomes invalid if your condition changes so that you would answer YES to any of the seven questions.

CSEP
SCPE © Canadian Society for Exercise Physiology   Supported by: [🍁] Health Canada   Santé Canada

continued on other side...

FIGURE 5.3   Physical Activity Readiness Questionnaire (PAR-Q).

Physical Activity Readiness Questionnaire (PAR-Q) © 2002. Reprinted with permission from the Canadian Society for Exercise Physiology. Http://www.csep.ca/form.asp

PAR-Q & YOU

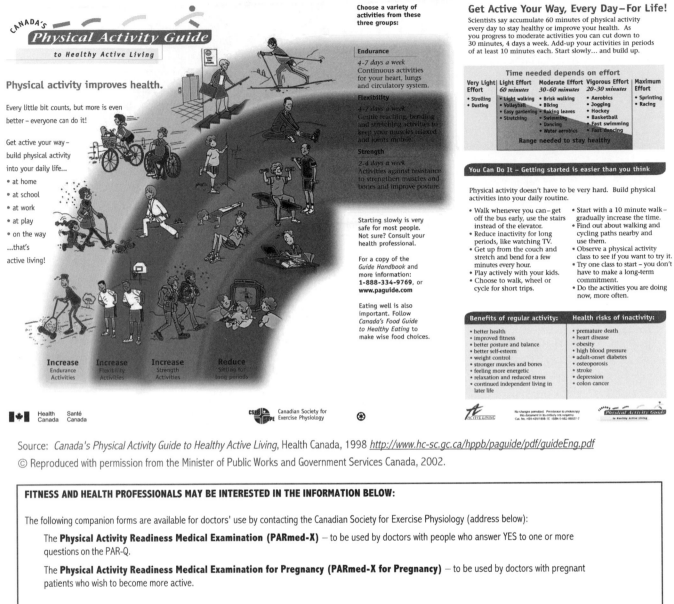

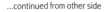

Source: *Canada's Physical Activity Guide to Healthy Active Living*, Health Canada, 1998 http://www.hc-sc.gc.ca/hppb/paguide/pdf/guideEng.pdf

© Reproduced with permission from the Minister of Public Works and Government Services Canada, 2002.

FITNESS AND HEALTH PROFESSIONALS MAY BE INTERESTED IN THE INFORMATION BELOW:

The following companion forms are available for doctors' use by contacting the Canadian Society for Exercise Physiology (address below):

The **Physical Activity Readiness Medical Examination (PARmed-X)** – to be used by doctors with people who answer YES to one or more questions on the PAR-Q.

The **Physical Activity Readiness Medical Examination for Pregnancy (PARmed-X for Pregnancy)** – to be used by doctors with pregnant patients who wish to become more active.

References:

Arraix, G.A., Wigle, D.T., Mao, Y. (1992). Risk Assessment of Physical Activity and Physical Fitness in the Canada Health Survey
Follow-Up Study. **J. Clin. Epidemiol.** 45:4 419-428.

Mottola, M., Wolfe, L.A. (1994). Active Living and Pregnancy, In: A. Quinney, L. Gauvin, T. Wall (eds.), **Toward Active Living: Proceedings of the International Conference on Physical Activity, Fitness and Health**. Champaign, IL: Human Kinetics.

PAR-Q Validation Report, British Columbia Ministry of Health, 1978.

Thomas, S., Reading, J., Shephard, R.J. (1992). Revision of the Physical Activity Readiness Questionnaire (PAR-Q). **Can. J. Spt. Sci.** 17:4 338-345.

To order multiple printed copies of the PAR-Q, please contact the:

Canadian Society for Exercise Physiology
202-185 Somerset Street West
Ottawa, ON K2P 0J2
Tel. 1-877-651-3755 • FAX (613) 234-3565
Online: www.csep.ca

The original PAR-Q was developed by the British Columbia Ministry of Health. It has been revised by an Expert Advisory Committee of the Canadian Society for Exercise Physiology chaired by Dr. N. Gledhill (2002).

Disponible en français sous le titre «Questionnaire sur l'aptitude à l'activité physique - Q-AAP (revisé 2002)».

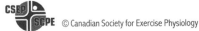

© Canadian Society for Exercise Physiology

Supported by: Health Canada Santé Canada

FIGURE 5.3   *(continued)*

Physical Activity Readiness Questionnaire (PAR-Q) © 2002. Reprinted with permission from the Canadian Society for Exercise Physiology. Http://www.csep.ca/form.asp

small number of adults for whom physical activity might be unsafe or who need medical advice regarding the most appropriate form of activity. It is a self-administered questionnaire that instructs participants to contact their personal physicians if they answer yes to more than one question.

The PAR-Q identifies symptoms associated with heart disease and musculoskeletal problems that should be evaluated before participation in performance testing or exercise because these conditions might require modification of the exercise program. It is recommended that you include this questionnaire as part of the screening to help identify individuals who are at risk. However, note that there are some limitations to the PAR-Q: Participants over the age of 69 who are not very physically active should check with their doctors prior to any type of physical activity. Although the phrase "very physically active" is quite subjective, a growing number of fitness professionals highly recommend obtaining a physician's consent for a client to participate in a structured exercise program. A physician's consent letter also helps to inform the client's doctor about the quality of your program and provides an opportunity for the physician to recommend exercise adaptations.

Step 3: Physician Consent

In addition to obtaining the consent of the participant, the international curriculum guidelines for preparing physical activity instructors recommend obtaining a physician's consent for the client to participate. The consent document for the physician should describe the exact nature of the performance testing to be conducted and the major components of the program. It should also include contact information so that the physician can contact you, or another responsible person such as the facility director, if he or she has any questions about the program. The document should have a place for the physician's endorsement of his or her patient's participation, with or without any conditions for participation, and a place for denial of endorsement with an option to state the reason or reasons. Figure 5.4 provides a sample physician's consent letter.

Step 4: Health History and Activity Questionnaire

One of the most important steps in the screening is to identify any contraindications to performance testing and exercise and to determine any risks or

limitations that may be relevant to the exercise program. This step is typically accomplished by administering a questionnaire. Typically, the participant completes the questionnaire on his or her own. After reviewing the information, you can then follow up with specific questions to gain further clarification where needed. The information gathered will help you to classify an individual's level of risk according to the ACSM screening guidelines that were described in table 5.1.

Figure 5.5 provides an excellent example of a health and activity questionnaire developed at California State University–Fullerton. The questionnaire asks for information about demographics (question 1); existing chronic or acute diseases (questions 2-8); assistive devices such as eyeglasses, hearing aids, canes (questions 9-11); perceived health status (question 12); family history of heart disease (question 13); medications (question 14); smoking behavior (question 15); fall history (questions 17-19); functional limitations and disability (questions 16, 20-22, and 30); current levels of activity (questions 23-26); work history (questions 27 and 28); and perceived quality of life (question 29). Question 22, the Composite Physical Function (CPF) scale, is used to evaluate a participant's ability to perform a wide range of activities, from basic activities of daily living such as dressing and bathing to advanced activities such as aerobic dance and other strenuous exercise (Rikli & Jones, 1998). The participant's functional ability can be classified by adding the scores on the 12 items of the CPF scale: 22 to 24 points indicate high function; 16 to 21 points, moderate function; and below 16 points, low function.

While health and activity questionnaires can be very extensive, they do not need to inquire about every disease and disorder that could possibly exist. They need only to help you categorize an individual's level of risk in more general terms. The participant's health and activity history enables you to identify conditions that may place him or her at risk and to detect any contraindications to performance testing and exercise. Relative contraindications are those for which the benefits of testing and exercise must be considered in light of the potential risk, and absolute contraindications are those that preclude testing or exercise participation altogether (review figure 5.1).

From your participants' questionnaire responses you can also identify whether they are taking any medications, such as beta-blockers, bronchodilators, or insulin, that could affect their ability to

Center for Physical Activity and Aging
Health Promotion Clinic of Healthy State University
Senior Fitness Program

Medical Clearance by Personal Physician

Your patient, _____, has expressed an interest in participating in the Senior Fitness Program, one of the programs offered by the Center for Physical Activity at Healthy State University. The center, under the direction of Kurt V. Trout, has offered exercise training programs for older adults for the past 10 years.

We would appreciate your medical opinion and recommendations concerning this individual's participation in exercise. If you feel that this individual might benefit from participation in the program, we would greatly appreciate your endorsement of his or her participation.

Assessments: The program participants are required to complete a medical and activity questionnaire, followed by a series of functional fitness assessments. This is done to identify weaknesses in physical parameters associated with activities of daily living and to more effectively prescribe appropriate exercise.

Physical Parameters	*Assessments*	*Approval*
Cardiovascular	Two-minute step-in-place	yes___ no___
	Six-minute walk	yes___ no___
Muscular strength and endurance	30-second chair stand	yes___ no___
	30-second arm curl	yes___ no___
Flexibility	Chair sit-and-reach	yes___ no___
	Back scratch	yes___ no___
Balance & gait	8-foot (2.4-meter) up-and-go	yes___ no___
	50-foot (15.2-meter) walking speed	yes___ no___

Exercise program: The intensity of the program is based on the individual capabilities of each participant. The class meets three times per week for 60 minutes. Each class will be instructed by trained students and supervised by personnel with extensive education and experience in exercise science and aging. The class will consist of a 10-minute warm-up; three 15-minute stations including aerobic, strength, and flexibility and mobility training; and a 5-minute cool-down.

Exercise class approval: yes _____ no _____

Please list any modifications or comments for testing and exercise class: _____
_____

Patient's last blood pressure reading: _____ / _____

Please indicate by your signature below that your patient is medically cleared to participate in the specific testing and training described. Please call Dr. Kurt Trout at 316-555-9595 if you have any questions concerning the program.

_____   _____   _____
Signature of physician   *Print name of physician*   *Date*

Physician's phone #: (____) _____ - _____

FIGURE 5.4   Sample physician's consent letter.

Health History and Activity Questionnaire

1.

Date _____

Name _____

Address _____ City _____ State _____ Zip _____

Home phone # _____ Sex: Male ___ Female ___

Age _____ Date of birth _____ Height _____ Weight _____

Highest level of education completed _____ Ethnicity _____

Whom to contact in a case of emergency _____ Phone # _____

Name of your physician _____ Phone # _____

2. Have you ever been diagnosed as having any of the following symptoms or conditions?

	Yes (✓)	Year it began (approximate)
Heart attack	_____	_____
Transient ischemic attack	_____	_____
Angina (chest pain)	_____	_____
Stroke	_____	_____
Peripheral vascular disease	_____	_____
Heart surgery	_____	_____
High blood pressure	_____	_____
High cholesterol	_____	_____
Diabetes	_____	_____
Respiratory disease	_____	_____
Osteoporosis	_____	_____
Joint replacement (site: _____)	_____	_____
Cancer (type: _____)	_____	_____
Cognitive disorder (type: _____)	_____	_____
Neuropathies (problems with sensations)	_____	_____
Parkinson's disease	_____	_____
Multiple sclerosis	_____	_____
Polio or postpolio syndrome	_____	_____
Epilepsy or seizures	_____	_____
Other neurological conditions	_____	_____

FIGURE 5.5   Health history and activity questionnaire.

(continued)

Rheumatoid arthritis _____ _____
Other arthritic conditions _____ _____
Visual or depth perception problems _____ _____
Inner ear problems or recurrent ear infections _____ _____
Cerebellar problems (ataxia) _____ _____
Other movement disorders _____ _____
Chemical dependency (alcohol or drugs) _____ _____
Depression _____ _____

Please describe any other health concerns: _____

_____

3. Do you currently have a medical condition that might limit your physical performance?

No ___ Yes ___ If YES, please describe the condition(s): _____

_____

4. Do you have a pacemaker? No___ Yes ___ Does it automatically resuscitate? No___ Yes ___

5. Do you currently suffer any of the following symptoms in your legs or feet?

Yes (✓)

Numbness ___
Tingling ___
Arthritis ___
Swelling ___

6. Do you currently have any medical conditions for which you see a physician regularly?

No ___ Yes ___ If YES, please describe the condition(s): _____

_____

_____

7. Have you required emergency medical care or hospitalization in the last **three years?**

No ___ Yes ___ If YES, please state when this occurred and briefly explain why:

_____

_____

8. In general, how depressed have you felt within the past four weeks?

Not at all ____ Slightly ____ Moderately ____ Quite a bit ____ Extremely ____

9. Do you require eyeglasses? No ___ Yes ___

10. Do you require hearing aids? No ___ Yes ___

11. Do you use an assistive device for walking? No ___ Yes ___ Sometimes ___ Type: _____

_____

12. How would you describe your health?

Excellent _____ Very good _____ Good _____ Fair _____ Poor _____

13. Have you had a close relative who had a heart attack before age 55 (father or brother) or before age 65 (mother or sister)? No _____ Yes _____

If YES, who and at what age: _____

FIGURE 5.5 (continued)

14. List the prescription medications that you currently take (by exact name or by type):

       Type of medication   For what condition

_____   _____

_____   _____

_____   _____

_____   _____

_____   _____

15. Do you currently smoke cigarettes?   No ____   Yes ____

     Number smoked on an average day   ____

     If NO, have you ever smoked?   No ____   Yes ____   How many years? _____

     How many years since you stopped?   ____

     Number formerly smoked on an average day   ____

16. In the past four weeks, to what extent did health problems limit your everyday physical activities (such as walking and household chores)?

     Not at all ___   Slightly ___   Moderately ___   Quite a bit ___   Extremely ___

17. How many times have you fallen **within the past year**? _____

     Did you require medical treatment?   No ____   Yes ____

     If you have fallen once or more in the past year, please list the approximate date of the fall, the medical treatment required, and the reason you fell **in each case** (e.g., uneven surface, going down stairs):

     _____

     _____

18. Have you ever had any condition or suffered any injury that has affected your balance or ability to walk without assistance?   No ____   Yes ____

     If YES, please list when this occurred and briefly explain the condition or injury:

     _____

     _____

19. Are you **worried** about falling? (circle appropriate number)

     1 - - - - - - - 2 - - - - - - - 3 - - - - - - - 4 - - - - - - - 5 - - - - - - - 6 - - - - - - - 7

     Not at all   A little   Moderately   Very   Extremely

20. In general, do you currently require household or nursing assistance to carry out daily activities?

     No ___   Yes ___   If YES, please check the reasons:

                 a. Health problems ___

                 b. Chronic pain ___

                 c. Lack of strength or endurance ___

                 d. Lack of flexibility or balance ___

                 e. Other reasons: _____

21. In a typical week, how often do you leave your house (to run errands or go to work, meetings, classes, church, social functions, etc.)?

     _____ less than once a week   _____ 3-4 times a week

     _____ 1-2 times a week   _____ almost every day

FIGURE 5.5   *(continued)*

22. Please indicate your ability to do each of the following (circle appropriate response).*

	Can do	Can do with difficulty or with help	Cannot do
a. Take care of own personal needs, such as dressing yourself	2	1	0
b. Bathe yourself, using tub or shower	2	1	0
c. Climb up and down a flight of stairs (e.g., to a second story in a house)	2	1	0
d. Walk outside one or two blocks	2	1	0
e. Do light household activities, such as cooking, dusting, washing dishes, sweeping a walkway	2	1	0
f. Do own shopping for groceries or clothes	2	1	0
g. Walk 1/2 mile (6-7 blocks, 0.8 kilometer)	2	1	0
h. Walk 1 mile (12-14 blocks, 1.6 kilometers)	2	1	0
i. Lift and carry 10 pounds (4.5 kilograms, a full bag of groceries)	2	1	0
j. Lift and carry 25 pounds (11.3 kilograms, a medium to large suitcase)	2	1	0
k. Do most heavy household chores, such as scrubbing floors, vacuuming, raking leaves	2	1	0
l. Do *strenuous* activities, such as hiking, digging in garden, moving heavy objects, bicycling, aerobic dance exercises, strenuous calisthenics, etc.	2	1	0

* Composite Physical Function Scale (Rikli & Jones, 1998)

23. Do you currently participate in regular physical activity (such as walking, jogging, sports, exercise classes, housework, yard work) that is strenuous enough to cause a noticeable increase in breathing, heart rate, or perspiration?

No ____ Yes ____ If YES, how many days per week? (circle appropriate number)

1 2 3 4 5 6 7

24. Do you go for walks on a regular basis? No ____ Yes ____

If YES, how many times per week on average? _____

How many minutes at a time usually? _____

How far do you usually walk?   _____

25. When you go for walks (if you do), which of the following best describes your usual pace:

Strolling (easy pace, takes 30 minutes or more to walk a mile [1.6 kilometers]) ____

Average or normal (can walk a mile [1.6 kilometers] in 20-30 minutes)   ____

Fairly brisk (fast pace, can walk a mile [1.6 kilometers] in 15-20 minutes)   ____

Do not go for walks on a regular basis   ____

26. Please list all other types of exercise activities (other than walking) that you usually do each week. Include activities such as exercise, light or heavy housework or yard work, and so on. Think through the past week (or a typical week in the past month); list **only** your **regular** physical activities.

FIGURE 5.5   *(continued)*

Activity	Number of days per week	Number of minutes or hours per day
_____	_____	_____
_____	_____	_____
_____	_____	_____
_____	_____	_____

27. What is your current occupational status?

    Working ____   Semiretired ____   Retired/not working ____

28. What have been your major occupations? How long were you in each occupation? How would you describe the physical demands of these jobs?

Occupations	From (age)	To (age)	Mostly sedentary	Light exercise	Moderate exercise	Heavy labor
_____	____	____	____	____	____	____
_____	____	____	____	____	____	____
_____	____	____	____	____	____	____

29. In general, how would you rate the quality of your life? (circle appropriate number)

    1 - - - - - - 2 - - - - - - 3 - - - - - - 4 - - - - - - 5 - - - - - - 6 - - - - - - 7

    Very low   Low   Moderate   High   Very high

30. Did you require assistance in completing this form?

    None (or very little) _____   Needed quite a bit of help _____

    Reason: _____

    Thank you!

FIGURE 5.5   *(continued)*

exercise or their response to exercise in general (e.g., heart rate or blood pressure). If an individual has a medical condition or is taking a medication that is unfamiliar to you, be sure to obtain more information from an appropriate medical or pharmaceutical resource before allowing that individual to participate in performance testing or exercise. (Refer to chapter 21 regarding exercise considerations for common medical conditions.)

The questionnaire provides you with the following additional information about your clients: (1) previous and current exercise activities, (2) ability to participate in an exercise program, (3) exercise preferences, (4) risk of suffering a medical emergency during exercise, and (5) risk of falls and disability. Depending on the purpose of your program and the staff available for health behavior counseling, you might ask for additional informa-

tion, such as alcohol and caffeine consumption, drug use, driving record, recreational pursuits, nutritional patterns, sleep habits, and stress levels. This information can identify participants who are at risk for heart attack, stroke, cancer, and other diseases and accidents such as falls.

Information gathered from preactivity screening, physical examination reports, clinical test results, and performance test scores (see chapters 6 and 7) also facilitates the development of realistic and achievable goals and a safer and more individualized physical activity program for your participants. Many chronic, degenerative diseases are related to lifestyle. Although it is impossible to change certain risk factors such as age, sex, and family history, many other factors can be positively affected by behavioral and lifestyle modifications. For example, many of the risk factors associated with coronary artery disease, including smoking, high blood pressure, elevated cholesterol, and a sedentary lifestyle, can be addressed through behavior modification techniques such as smoking cessation, reduction of fat intake, and regular exercise. Although helping your clients with behavioral modification may not be feasible because of time constraints or lack of expertise, you can suggest that they ask their physicians for a referral.

Step 5: Feedback to Clients and Confidentiality

Once you have gathered and interpreted the information from the preactivity screening, you should share the results with the client. This feedback is very valuable. It allows you to educate the client about his or her health and disability status. It also enables you and the client to establish goals and discuss how participation in specific activities can help meet those goals.

Screening information should be discussed privately with each client. The results and interpretation of the client's screening assessment should be explained in language that is easily understood by the client. Be sure to avoid technical terms with which the client might not be familiar. Telling a client that he or she is at increased risk of disease is never good news for the client. To motivate the client to participate in an activity program, explain the results in a positive manner that does not scare or intimidate him or her. Share the good news: Many things can be done to improve the client's current health. Identifying appropriate, low-risk activities and periodically reevaluating his or her health status are encouraging and help to convince the client that better health can be achieved.

A separate folder containing each client's health and medical information should be permanently maintained. This allows you to refer to previous screening results and compare assessments over

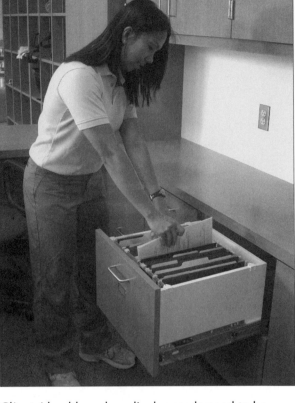

Clients' health and medical records need to be filed and kept confidential.

time. A good filing system allows you to easily update information when necessary, such as a change in medications. Remember, the information that you collect during screening is confidential. It is to be shared only with the client and the appropriate staff members as needed for risk identification and program management. You may choose to give a copy of the results to the client so that he or she can share them with his or her physician. However, the information is not to be shared with other clients, even if requested by another client. The information must be kept secure and not left in an area with unrestricted access. Folders containing this confidential information should be kept in a locked cabinet that is accessible only to you and other designated staff members.

Additional Screening Tools

It is not feasible, or necessary, to conduct a thorough battery of laboratory tests on every individual who wishes to join an exercise program. However, relatively easy-to-use screening tools can provide

The five pre-screening exercise steps are the following:

1. Informed consent
2. Physical Activity Readiness questionnaire
3. Physician's consent
4. Health history and activity questionnaire
5. Feedback to clients and confidentiality

valuable information about clients' blood pressure and body composition.

Blood Pressure

When possible, measuring a client's blood pressure should be part of the screening. Because high blood pressure is an important risk factor to recognize before performance testing or exercise participation begins, measuring a client's blood pressure can help you assess a participant's health and risk of an exercise-related medical event. If a client's blood pressure reading is high, he or she should be immediately referred to a physician for further consultation before any performance testing or exercise participation.

Blood pressure is measured in millimeters of mercury (mmHg). The reading typically is recorded as two numbers or a ratio: Systolic pressure (the pressure while the heart contracts) is expressed first, or on top, and the diastolic pressure (the pressure while the heart relaxes between beats) is given second, or on the bottom. Resting systolic blood pressure usually varies between 110 and 140 mmHg, while resting diastolic values range from 60 to 80 mmHg. A person is considered to

be hypertensive when the systolic pressure is 140 mmHg or higher or the diastolic pressure is 90 mmHg or higher on two separate occasions. The classification system for the severity of hypertension is shown in table 5.2. Older adults with hypertension should have their blood pressure monitored using either an automatic or manual blood pressure cuff, during and after exercise to ensure that it is under control.

Body Mass Index

A commonly used measurement that provides a rough indication of obesity is the body mass index (BMI). The BMI is a quick and easy method of determining the appropriateness of a client's body weight in relation to his or her height. The BMI can be calculated by dividing body weight in kilograms (kg) by height in meters squared (m²):

$$BMI = kg/m^2$$

To convert body weight to kilograms, divide the body weight in pounds by 2.2. To determine height in meters, divide the height in inches by 39.4. For

TABLE 5.2   Classification of Blood Pressure for Adults Ages 18 Years and Older

Systolic (mmHg)		Diastolic (mmHg)	Category
Less than 130	and	Less than 85	Normal blood pressure
130-139	or	85-89	High-normal blood pressure
140-159	or	90-99	Stage 1 (mild) hypertension
160-179	or	100-109	Stage 2 (moderate) hypertension
180-209	or	110-119	Stage 3 (severe) hypertension
210 or higher	or	120 or higher	Stage 4 (very severe) hypertension

Reprinted from the Sixth Report of the Joint National Committee on Detection, Evaluation and Treatment of High Blood pressure, Public Health Service, National Institutes of Health, National Heart, Lung and Blood Institute. NIH Publication 98-4080, 1997.

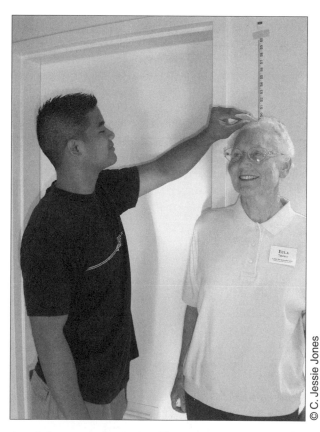

© C. Jessie Jones

A quick way to determine if someone is overweight or obese is to measure their body mass index (BMI).

example, if an individual weighs 160 pounds (160 pounds/2.2 = 72.7 kilograms) and is 5 feet 6 inches tall (66 inches/39.4 = 1.7 meters), you would divide 72.7 kilograms by 2.89 square meters, resulting in a BMI of 25.2 kilograms per square meter.

A BMI between 18.5 and 24.9 kilograms per square meter for men or women is desirable (Expert Panel on the Identification, Evaluation, and Treatment of Overweight and Obesity in Adults, 1998). When the BMI is between 25 and 29.9 kilograms per square meter, an individual is considered overweight and is at a slightly elevated risk of developing obesity-related medical conditions, including heart disease, hypertension, and diabetes. It is recommended that individuals in this category who have no other cardiovascular disease risk factors not gain additional weight. Those with two or more obesity-related risk factors, such as hypertension and diabetes, should be advised to lose weight. A BMI above 30 kilograms per square meter indicates obesity and is associated with a significantly higher risk of developing obesity-related disorders. Individuals with a BMI over 30 kilograms per square meter should also lower their weight.

The BMI is a good starting point for determining body composition because it is easy to calculate and can be used to evaluate change. However, it should be used in conjunction with the waist-to-hip ratio or waist circumference (discussed in the following section), or even visual inspection, since the BMI does not discriminate between fat and nonfat tissue. As a result, the BMI for those with high muscle mass must be interpreted with caution since their BMI may incorrectly indicate that they are overweight, or even obese. Although this is rarely an issue in older adult populations, it may apply to some master-level athletes, especially those involved in heavy resistance exercise.

Waist-to-Hip Ratio and Waist Circumference

Two other methods to evaluate obesity are waist-to-hip ratio and waist circumference. These measures indicate an individual's amount of abdominal fat (android obesity), high levels of which are associated with greater risk of heart disease, type 2 diabetes, and hypertension. To determine the **waist-to-hip ratio,** simply divide the client's waist circumference by hip circumference. The **waist circumference** is measured at the narrowest part of the trunk between the bottom of the sternum and the belly button. The hip measurement is taken at the largest circumference around the buttocks. Waist-to-hip ratios above 0.97 for men 50 to 59 years old and 0.82 for women the same age are associated with chronic disease risk. For adults ages 60 to 69 years, the high-risk category is indicated by a waist-to-hip ratio above 0.99 for men and 0.84 for women (Heyward & Stolarczyk, 1996).

Waist circumference alone, without hip circumference, can also be used to evaluate abdominal fat content. The Expert Panel on the Identification, Evaluation, and Treatment of Overweight and Obesity in Adults (1998) has indicated that men with waist circumferences greater than 102 centimeters (40 inches) and women with waist circumferences greater than 88 centimeters (35 inches) who have a BMI of 25 to 29.9 have a high risk of coronary artery disease, while those with BMIs of 30 or higher have a very high risk.

- The BMI is based on a client's body weight in relation to his or her height.
- The BMI can be calculated by dividing body weight in kilograms by the square of height in meters.
- A BMI between 18.5 and 24.9 kilograms per square meter is desirable for men and women.
- A BMI above 30 kilograms per square meter indicates obesity and is associated with a significantly higher risk of developing obesity-related medical conditions, including heart disease, hypertension, and diabetes.

- Waist-to-hip ratio and waist circumference can be used to evaluate abdominal fat, high levels of which are associated with greater risk for heart disease, type 2 diabetes, and hypertension.
- For adults ages 60 to 69 years, waist-to-hip ratios above 1.03 for men and 0.90 for women are associated with substantially greater risk of heart disease.
- Men with waist circumferences greater than 102 centimeters (40 inches) and women with waist circumferences greater than 88 centimeters (35 inches) who have BMIs of 30 or more have a very high risk of coronary artery disease.

Implications for Program Design and Management

Preactivity screening provides information about individuals *before* they participate in performance testing or exercise classes. Clearly, many factors that can affect, for better or worse, an individual's health status, require a change in the exercise program. How often should the information gained from screening be updated? A basic rule of thumb is that whenever a client has a recognized decline in health or function that suggests an elevation in risk, he or she should be reevaluated. For example, if a client experiences acute symptoms such as dizziness or fatigue, the exercise intensity should be lowered to a level that does not produce the symptoms. If a client begins to experience chronic symptoms (e.g., chest pain indicative of heart disease) that are aggravated by exercise, he or she should be referred to a physician and reevaluated before resuming the exercise program. In addition, each client's health information should also be updated whenever there is a recognized change in care or status. For example, if the physician prescribes a new medication, the individual's confidential, permanent health information should be updated to reflect that change. Clients are recommended to have an annual medical examination, regardless of health status, and all preactivity screening tests and forms should be repeated or renewed annually, including the physician's consent form, the health and activity questionnaire, BMI measurement, blood pressure measurement, and so on.

One challenge that instructors of community-based programs face is dealing with walk-ins, people who would like to participate immediately but have not been screened. Although it is recommended that you screen all participants following the steps in this chapter, it is not always possible to do this in some exercise class settings. In such cases, have the participants complete the PAR-Q to quickly identify those at the greatest risk of injury. As for any client, if a walk-in answers yes to any of the questions, his or her participation should be delayed until further screening can be performed.

Screening is an essential component of all exercise programs for older adults. Not only is screening a legal responsibility, but the client's safety and the program's effectiveness depend on it. Some people are reluctant to provide health or personal information. An open line of communica-

tion between you and each participant is extremely important. You should do your best to educate all prospective clients about the importance of providing accurate information during screening and the need for further medical screening if it is indicated. Without this information, it is impossible to determine whether a person is at a high risk of injury or death while participating in performance testing or exercise. If you feel you need more information as you conduct the screening process, do not hesitate to refer clients to their physicians. Because safety is paramount, you should exclude from participation those individuals with cardiovascular disease who do not complete recommended medical evaluations and those who fail to complete the screening questionnaires.

Summary

An initial screening of participants to identify those with symptoms of disease and those at increased risk of disease is essential to optimize safety during performance testing and exercise and to develop an effective exercise prescription. In addition, screening establishes a baseline of health and fitness parameters that can be used to monitor future progress. Thus it is also an invaluable motivational tool for older adults. By following the five steps of the screening process described in this chapter, you can identify those individuals who need a medical check-up before participating in performance testing or exercise.

The basic tools required for preactivity screening include consent forms for the participant and his or her physician and questionnaires for the participant to complete. Several items must be covered by the participant's consent form, including a description of the risks, benefits, and procedures of the exercise program. The PAR-Q can serve as an evaluation tool for minimal screening of individuals before a low- to moderate-intensity exercise program or for initial screening of walk-ins. In addition, the health and activity questionnaire provides you with information about an individual's health history, lifestyle, and physical activity.

Other screening tools, such as blood pressure and BMI, can improve your understanding of a client's health status. Guided by the information that you obtain during the preactivity screening, you can recognize conditions that put an individual at risk during performance testing or exercise and conditions that require medical referral before participation. Furthermore, documenting the information that you gather during screening reduces your risk of liability and improves your ability to individualize each participant's exercise prescription. Updating this information at least yearly allows you to gauge progress and determine whether an individual's exercise program should be modified.

Key Terms

Recommended Readings

American College of Sports Medicine. (2000). *ACSM's guidelines for exercise testing and prescription* (6th ed.). Philadelphia: Lippincott Williams & Wilkins.

Howley, E.T., & Franks, B.D. (1997). *Health fitness instructor's handbook* (4th ed.). Champaign, IL: Human Kinetics.

Study Questions

1. Which of the following individuals should have a medical exam prior to starting a moderate walking program?
   a. 22-year-old male student with a father who died at age 50 from a heart attack
   b. 35-year-old sedentary woman with high blood pressure
   c. 52-year-old man who smokes, has high serum cholesterol, and has chest pain and difficulty breathing when climbing stairs
   d. all of the above

2. Which of the following factors should be considered when classifying an individual's risk status prior to exercise?
   a. diagnosed high blood pressure
   b. serum cholesterol over 240 milligrams per deciliter
   c. family history of heart disease in parents or siblings before age 55 for male relatives and age 65 for female relatives
   d. all of the above

3. The Physical Activity Readiness Questionnaire (PAR-Q)
   a. can be used as a minimal screening for entry into a low- to moderate-intensity exercise program
   b. can be used as a minimal screening for entry into a high-intensity exercise program
   c. is recommended for screening people of any age
   d. should never be used for walk-ins

4. According to the ACSM risk stratification, an individual with two positive risk factors for heart disease is classified as
   a. apparently healthy
   b. low risk
   c. moderate risk
   d. more information is needed to answer the question

5. Which is *not* a positive risk factor for heart disease in men?
    a. blood pressure of 146/95 mmHg
    b. waist circumference of 90 centimeters
    c. father died of heart attack at age 58
    d. HDL cholesterol of 25 milligrams per deciliter

6. Which of the following does *not* need to be included as part of an informed consent document?
    a. explanation of risks and benefits
    b. name of a physician to contact in case an injury occurs
    c. statement that participation is voluntary
    d. contact information of someone who can answer questions

7. The BMI indicates a client's
    a. body weight in relation to height
    b. percentage body fat
    c. blood cholesterol
    d. waist circumference

8. An individual with a resting blood pressure of 165/85 mmHg has
    a. high-normal blood pressure
    b. stage 1 (mild) hypertension
    c. stage 2 (moderate) hypertension
    d. stage 3 (severe) hypertension

9. Which of the following is *not* an absolute contraindication to exercise?
    a. acute myocarditis
    b. high-risk unstable angina
    c. suspected dissecting aneurysm
    d. acquired immune deficiency syndrome (AIDS)

Application Activities

1. George is a 72-year-old man who is 5 feet 9 inches tall and weighs 210 pounds. Determine his BMI. In which category does this place him: desirable body composition, overweight, or obese?

2. While reviewing a female client's health history and activity questionnaire, you note that she has reported on the Composite Physical Function scale that she can dress and bathe independently, walk up and down stairs, walk a block outside, cook and dust, go shopping, and walk six blocks. However, she finds it difficult to walk a mile, lift and carry a bag of groceries or a large suitcase, and rake leaves. In addition, she cannot perform strenuous activities such as hiking or bicycling. Based on this information, how would you classify her functional ability?

3. The following individuals are interested in joining your exercise program. Based on their following results of preexercise screening, evaluate their eligibility to participate in your physical activity program and any further actions that should be taken.
    a. Phil is a 50-year-old postal letter carrier. He estimates that he walks approximately 90 minutes while delivering the mail on five days each week. He is 5 feet 8 inches (173 centimeters) tall and weighs 142 pounds (64 kilograms). He smokes one pack of cigarettes a day. His blood pressure is 130/84 mmHg, his cholesterol level is 190 milligrams per deciliter, and his HDL is 60 milligrams per deciliter. He has no family history of heart disease or any other metabolic disorders.

(continued)

b. Nancy is a 67-year-old retired secretary who is 5 feet 6 inches (168 centimeters) tall, weighs 180 pounds (82 kilograms), and has never smoked. She recently retired from her job and wants to begin an exercise program to improve her health. Her blood pressure is 120/70 mmHg, her cholesterol level is 180 milligrams per deciliter, and her HDL is 44 milligrams per deciliter. She has no family history of heart disease or any other metabolic disorders.

c. Maria is a 71-year-old retired retail store manager who is 5 feet 9 inches tall (175 centimeters) and weighs 206 pounds (93 kilograms). She has been a heavy smoker all of her life, smoking a pack a day. She has type 2 diabetes, a resting blood pressure of 160/90 mmHg, a cholesterol level of 250 milligrams per deciliter, and an HDL level of 28 milligrams per deciliter. Maria's mother had a heart attack when she was 63.

6

Field-Based Physical and Mobility Assessments

C. Jessie Jones
Roberta E. Rikli

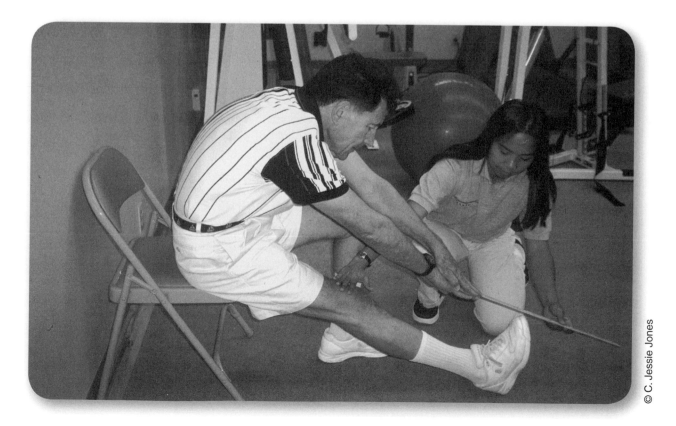

Safe and effective physical activity programming depends on a multifaceted approach to screening and assessment. No single assessment tool can measure all factors related to disease and disabilities, physical limitations, balance and mobility problems, and fall risks. In addition to preexercise screening to learn more about each client's medical and physical activity history, cardiovascular risk factors, and disability status (see chapter 5), an assessment of clients' **physical impairments** (i.e., declines in specific body systems such as the musculoskeletal, cardiovascular, and neurological systems) and **functional limitations** (i.e., restrictions in physical behaviors such as rising from a chair, lifting, or climbing stairs) is also critical before clients begin an exercise program.

Improving functional mobility and delaying the onset of physical frailty in older adults are two of the most important goals of a physical activity instructor. As discussed in previous chapters, much of the physical decline that leads to disability is preventable and even reversible through the early detection of impairments and functional limitations and the initiation of targeted physical activity programs. Specific assessments can also help you to (1) identify and predict who is or will be at risk for mobility problems and disability, (2) determine if your program is appropriate for a particular older adult, (3) motivate your clients to set personal behavioral goals, (4) select exercises that address an older adult's specific needs, (5) provide meaningful feedback to participants, (6) determine if a

referral to the client's physician is indicated, and (7) document the benefits of your physical activity or fitness program.

Unfortunately, very few physical activity instructors actually conduct the types of assessments needed to appropriately individualize programs for their clients. Common reasons reported for this omission include (1) lack of time, space, and budget; (2) absence of a requirement by facility management; (3) insufficient personnel; (4) lack of appropriate assessment tools to address the wide range of functional levels; and (5) lack of training in administering tests and interpreting their results. The purpose of this chapter is to provide the knowledge and skills necessary to select and use appropriate assessment tools to measure important physical and functional performance variables, including fall risk, in older adults.

Functional Fitness Framework

The Functional Fitness Framework (Rikli & Jones, 1997; 1999; 2001) identifies the physical fitness parameters associated with functional mobility that are required for the performance of various activities of daily life. Some common activity goals are listed in the last column of figure 6.1 (e.g., personal care, shopping, housework). These activity goals cannot be achieved unless certain motor func-

Physical parameters	Functions	Activity goals
Muscle strength/endurance	Walking	Personal care
Aerobic endurance	• Stair climbing	• Shopping/Errands
Flexibility	Standing up from chair	Housework
Motor ability	Lifting/reaching	Gardening
• Balance	Bending/kneeling	Sports
• Coordination	Jogging/running	Traveling
• Speed/agility		
• Power		
Physical impairment →	Functional limitation →	Physical disability/dependence

FIGURE 6.1 Functional Fitness Framework. A physical performance framework demonstrating the progressive relationship between physiological performance, functional performance, and activity goals.

Adapted, by permission, from R.E. Rikli and C.J. Jones, 1997, "Assessing physical performance in independent older adults: Issues and guidelines," *Journal of Aging and Physical Activity* 5(3): 246.

tions, listed in the middle column (e.g., walking, stair climbing, lifting), can be performed. These functions in turn require an adequate level of one or more of the physical fitness parameters identified in the first column (e.g., strength, endurance, flexibility).

Disability is defined as difficulty in the performance of socially defined roles and tasks, such as personal care, household chores, socializing with friends, working, and recreation (Rikli & Jones, 1997). The Functional Fitness Framework can also be used as a guide in selecting appropriate assessment tools to identify physical impairments or functional limitations that may affect your clients' ability to perform activities of daily living or engage in recreational pursuits.

Considerations for Test Selection and Evaluation

Although numerous scales and tests have been developed to measure physical disabilities in frail older adults, far fewer assessment tools have been developed that can also be used to measure physical performance and functional ability levels in the healthier, community-dwelling older adult population (VanSwearingen & Brach, 2001). Before we describe recommended assessment tools, it is important that you become familiar with the criteria used to select sound measurement tools. Unfortunately, not all published assessment tools

currently have the scientific rigor necessary to ensure their reliability and validity for the intended population. The following sections discuss two major categories of criteria for the selection and evaluation of test instruments: (1) practicality of use and (2) psychometric properties (the degree to which tests meet established test construction guidelines.

Practicality

Practicality, also referred to as the usability or feasibility of the test, should be considered when selecting an assessment tool. A practical test is one that is usable within the conditions at hand. Many factors influence the usability of a test item, including (1) whether medical permission or supervision is required and is available, (2) the time needed to administer and score the test, (3) the personnel and expertise needed to conduct the test, (4) the type of equipment and space needed, (5) the level of fatigue caused by a particular test or test item, and (6) whether the test is socially acceptable and meaningful to your clients. For example, although a preferred means of measuring lower-body strength might be using a Cybex leg press, this may not be practical for use in most field settings because of the cost of this specialized equipment or because of the time it would require to measure a large number of clients on the same day. Similarly, a strenuous test that requires physician approval would not be practical in settings when participants do not have easy access to physicians.

Psychometric Properties

The selection and evaluation of a test item should also be based on its **psychometric properties** (i.e., the degree to which the test meets test construction guidelines with respect to reliability, validity, discrimination power, and performance standards). For example, in assessing older adults, it usually is important that test items be able to provide accurate (reliable) measures of current ability and be able to assess the current or future risk for mobility problems, falls, or disability.

Reliability

Reliability indicates the degree to which two test scores would be similar if the test were repeated under identical conditions, meaning that the test is relatively free of measurement error and provides dependable and consistent scores. This type of consistency in a score is also referred to as *test–retest reliability*. Test reliability (i.e., the correlation between two sets of scores) should be greater than .80. In collecting baseline measures, it is especially important that a test provide a reliable baseline score; otherwise you can never be sure that a change in score reflects an actual change in performance over time. The reliability of a test item is always determined using trained test administrators. Therefore, it is extremely important that all testers are trained to administer each test item according to its published protocol. If more than one tester will administer the same test item, then each tester should practice administering and scoring the test item with the same small set of clients. The scores obtained by each tester for the same clients should be compared for accuracy. When scores obtained by multiple testers are very similar (are highly correlated), the test is considered to have good **interrater reliability.**

Validity

The most important characteristic of any test is its **validity.** A valid test is one that has been shown to measure what it is intended to measure. One way to evaluate a test's validity is by comparing its scores with scores on another criterion measure that is already known to be valid (sometimes referred to as a *gold standard*). For example, a test to measure lower-body strength such as the 30-sec chair stand test (see figure 6.2), discussed later in this chapter, was validated by comparing an older adult's performance on it with his or her performance on a common laboratory-based measure of

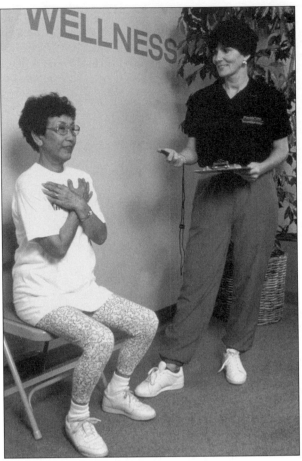

© Human Kinetics

FIGURE 6.2   The chair stand is a field-based measure of lower-body strength.

lower-body strength, a one-repetition maximum (1RM) leg press. The scores of the two tests were statistically compared using correlation analysis. Tests are generally considered to have acceptable **criterion-related validity** when the correlation values are greater than .70.

A test's validity can also be assessed through content analysis. **Content validity,** often referred to as *face* or *logical validity,* is the degree to which a test measures the domain of interest. No statistical procedures are needed to determine whether a test has content validity; experts in the field only need to agree that the test measures a particular domain of interest. For example, the domain of interest of the Berg Balance Scale is balance (BBS; Berg, Wood-Dauphinee, Williams, & Gayton, 1989; Berg, Wood-Dauphinee, & Williams, 1992). Experts in the field have agreed that the items on the BBS do indeed measure different dimensions of balance.

When a test can predict future conditions or behaviors, such as falling or disability, the test is said to have **predictive validity.** For a test to have predictive validity, research findings must demonstrate statistically that its score is highly related to a future outcome, such as falls, loss of functional mobility, or disability. For example, people who score below 46 points out of 56 on the Berg Balance Scale have been shown statistically to have high risk of falls. Predictive validity also provides a meaningful standard for expected performance, which can be used to evaluate the program outcome (Guralnik et al., 2000).

Discrimination Power

When a test is able to discriminate among different levels of an attribute or ability, it is said to have **discrimination power.** To assess a change in performance over time or in relation to a particular intervention, a test needs to measure performance levels on a continuum, with minimal floor or ceiling effects. A **floor effect** occurs when a test is too difficult for many of the clients performing it (e.g., using the 1-mile [1.6-kilometer] walk or run for frail older adults). A **ceiling effect** occurs when a test is too easy for most clients. For example, the Berg Balance Scale tends to exhibit ceiling effects when administered to high-functioning older adults. Many community-residing older adults achieve the maximum score of 56 points on that test, despite reporting balance problems. A subcomponent of discrimination power is the **responsiveness** of a measure, which is its ability to detect meaningful change over time. The smaller the change in performance detected by the measure, the higher the responsiveness and the more confident the instructor can be about detecting changes at the end of the exercise program. Tests that use continuous scoring systems (e.g., the timed eight-foot [2.4-meter] up-and-go, which is reported in seconds) are inherently more sensitive to changes in performance than tests that use only categorical scores (e.g., good, average, and poor) or a numerical rating scale (e.g., 1, 2, 3).

Performance Standards

After clients are tested, it is important to have a way of interpreting their score to them. Performance standards provide a useful way of evaluating test results. There are two types of performance standards: norm referenced and criterion referenced. The scores of a test with **norm-referenced standards** can be evaluated in comparison to others of the same age and sex. **Criterion-referenced standards** provide a means of evaluating performance in relation to a particular reference point or goal of interest, such as having the fitness level needed to climb stairs or to remain functionally independent. Although both types of standards provide important comparison information, criterion standards are especially helpful in identifying people at risk for mobility problems. For example, if an older adult is unable to complete eight chair stands in 30 seconds without using his or her hands, studies have shown that he or she may be at risk for loss of functional mobility (Rikli & Jones, 1999).

Reliability: The degree to which two test scores are similar when the test is repeated under similar conditions.

Interrater reliability: The degree to which two or more test administrators are able to produce the same scores for the same clients.

Validity: The ability of a test to measure what it is intended to measure.

Criterion-related validity: The degree to which a test correlates with a criterion measure (the gold standard).

Content validity: The degree to which a test measures the intended domain of interest.

Predictive validity: The ability of a test to predict future outcomes.

Discrimination power: The ability of a test to distinguish different performance or attribute levels.

Floor effect: Occurs when a test is too difficult for much of the population of intent, thus making it impossible for these people to receive a score.

Ceiling effect: Occurs when a test is too easy for a large part of the population, causing many people to "top out" in the scoring scale, which limits the discrimination ability of the test.

Performance standards: Can be either norm-referenced (where individuals scores are compared to others within a particular group) or criterion-referenced (where scores are compared to some point of interest, such as ability to climb stairs).

Recommended Assessment Tools

This section briefly describes two field-based assessment tools designed to measure physical impairments and functional limitations in older adults. Both tests are designed to meet the basic criteria for sound tests discussed in the previous section. The tests described in this section are capable of measuring various aspects of the physical fitness parameters or motor functions needed to achieve the activity goals described in the Functional Fitness Framework presented earlier (see figure 6.1). Based on feedback from hundreds of practitioners in the field, these tests are practical and easy to use in terms of training, equipment, space, and time requirements.

The Senior Fitness Test

The Senior Fitness Test (SFT) was developed not only to measure the underlying physical parameters of functional mobility but also to assess the ability to perform functional tasks of daily living (e.g., ambulation, reaching, rising from a chair, climbing stairs); hence the test battery was originally titled the Functional Fitness Test (Rikli & Jones, 1999). For example, instead of measuring just lower-body strength, the 30-second chair stand also measures the ability to perform the common task of standing up from and sitting back down on a chair. Because each of the SFT items is practical and relevant, participants who com-

plete the test find the experience meaningful and motivating. A brief description of each test item is presented in figure 6.3. The SFT manual (Rikli & Jones, 2001) provides detailed information on administering and scoring the test in individual and group settings and explains how to provide feedback to participants about their results using a provided set of U.S. national norms. The appendix of the SFT manual includes reproducible sample forms, charts, tables, and posters for instructors to use in their programs. An instructional video and computer software for recording and analyzing the results are also available for use with the SFT.

- This test battery was designed to meet the practical and psychometric properties (reliability, validity, and discrimination) conditions previously discussed.
- It is convenient and practical to use in terms of equipment, training, space, and time requirements.
- Its norm-referenced standards increase the interpretability of the test items in the United States.
- It is currently used in several countries.
- It assesses a wide range of physical abilities.
- It uses continuous-scale scoring so that significant differences can be detected in functional levels and over time.
- Older adults can perform test items safely without the need for a medical release in most cases.

Exercise	Purpose	Description	Risk zone
30-Second Chair Stand	To assess lower body strength needed for numerous tasks such as climbing stairs; walking; and getting out of a chair, tub, or car	Number of full stands that can be completed in 30 seconds with arms folded across chest	Less than 8 unassisted stands for men and women

FIGURE 6.3   Brief summary of the Senior Fitness Test items.

Adapted, by permission, from R.E. Rikli and C.J. Jones, 2001, *Senior fitness test manual* (Champaign, IL: Human Kinetics), 61, 63, 65, 67, 69, 71, 72.

Exercise	Purpose	Description	Risk zone
Arm Curl	To assess upper-body strength needed for performing household tasks and other activities involving lifting and carrying things such as groceries, suitcases, and grandchildren	Number of biceps curls that can be competed in 30 seconds holding a hand weight of 5 lbs (2.27 kg) for women; 8 lbs (3.63 kg) for men	Less than 11 curls using correct form for men and women
6-Minute Walk	To assess aerobic endurance, which is important for such tasks as walking distances, climbing stairs, shopping, and sightseeing	Number of yards/meters that can be walked in 6 minutes around a 50-yard (45.7-meter) course (5 yards = 4.57 meters)	Less than 350 yards for both men and women
2-Minute Step Test	Alternate aerobic endurance test for use when space limitations or weather prohibits taking the 6-Minute Walk Test	Number of full steps completed in 2 minutes, raising each knee to a point midway between the patella (kneecap) and iliac crest (top hip bone); score is number of times right knee reaches the required height	Less than 65 steps for both men and women
Chair Sit-and-Reach	To assess lower-body flexibility, which is important for good posture, normal gait patterns, and various mobility tasks such as getting in and out of a bathtub or car	From a sitting position at the front of a chair, with leg extended and hands reaching toward toes, the number of inches (cm) (+ or -) between extended middle fingers and tip of toe	**Men:** Minus (–) 4 inches or more **Women:** Minus (–) 2 inches or more
Back Scratch	To assess upper-body (shoulder) flexibility, which is important in tasks such as combing hair, putting on overhead garments, and reaching for a seat belt	With one hand reaching over the shoulder and one up the middle of the back, the number of inches (cm) between extended middle fingers (+ or –)	**Men:** Minus (–) 8 inches or more **Women:** Minus (–) 4 inches or more
8-Foot Up-and-Go	To assess agility and dynamic balance, which are important in tasks that require quick maneuvering such as getting off a bus in time, getting up to attend to something in the kitchen, or getting up to go to the bathroom or to answer the phone	Number of seconds required to get up from a seated position, walk 8 feet (2.44 meters), turn, and return to seated position	More than 9 seconds

FIGURE 6.3 *(continued)*

Adapted, by permission, from R.E. Rikli and C.J. Jones, 2001, *Senior fitness test manual* (Champaign, IL: Human Kinetics), 61, 63, 65, 67, 69, 71, 72.

TABLE 6.1   Fullerton Advanced Balance (FAB) Scale

Test item	Dimension of balance measured
1. Stand with feet together, eyes closed	Sensory organization (use of somatosensory inputs)
2. Reaching forward to retrieve object	Forward limits of stability
3. Turning in a full circle to right and left	Sensory organization, dynamic balance
4. Stepping up and over bench	Anticipatory postural control, dynamic balance
5. Tandem walk	Dynamic balance on reduced base of support
6. Standing on one leg, eyes open	Static balance on reduced base of support
7. Standing on foam, eyes closed	Sensory organization (use of vestibular inputs)
8. Two-footed jump for distance	Dynamic balance, whole-body motor coordination
9. Walk with head turns	Sensory organization (visual-vestibular inputs)
10. Unexpected backward release	Reactive postural control

Adapted from D.J. Rose 2003.

Fullerton Advanced Balance Scale

The Fullerton Advanced Balance (FAB) Scale is a newly developed test to measure multiple dimensions of balance in different sensory environments (Rose, 2003). The test was developed for higher-functioning older adults. The FAB Scale comprises 10 items that are scored using a 0-to-4 ordinal scale (see table 6.1). The highest score possible on the test is 40 points. Items include standing on foam with eyes closed, walking with head turns, stepping up and over an obstacle (figure 6.4), and jumping for distance. The FAB Scale has demonstrated high test–retest reliability, intra- and interrater reliability (with trained professionals), and construct validity. The procedures for administering and scoring the test are described in *FallProof* (Rose, 2003).

Guidelines for Group Testing

This section provides some basic guidelines to help ensure safe, reliable, and efficient assessments in a group setting. Before assessment day a number of tasks must be completed. Two important tasks are the training of test administrators and the scheduling of testing for clients.

Administrator Training

Once you have selected the test items that are appropriate for your setting, you need to pur-

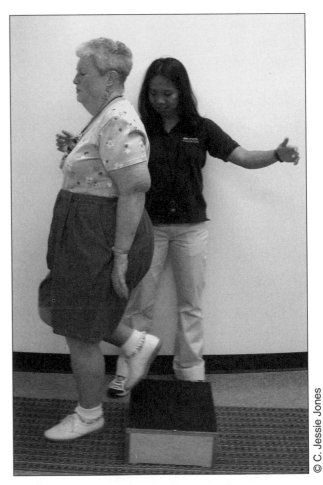

© C. Jessie Jones

FIGURE 6.4   Participant steps up and over a 6-inch high bench, an item on the FAB Scale that measures anticipatory postural control and dynamic balance.

chase the necessary equipment and tools and then become very familiar with how to administer the test. It is best to practice administering and scoring the tests with a group of clients you know well. After you are comfortable with your skills in administering the test items, you have to decide how many assistants you need to administer the test items efficiently and effectively in a group setting. The next step is to train each test administrator until he or she can conduct the test and record the score reliably. It is best for you and your assistants to practice measuring the same group of clients and then comparing scores to check their accuracy. It is extremely important to follow the test protocol exactly as written and to treat all clients the same. However, if a client is unable to perform a test item using the exact protocol, allow him or her to complete the test, but note the adaptation on the scorecard.

Assessment Day

Before scheduling the assessments, you need to establish how many clients you can accommodate in a single testing period. Whether you conduct individual or group assessments, each participant needs to complete a health and physical activity questionnaire and an informed consent form and receive medical clearance if necessary before the assessment (see chapter 5).

Before performing a Senior Fitness Test item that measures aerobic endurance (the six-minute walk or the two-minute step test), a client requires medical clearance in any of following conditions:

- A physician has previously advised the client not to exercise because of a medical condition.

- The client currently is experiencing chest pain or dizziness or has angina (chest tightness, pressure, pain, heaviness) following exertion or during exercise.

- The client has experienced congestive heart failure.

- The client has high and uncontrolled blood pressure (160/100 mmHg or above).

Participants should also be reminded on the informed consent form to monitor their physical exertion level, to perform all test items within their comfort zone (i.e., never to a point of overexertion or beyond what feels safe), and to notify the instruc-

tor if they feel any discomfort or experience any unusual symptoms. In addition, before assessment day, participants should be given written instructions to avoid heavy exertion and alcohol use for 24 hours before testing, to eat a light meal one hour before testing, to wear clothing and shoes appropriate for physical activity, and to bring a hat and sunglasses for walking outside. As a reminder, the assessment date and time can also be written on the top of the instruction sheet.

Arrive early on assessment day to make sure that each test station is set up correctly, scorecards are ready, and all equipment is in working order. Double-check that your assistants understand their responsibilities. Clients should not be allowed to participate in any assessments if their health and activity questionnaires or informed consent forms have not been completed. Before conducting the assessments, you or another physical activity instructor should lead the participants through 8 to 10 minutes of general warm-up and flexibility exercises. The measures of functional status described in this chapter do not require a warm-up period longer than this. Before starting, participants should be instructed to do the best they can but never to push themselves to overexertion or beyond what they feel is safe for them. The participants can then be evenly divided and sent to one of the stations to begin testing (see figure 6.5). Testing stations should be planned so that one test item does not

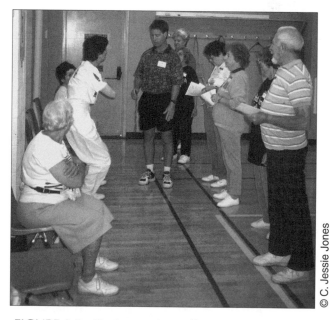

FIGURE 6.5 Testing stations allow you to measure more people at one time.

overly fatigue the participant prior to the next test item. It is ideal for you not to be responsible for a test station so that you can spot-check your assistants' accuracy in test administration and scoring.

After all testing is completed, check each recorded score for readability and completeness. It is extremely important that you treat all data (client information and scores) as confidential and store it in a cabinet that locks. Detailed information for group testing and interpreting SFT scores can be found in the SFT manual (Rikli & Jones, 2001). Information about interpreting scores on the Fullerton Advanced Balance Scale has been published in *FallProof* (Rose, 2003).

Interpreting Test Results

After testing your clients, they are almost certainly going to ask "How did I do?" There is no single best way to share test results with your clients, but you need to consider the individual and inspire hope no matter how poorly she or he performed on the test. You need to communicate that everyone can improve with exercise and that it is never too late to improve. Refer to the test manuals to see whether performance norms and criterion standards are available for interpreting scores. Depending on the test item, there are three basic ways to interpret scores:

- Pre- and posttesting. If performance norms or criterion standards for a test item are not available, you must use your professional judgment to interpret the initial scores. After your clients have participated in your program for a certain period of time (at least eight weeks), you can administer the same test again (posttest) and compare the scores from before and after your program. You can express the difference in scores as a percentage and share that information with each participant. Pre- and post-testing also let you know how effective your program intervention is at improving the physical and functional status of your clients.

- Performance norms. Very few tests have performance norms that allow comparisons with others of the same age and sex. It is important to remember when interpreting scores that norms are based on average scores for a particular group of people. For example, the norms for the SFT battery are based on the scores of over 7,000 community-dwelling older adults in the United States

between 60 and 94 years of age who volunteered to be tested at a local facility. The volunteers were 89 percent white and 11 percent nonwhite, fairly well-educated, and generally active individuals (about 60 percent reporting that they exercised at least three times per week for at least 30 minutes per day in moderate physical activity). Although you should be able to generalize the normative values to scores of similar older adults, you must take care in interpreting scores for individuals who are different from those represented in the normative study. Table 6.2 provides normal range scores for men and women, with *normal* defined as the middle 50 percent of the population. Participants scoring above the normal range would be considered *above average* for their age and gender, while those scoring below the range would be *below average*.

- Criterion standards. If a test item has a criterion standard, scores can be compared to a threshold score that helps to identify people at risk for mobility problems, falls, or disability. For example, figure 6.6 illustrates the criterion score for men who completed the eight-foot up-and-go. If a male client anywhere between 64 and 90 years old takes longer than nine seconds to complete this test, he is at risk for mobility problems. Threshold scores, that is, individuals "at risk" for mobility problems, have been provided in the last column for each test item in figure 6.3.

Summary

Being able to select, administer, and interpret tests to identify physical impairments and functional limitations is a necessary skill for all physical activity instructors of older adults. The benefits of assessments include the ability to (1) identify and predict which clients are at risk for mobility problems, (2) determine if your physical activity program is appropriate for particular clients, (3) motivate clients, (4) individualize the physical activity program, (5) provide meaningful feedback to clients, (6) determine if a medical referral is necessary, and (7) evaluate program outcomes.

The selection and evaluation of test items or test batteries should be based on their practicality of use and their psychometric properties (reliability, validity, and discrimination power). The availability of performance standards further aids in the interpretation of the scores. When a test has

TABLE 6.2 Normal Range of Scores for Men and Women

Exercise	NORMAL RANGE OF SCORES—MEN						
	60-64 yrs	65-69 yrs	70-74 yrs	75-79 yrs	80-84 yrs	85-89 yrs	90-94 yrs
Chair stands (no. of stands)	14-19	12-18	12-17	11-17	10-15	8-14	7-12
Arm curls (no. of reps)	16-22	15-21	14-21	13-19	13-19	11-17	10-14
6-Minute Walk Test (no. of yards)	610-735	560-700	545-680	470-640	445-605	380-570	305-500
2-Minute Step Test (no. of steps)	87-115	86-116	80-110	73-109	71-103	59-91	52-86
Chair Sit-and-Reach (inches + or −)	−2.5-+4.0	−3.0-+3.0	−3.5-+2.5	−4.0-+2.0	−5.5-+1.5	−5.5-+0.5	−6.5-+0.5
Back Scratch (inches + or −)	−6.5-+0.0	−7.5-−1.0	−8.0-−1.0	−9.0-−2.0	−9.5-−2.0	−10.0-−3.0	−10.5-−4.0
8-Foot Up-and-Go (seconds)	5.6-3.8	5.7-4.3	6.0-4.2	7.2-4.6	7.6-5.2	8.9-5.3	10.0-6.2
Exercise	NORMAL RANGE OF SCORES—WOMEN						
	60-64 yrs	65-69 yrs	70-74 yrs	75-79 yrs	80-84 yrs	85-89 yrs	90-94 yrs
Chair stands (no. of stands)	12-17	11-16	10-15	10-15	9-14	8-13	4-11
Arm curls (no. of reps)	13-19	12-18	12-17	11-17	10-16	10-15	8-13
6-Minute Walk Test (no. of yards)	545-660	500-635	480-615	430-585	385-540	340-510	275-440
2-Minute Step Test (no. of steps)	75-107	73-107	68-101	68-100	60-91	55-85	44-72
Chair Sit-and-Reach (inches + or −)	−0.5-+0.5	−0.5-+4.5	−1.0-+4.0	−1.5-+3.5	−2.0-+3.0	−2.5-+2.5	−4.5-+1.0
Back Scratch (inches + or −)	−3.0-+1.5	−3.5-+1.5	−4.0-+1.0	−5.0-+0.5	−5.5-+0.0	−7.0-−1.0	−8.0-−1.0
8-Foot Up-and-Go (seconds)	6.0-4.4	6.4-4.8	7.9-4.9	7.4-5.2	8.7-5.7	9.6-6.2	11.5-7.3

Normal is defined as the middle 50 percent of the population. Those scoring above this range would be considered above average for their age and those below the range as below average.

norm-referenced standards, an individual's score can be compared to scores of others of the same age and sex. A criterion-referenced standard is a threshold score that has been determined to signify risk of disease, mobility problems, or falls, to which an individual's score can be compared.

Although several measurement instruments are available, we recommend two test batteries for assessing independent, community-dwelling older adults: the Senior Fitness Test (SFT), and the Fullerton Advanced Balance (FAB) Scale. Specific guidelines for group testing include obtaining necessary equipment, practicing administering and scoring test items, training assistants, scheduling assessments, having clients complete the necessary paperwork, preparing scorecards, and setting up test stations. Three basic ways to interpret scores or determine clients' improvement include pre-

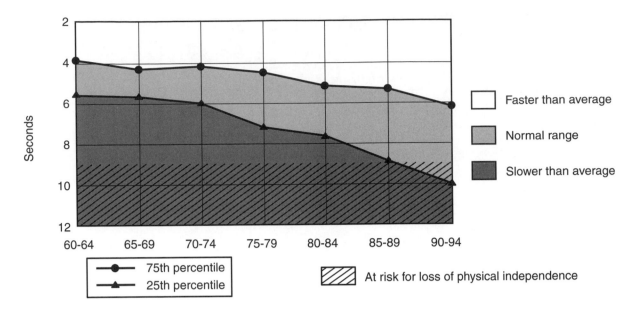

FIGURE 6.6 Men's criterion standards and normative standards for the 8-Foot Up-and-Go.

Reprinted, by permission, from R.E. Rikli and C.J. Jones, 2001, *Senior fitness test manual* (Champaign, IL: Human Kinetics), 140.

and posttest comparisons, performance norms, and criterion standards.

Key Terms

Recommended Readings

Rikli, R., & Jones, C.J. (2001). *Senior fitness test manual.* Champaign, IL: Human Kinetics.

Rose, D. (2003). *FallProof: A comprehensive balance and mobility program.* Champaign, IL: Human Kinetics.

Study Questions

1. Most older adults
   a. are not interested in their functional ability
   b. dislike having any physical attribute assessed
   c. are anxious to learn how they can improve their performance after testing is completed
   d. do not care how they perform relative to other people their own age

2. When two or more test administrators obtain very similar scores for the same clients, the test is said to have acceptable
   a. interrater reliability
   b. validity

c. discrimination power
d. predictability

3. _____ is/are a means of evaluating performance against a particular standard or goal of interest, such as functional independence.
   a. Criterion standards
   b. Normative standards
   c. Pre- and posttesting
   d. Practicality

4. If you wanted to compare your client's performance with what is expected for someone of the same age and sex, you would use
   a. criterion standards
   b. normative standards
   c. pre- and posttesting
   d. practicality
   e. discrimination

Application Activities

1. Develop a short presentation to deliver to an activity program director at a senior center to explain the potential benefits of offering an assessment program for clients.

2. Plan and administer one of the test batteries discussed in this chapter to a small group of older adults at different functional levels. Provide them with feedback about their results, and explain how they might use these results to improve their fitness and mobility.

7

Laboratory-Based Physiological Assessment of Older Adults

Gareth R. Jones
Anthony A. Vandervoort
Thomas J. Overend

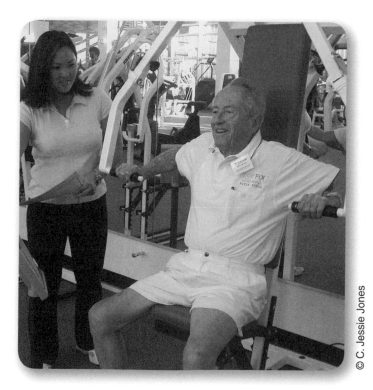

Objectives

After completing this chapter, you will be able to

1. understand the physiological basis for various laboratory-based assessments of cardiorespiratory function, muscle strength, body composition, and balance;

2. describe the key tests and equipment commonly used in an exercise physiology laboratory to conduct fitness assessments;

3. correctly administer and interpret results of selected tests of cardiorespiratory function, muscle strength, and balance; and

4. provide meaningful feedback to clients about laboratory test results.

The primary goal of exercise programs designed for older adults should be to improve or maintain all components of health-related and motor-skill-related physical fitness. The previous chapter described field-based assessments that are commonly used to measure several components of physical fitness. In settings that have more advanced equipment and professional staff, laboratory-based physical fitness assessments can provide objective and accurate information regarding older adults' strengths and weaknesses. These assessments, when performed by trained professionals, provide an accurate portrait of the overall health-related fitness of the older adult. The results can then be used to determine appropriate and safe exercise intensities (e.g., target heart rates, resistance), types of activities (e.g., aerobic endurance, strength, flexibility), and exercise settings (e.g., aquatic) most appropriate for the older adult who is interested in starting an exercise program.

The purpose of this chapter is to describe a selection of laboratory-based assessment tools to measure three health-related physical fitness components—cardiorespiratory function, muscular strength, and body composition—and one skill-related fitness component, balance.

Cardiorespiratory Function

Cardiorespiratory function (CRF) can be defined as the overall function of the cardiovascular (heart and blood vessels) and respiratory (lungs and airways) systems. Synonyms include *aerobic fitness*, *aerobic endurance*, and *cardiorespiratory endurance*. There are two good reasons that the function of

these systems should be tested in older adults. First, CRF is a key determinant of maintaining independent living. Accomplishing routine activities of daily living become difficult below certain CRF thresholds. It has been suggested that older men and women must consume a minimum of 18 milliliters of oxygen per kilogram of body weight per minute and 15 milliliters per kilogram per minute, respectively, in order to perform basic activities of daily living (BADLs; defined as fundamental activities required for self care, e.g., eating, toileting, dressing, taking medication) and instrumental activities of daily living (IADLs; defined as activities not necessary for fundamental functioning but still useful in the community, e.g., making beds, vacuuming, shopping) (Paterson, Cunningham, Koval, & St. Croix, 1999). If the cardiorespiratory system cannot provide this minimal level of oxygen to working muscles, activities of daily living (ADLs) become too difficult to perform. Thus, CRF screening can provide information regarding the functional status and potential of an older person to maintain an independent lifestyle. The second reason that CRF should be tested in older adults is to establish a baseline, or initial, cardiorespiratory fitness level before an exercise program is started. This is essential for proper prescription of work rate or intensity of aerobic endurance exercise. Subsequent tests are required to assess improvement in CRF so that the exercise intensity can be adjusted to maintain the proper training stress.

How to Measure CRF

There are two methods in which to measure CRF in a laboratory. The direct method involves measurements during maximal-intensity exercise tests. The indirect method requires measurements at one or more submaximal exercise intensities and then extrapolating, or predicting, what the measurement would be if exercise intensity had progressed to the maximum. Direct measurements are more accurate (typical error is ±3 to 5 percent) and hence provide a more precise estimation of the desired exercise intensity. Unfortunately, direct measurements also require sophisticated and expensive equipment, place greater stress on the person being tested, and are associated with a higher risk of adverse events. Physician supervision is therefore required for direct tests of CRF. Direct methods are appropriate for younger, healthy people or athletes, but relative risks, costs, and benefits must be considered when contemplating use of these tests for older adults or any individuals with moderate- or high-risk cardiac profiles. It is beyond the scope of this chapter to teach you how to perform maximal CRF tests; the focus in this section is how to conduct indirect tests of CRF.

Indirect measurements of CRF are less accurate, with typical errors of approximately 10 to 20 percent in maximal CRF prediction. This degree of error therefore makes them unsuitable for predictive purposes. It is preferable to calculate oxygen consumption from the highest submaximal work rate attained using validated equations (Franklin, Whaley, & Howley, 2000) or simply to measure heart rate (HR) at a given work rate. On the positive side, indirect measurements are generally easier to make, require less-sophisticated equipment, and involve lower risks to the person being tested. Indirect methods can be used with many types of clients but are particularly appropriate for older adults and individuals with known cardiac risk factors.

People with absolute contraindications (see chapter 5) should not be tested, and the benefits and risks must be carefully weighed in the case of individuals with relative contraindications. If the benefits outweigh the risks, exercise testing can be conducted with caution, but the test should be terminated at a submaximal rather than maximal level of exertion. Of course, no exercise test should be conducted before the older adult has received the appropriate screening for risk factors (see chapter 5). All tests described in this chapter are based on the assumption that the clients being tested have already been screened and cleared for exercise.

Equipment Required for Submaximal CRF Tests

The two types of exercise testing equipment commonly used to conduct indirect tests of CRF are treadmills and exercise bicycles (also called cycle ergometers). The primary disadvantages of treadmills for this type of test are that they are expensive and not portable, they make it difficult to obtain some measurements (e.g., blood pressure), and they are not appropriate for older adults with balance or gait disorders. It is also difficult to determine work in standardized units (e.g., watts) on a treadmill, as there is no way to measure resistance accurately. However, treadmills are the most functionally relevant type of equipment to use because walking is a very common activity.

Leg cycle ergometers are preferred for testing older adults with balance, gait, or weight problems. They also make it easy to obtain additional measures such as blood pressure because the upper body is stationary during the test. They can be adapted so that testing can be conducted in an upright or a recumbent position, they cost less than treadmills, and they are generally more portable. Because resistance to pedaling can be accurately set, it is also easy to calculate work rate in standardized units. However, cycling is not always a functional activity, especially for older adults, because only the leg muscles work during the test. Localized muscle fatigue is therefore more likely and may lead to premature curtailment of the test before a true maximal performance is achieved.

Arm cycle ergometers (see figure 7.1) are used to assess CRF in people who have little or no ambulatory ability. They are particularly useful for people with spinal cord injuries or older adults who may be confined to a wheelchair or bed. They are portable and relatively inexpensive and allow precise calculation of work rate. Their disadvantages include the increased likelihood of localized muscle fatigue because only the smaller arm muscles work during the test, the lack of functional specificity, and the difficulty in taking blood pressure measurements during the test.

Recommended Tests of CRF

Many testing protocols can be used to measure CRF in a laboratory setting, and there is no single best protocol for testing older adults because their CRF varies greatly. Three test protocols are

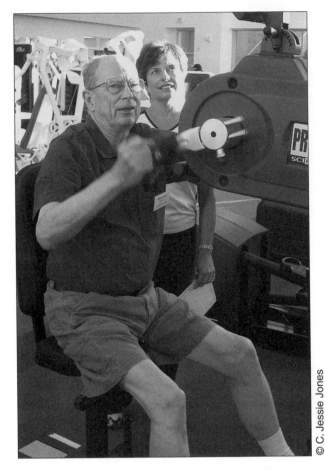

© C. Jessie Jones

FIGURE 7.1   One way to measure the cardiorespiratory fitness of participants with mobility problems is with the arm cycle ergometer.

described. The first involves a treadmill, the second a leg cycle ergometer, and the final test the arm ergometer. Either of the first two tests is appropriate for older adult clients. The final test is appropriate for older adults with certain types of disabilities. Each of the three test protocols described involves indirect measurement or estimation of the volume of oxygen consumed per minute $(VO_2 \, l \cdot min^{-1})$ using the heart rate at a given workload. These are tests that a physical activity instructor, after supervised practice, can administer without a physician in attendance.

Submaximal exercise tests require a client to work only until he or she reaches about 75 percent of maximum age-predicted heart rate. The accuracy of these tests for predicting VO_2max relies heavily on one critical assumption: that heart rate rises at the same rate as work rate during an exercise test. If this assumption were true, then submaximal test results for heart rate and work rate could be extrapolated to maximal values, allowing predic-

tion of VO_2max. However, this assumption is not completely accurate; thus there is an error of 10 to 20 percent in maximal results predicted from submaximal test values. Submaximal exercise tests are therefore better used without this extrapolation. Simply comparing the heart rate at a given work rate or oxygen consumption at a given heart rate from test to test provides an excellent indication of changes in CRF over time.

Conditions for CRF Measurement

Before conducting any CRF test, you should standardize both the test conditions (see figure 7.2) and the verbal instructions provided to the client (see figure 7.3) in order to improve the reproducibility and accuracy of the test results. Many factors affect heart rate (HR), blood pressure (BP), and rating of perceived exertion (RPE), the three most common measurements taken during exercise testing. Standardizing the instructions to the client and the test conditions makes it more likely that changes in these measurements from one test to the next are due to actual changes in CRF. Adopting a professional approach, providing a full explanation of all procedures, and allowing adequate time for older adults to ask questions and familiarize themselves with the exercise equipment assist in reducing their test anxiety.

Rating of perceived exertion (RPE) is an important measure to obtain. To increase reliability and validity of the RPE, clients should be taught how to judge their effort using this scale before any testing begins (see figure 7.4). Standardized instructions for using the RPE scale can be provided to clients in written form: "During the exercise test we want you to pay close attention to how hard you feel the exercise work rate is.

- Temperature (21-23 degrees Celsius, or 70-73 degrees Fahrenheit) and humidity (less than 60 percent) in the testing room
- Time of day of the test
- Psychological environment for the test
- Seat height on the cycle ergometer
- Type of treadmill or ergometer (arm bike or leg bike)

FIGURE 7.2   Factors to standardize before cardiorespiratory testing.

- Get a good night's sleep before the test.
- Do not eat or drink alcohol for at least three hours before the test.
- Do not drink coffee, tea, or other caffeine-containing beverages for three hours before the test.
- Do not smoke for three hours before the test.
- Take any medications at the usual time before the test.
- Do not do any heavy or moderate exercise on the day of the test.
- Wear loose-fitting clothing (T-shirt, shorts or sweatpants) that permits freedom of movement for either walking on a treadmill or arm or leg cycling.
- Wear good walking or running shoes.
- Void bladder and bowels before the test.
- Drink water as necessary for hydration.

FIGURE 7.3 Instructions to clients before cardiorespiratory testing.

6	No exertion at all
7	
8	Extremely light
9	Very light
10	
11	Light
12	
13	Somewhat hard
14	
15	Hard (heavy)
16	
17	Very hard
18	
19	Extremely hard
20	Maximal exertion

Borg RPE scale
© Gunnar Borg, 1970, 1985, 1994, 1998

FIGURE 7.4 Rating of perceived exertion (RPE) scale.

Reprinted, by permission, from G. Borg, 1998, *Borg's perceived exertion and pain scales* (Champaign, IL: Human Kinetics), 47.

This feeling should reflect your total amount of exertion and fatigue, combining all sensations and feelings of physical stress, effort, and fatigue. Don't concern yourself with any one factor such as leg pain, shortness of breath, or exercise intensity, but try to concentrate on your total, inner feelings of exertion. Try not to underestimate or overestimate your feelings of exertion; be as accurate as you can" (Franklin et al., 2000).

Treadmill Test

Treadmills are an effective and functional method to assess cardiorespiratory function in ambulatory older adults. The American College of Sports Medicine (Franklin et al., 2000) recommends that a modified Balke-Ware treadmill test be used for older adults, because it uses a slow and constant walking speed with small increases in grade every couple of minutes. This graded exercise test (GXT) is most appropriate for older adults with good ambulatory ability. The one potential problem with this test is that it may go on too long for fit older adults. However, the test can easily be modified for these clients by increasing the constant walking speed or the grade increments. Your judgment is required to determine what modifications are most appropriate for your client. Knowledge of your client's past and present physical capabilities based on completed physical activity questionnaires can help you make

these modifications. Instructions for conducting a modified Balke-Ware treadmill test are provided in table 7.1. Reasons for stopping a test, besides reaching the target HR, include these:

- Client experiences angina-like symptoms.
- Client's BP drops below 20 mmHg from the BP value recorded at rest or shows no increase in systolic BP with increased exercise intensity.
- Client has an excessive rise in systolic BP over 260 mmHg and/or a diastolic BP over 115 mmHG.
- Client is not sweating; feels light-headed, confused, or unsteady; looks pale; or has blue lips.
- Client's heart rate does not rise with increased exercise intensity.
- Client has a noticeable change in heart rhythm.
- Client requests to stop.
- Client shows physical or verbal signs of severe fatigue.
- Failure of the testing equipment.

Adapted from ACSM's Guidelines for Exercise Testing and Prescription 6th Ed, 2000.

You can calculate oxygen consumption in milliliters per kilogram per minute at the target HR (75 percent of predicted maximal HR) using the following equation (Franklin et al., 2000):

$$\dot{V}O_2 = 0.1 \times \text{speed} + 1.8 \times \text{speed} \times \text{grade} + 3.5$$

In this equation, speed is expressed in meters per minute (1 mile per hour = 26.8 meters per minute), and treadmill grade is expressed as a decimal fraction (e.g., 10 percent grade = 0.1). The value 3.5 is added to account for the resting oxygen consumption (3.5 milliliters per kilogram per minute = 1 MET):

For example, a client is 75 years old and weighs 165 pounds (75 kilograms). His target HR (75 percent of predicated maximal HR) is (207 − 0.7 × 75) × 0.75 = 116 beats per minute.

TABLE 7.1   Recommended Protocol for the Balke-Ware Treadmill Test

Before the test*	During the test	After the test
1. Make sure you have all required equipment: heart rate monitor, blood pressure cuff, RPE chart, water, towel, data collection forms, and supplies. 2. Ensure that the treadmill is working properly. 3. Greet the client, and provide a full explanation of the test procedures and measurements to be taken (HR, BP, RPE). 4. Verify that the client is dressed appropriately. 5. Record baseline HR and BP. 6. Record basic demographic information (age, height, weight, sex). 7. Calculate and record predicted HRmax (207 − 0.7 × age) and 75% of HRmax. 8. Lead the client in some stretching exercises for the leg muscles (calf, front and rear thigh muscles). 9. Let the client get used to walking on the treadmill. Instruct client to • straddle the belt while holding on to the railing; • start the belt moving at 2 miles (3.2 km) per hour; • let one foot get the feel of the belt speed while keeping the other foot off the belt; • while holding on to the railings, step on with both feet, stand tall, and look forward; • try to walk heel to toe with a normal gait pattern; and • use fingertip support on the handrails until comfortable on the treadmill. 10. Review test instructions and procedures for stopping the test.	1. Set the treadmill speed at 2 miles (3.2 kilometers) per hour. Speed can be 2.5 or 3 miles (4 or 4.8 kilometers) per hour for better-conditioned clients. 2. Set the initial grade at 0%. 3. Instruct the client to start walking. Watch for correct walking form. 4. Increase the grade by 1% every minute (2% for better-conditioned clients). 5. Record HR and RPE near the end of every minute. If possible, record BP every second minute. Monitor the client's physical appearance, facial expressions, and symptoms. 6. Stop the test when • client reaches 75% of HRmax, • client requests that the test be stopped, or • any indications for stopping an exercise test are apparent (see page 99). 7. Record the HR and RPE immediately upon stopping the test.	1. Reduce grade to 0%, and have client keep walking comfortably for 4 minutes and monitor the client closely. Record HR and RPE near the end of every minute; record BP at the end of the fourth minute.** If the test is terminated early due to a health event, remove client immediately from the treadmill and assess their vital signs. 2. After the cool-down period, assist the client off the treadmill, and give him or her a drink of water and a towel; verbally check that the client has recovered from the test. 3. Calculate $\dot{V}O_2$ at the final stage of the test using the ACSM uphill-walking equation on page 100. 4. Provide meaningful feedback to the client about test results.

* Pretest screening should be conducted before this protocol.
** If HR and BP are still near exercise levels at the end of the first 4 minutes extend the cool-down period for an additional 4 minutes
Adapted from ACSM 2000.

Predicted target HR at 75% of maximum = (207 – 0.7 × age) 0.75

He reached his target HR at a grade of 8 percent and a speed of two miles per hour.

Step 1. Calculate speed in meters per minute:

2 miles per hour × 26.8 = 53.6 meters per minute

Step 2. Express grade as a decimal fraction:

8 percent grade = 0.08

Step 3. Calculate $\dot{V}O_2$:

$\dot{V}O_2$ = 0.1 × speed + 1.8 × speed × grade + 3.5

= 0.1 × 53.6 + 1.8 × 53.6 × 0.08 + 3.5

= 5.36 + 7.72 + 3.5

= 16.58 milliliters per kilogram per minute

The $\dot{V}O_2$ value obtained from indirect measurement does not by itself mean very much because there is very little information available on average CRF levels in older adults. Most exercise tests and exercise-related research are conducted with younger men and women. However, this calculation does indicate approximately 75% of your client's predicted maximal HR and whether his or her $\dot{V}O_2$ is comfortably higher than the theoretical threshold for accomplishing activities of daily living (between 15 and 18 milliliters per kilogram per minute; Paterson et al., 1999). More important, you can use this value as a baseline against which to compare subsequent $\dot{V}O_2$ values after an exercise program has been initiated. Over time you should see an increase in $\dot{V}O_2$ at the same HR level, which indicates that your client's CRF is improving. Repeating this treadmill test at regular intervals provides an excellent indication of changes in CRF as a result of regular participation in an exercise program.

Cycle Ergometer Test

In contrast to the treadmill test just described, the starting level in most cycle ergometer tests represents a moderate work rate for many older adults, leaving little room for safe progression to higher work rates. Perhaps the easiest test to administer is a simple six-minute cycle ergometer test known as the Astrand-Ryhming test. This test can be used either to predict $\dot{V}O_2$max or to compare heart rate and $\dot{V}O_2$ at a given work rate from test to test. The test can be conducted with any cycle ergometer on which work rate can be accurately calculated (in watts, or kilopond-meters per minute). The most

common cycle ergometer used for this type of test is the Monark ergometer. The recommended test protocol for the Astrand-Ryhming ergometer test is provided in table 7.2.

The oxygen consumption at the target HR (approximately 75 percent of predicted maximal HR) can be calculated using the following equation (Franklin et al., 2000):

$\dot{V}O_2$ = 1.8 × work rate × constant/body mass + 7

In this equation, body mass is measured in kilograms, and work rate is given as revolutions per minute (50 revolutions per minute in the Astrand-Ryhming test) multiplied by the bike resistance setting and is multiplied by a constant that represents how far the bike would travel for each pedal revolution if it were able to roll freely. For a Monark cycle ergometer, the constant is 6. For Tunturi or BodyGuard ergometers, the constant is 3. The number 7 is added to account for the oxygen consumption during unloaded cycling and at rest (7 milliliters per kilogram per minute = 2 METs). For example, your client is a 70-year-old woman who weighs 110 pounds (50 kilograms). She pedaled at a speed of 50 revolutions per minute at a bike (Monark cyle ergometer) resistance setting of 1.0 and achieved a steady-state HR near her target of 75 percent maximal HR, (207 – 0.7 × 70) × 0.75 = 119 beats per minute.

Step 1. Calculate the work rate times the ergometer constant:

Work rate = revolutions per minute × bike resistance setting × constant

= 50 revolutions per minute × 1 kilopond × 6 meters per revolution

= 300 kilopond-meters per minute

Step 2. Calculate $\dot{V}O_2$:

$\dot{V}O_2$ = 3 × work rate/body mass + 3.5

= 3 × 300/50 + 3.5

= 21.5 milliliters per kilogram per minute

Just as the $\dot{V}O_2$ value calculated for the treadmill test was not meaningful in and of itself, the $\dot{V}O_2$ value from a single cycle ergometer test does not yield much information either. This score also indicates whether, at an HR of about 75 percent predicted maximal HR, your client's CRF is comfortably greater than the theoretical threshold for accomplishing activities of daily living (15-18

TABLE 7.2　Recommended Protocol for the Astrand-Ryhming Leg Cycle Ergometer Test

Before the test*	During the test	After the test
1. Make sure you have all required equipment: heart rate monitor, blood pressure cuff, RPE chart, water, towel, data collection forms, metronome, and supplies.	1. Instruct the client to start pedaling in time to the metronome beat.	1. Reduce the resistance to near 0, and instruct the client to keep pedaling slowly for 4 minutes and monitor them carefully. If the test is terminated early due to a health event, remove client immediately from the cycle ergometer and assess their vital signs. Record HR and RPE near the end of every minute; record BP at the end of the fourth minute.**
2. Ensure that the cycle ergometer is working properly and has been calibrated.	2. When the proper speed is attained, set the initial work rate to 150 kp · m/min (bike setting of 0.5) for women or 300 kp · m/min (bike setting of 1.0) for men, and start the timer for the test.	
3. Greet the client, and provide a full explanation of the test procedures and measurements to be taken (HR, BP, RPE).	3. Record HR and RPE near the end of every minute. If possible, record BP every second minute. Continually monitor the client's physical appearance, facial expressions, and symptoms.	
4. Verify that the client is dressed appropriately for bike riding.	4. Ensure that the resistance setting does not drift up or down and that the client is keeping time with the metronome.	
5. Record baseline HR and BP.	5. The goal of the test is to have the client work for 2 or 3 minutes at an HR close to 75% of HRmax. If, after the first 2 minutes, HR is still below 110 beats per minute, increase the resistance setting on the bike by 0.5 unit.	2. After the cool-down period, assist the client off the exercise bike, and provide him or her with water and a towel; verbally check that the client has recovered from the test.
6. Record basic demographic information (age, height, weight, sex).		
7. Calculate and record predicted HRmax (207 − 0.7 × age) and 75% of HRmax.	6. Check the HR at minute 5 and minute 6. If the difference between these heart rates exceeds 5 beats per minute, extend the test until a steady state (difference less than 5 beats per minute) is reached.	
8. Lead the client in some stretching exercises for the leg muscles (calf, front and rear thigh muscles).	7. Stop the test when	3. Calculate $\dot{V}O_2$ at the final stage of the test using the ACSM equation for leg cycle ergometry on page 101.
9. Adjust the seat height to a comfortable level for the client (knee should be almost straight when the pedal is at the bottom of the stroke), and record that level for subsequent testing.	• client achieves a steady state over the final 2 minutes at an HR close to 75% of predicted HRmax,	
	• client requests to stop,	
10. Set a metronome to 100 beats per minute for a pedaling rate of 50 revolutions per minute.	• any indications for stopping an exercise test are apparent (see page 99).	4. Share the test results with the client.
11. Let your client warm up on the exercise bike, keeping time with the metronome.	8. Record RPE and BP at the end of the test.	
12. Review test instructions and procedures for stopping the test.		

* Pretest screening should be conducted before this protocol.

** If HR and BP are still near exercise levels at the end of the first 4 minutes, extend the cool-down period for an additional 4 minutes.

milliliters per kilogram per minute). A score of 12 milliliters per kilogram per minute or lower indicates that the client's ability to live independently is likely to be compromised (Paterson et al., 1999). An appropriately designed exercise program should result in an increase in $\dot{V}O_2$ at the same HR level, indicating an improvement in your client's CRF. (See chapter 21 for a discussion of specific program components to improve CRF.) As was the case for the treadmill test, repeating the Astrand-Ryhming cycle ergometer test at regular intervals during an exercise program provides a good indication of changes in CRF.

Arm Cycle Ergometer Test

For older adults with lower-limb disabilities, an arm ergometer test may be a more suitable test of CRF. There is no standard arm cycle ergometer test, but a protocol can be adapted from the six-minute Astrand-Ryhming test discussed in the previous section. The test principles remain the same: the older adult being tested should reach a steady-state HR corresponding to about 75 percent of the predicted maximal HR. Improvement in CRF is indicated by increases in $\dot{V}O_2$ at the same heart rate or by decreases in HR at the same work rate with repeated testing. The test can use any arm ergometer on which the work rate can be accurately determined. The most commonly used arm ergometer is made by Monark. Compared to the leg cycle ergometer test, HR is higher for the same work rate on arm cycle ergometers because smaller muscles do the work. Instructions for conducting an arm cycle ergometer test are provided in table 7.3.

You can calculate the oxygen consumption at the target HR (approximately 75 percent of predicted maximal HR) using the following equation (Franklin et al., 2000):

$$\dot{V}O_2 = 3 \times \text{work rate} \times \text{constant/body mass} + 3.5$$

In this equation, work rate is calculated as revolutions per minute (50 revolutions per minute in the

TABLE 7.3 Procedures for an Arm Cycle Ergometer Test

Before the test*	During the test	After the test
1. Make sure you have all required equipment: heart rate monitor, blood pressure cuff, RPE chart, water, towel, data collection forms, metronome, and supplies. 2. Ensure that the arm cycle ergometer is working properly and has been calibrated. 3. Greet the client, and provide a full explanation of the test and stopping procedures and the measurements to be taken (HR, BP, RPE). 4. Verify that the client is dressed appropriately for arm cycle exercise. 5. Record baseline HR and BP. 6. Record basic demographic information (age, height, weight, sex). 7. Calculate and record predicted HRmax (207 − 0.7 × age) and 75% of HRmax. 8. Lead the client in some stretching exercises for the arm muscles (shoulders, front and rear arm muscles). 9. Adjust the chair height to a comfortable level for the client. Arms should be parallel to the floor when extended and almost straight when the pedal is at its farthest position. 10. Set a metronome to 100 beats per minute for a pedaling rate of 50 revolutions per minute. 11. Let the client warm up on the arm ergometer, keeping time with the metronome. 12. Review test instructions and procedures for stopping the test.	1. Instruct the client to start arm cycling in time to the metronome beat. 2. When the proper speed is attained, set the initial work rate of 60 kp · m/min (ergometer setting of 0.5) for women or 120 kp · m/min (setting of 1.0) for men, and start the timer for the test. 3. Record HR and RPE near the end of every minute. Continually monitor the client's physical appearance, facial expressions, and symptoms. 4. Ensure that the resistance setting does not drift up or down and that the client is keeping time with the metronome. 5. The goal of the test is to have the client work for 2 or 3 minutes at an HR close to 75% of HRmax. If, after the first 2 minutes, HR is still below 110 beats per minute, increase the resistance setting on the ergometer by 0.25 or 0.5 unit. 6. Check the HR at minute 5 and minute 6. If the difference between these heart rates exceeds 5 beats per minute, extend the test until a steady state (difference less than 5 beats per minute) is reached. 7. Stop the test when • client achieves a steady state over the final 2 minutes at an HR close to 75% of predicted HRmax, • client requests that the test be stopped, • any indications for stopping an exercise test are apparent (see page 99). 8. Record RPE and BP at the end of the test.	1. Reduce the resistance to near 0, and instruct the client to keep arm pedaling slowly and comfortably for 4 minutes. If the test is terminated early due to a health event, remove the client immediately from the ergometer and assess their vital signs. Record HR and RPE near the end of every minute; record BP at the end of the fourth minute.** 2. After the cool-down period, provide the client with water and a towel; verbally check that the client has recovered from the test. 3. Calculate $\dot{V}O_2$ at the final stage of the test using the ACSM equation for arm cycle ergometry given on page 103. 4. Share the test results with the client.

* Pretest screening should be conducted before this protocol.

** If HR and BP are still near exercise levels following the first 4 minutes, extend the cool-down period for an additional 4 minutes.

Astrand-Ryhming test) multiplied by the resistance setting, which is multiplied by a constant that represents how far the wheel would travel for each pedal revolution if it were able to roll freely. For a Monark arm cycle ergometer, the constant is 2.4. The number 3.5 is added to account for the oxygen consumption at rest (3.5 milliliters per kilogram per minute = 1 MET). Body mass is measured in kilograms.

For example, your subject is 70 years old and weighs 165 pounds (75 kilograms). His target HR (75 percent of predicted maximal HR) is $(207 - 0.7 \times 70) \times 0.75 = 119$ beats per minute. He reached his target HR at a resistance setting of 1.0 and a cadence of 50 revolutions per minute.

Step 1: Calculate the work rate times the ergometer constant:

Work rate = revolutions per minute × resistance × constant

= 50 revolutions per minute × 1 kilopond × 2.4 meters per revolution

= 120 kilopond-meters per minute

Step 2: Calculate $\dot{V}O_2$:

$\dot{V}O_2$ = 3 × work rate/body mass + 3.5

= 3 × 120/75 + 3.5

= 8.3 milliliters per kilogram per minute

Equations for calculating oxygen consumption ($\dot{V}O_2$)

Treadmill

$\dot{V}O_2$ = 0.1 × speed + 1.8 × speed × grade + 3.5

1 mile per hour = 26.8 meters per minute

Cycle ergometer

$\dot{V}O_2$ = 1.8 × work rate/body mass + 7

Work rate = revolutions per minute × bike resistance setting × bike constant

Monark constant = 6

Tunturi or BodyGuard constant = 3

Arm ergometer

$\dot{V}O_2$ = 3 × work rate/body mass + 3.5

Work rate = revolutions per minute × resistance setting × ergometer constant

Monark constant = 2.4

Scores on arm ergometer tests are lower than scores on either treadmill tests or leg cycle ergometer tests because $\dot{V}O_2$ depends on the amount of working muscle mass, and the arms have less mass than the legs. To date, no norms or average values are available for arm cycle ergometer tests for older adults. Obviously, someone who can only be tested using an arm ergometer already has limited ability to perform activities of daily living. The initial value obtained, however, can be used as a baseline against which to compare subsequent test results obtained at regular intervals during an exercise program.

Muscular Strength

There are many different ways to measure muscle strength in the laboratory, but all measures can be grouped into two basic categories: **isometric,** in which the body and limbs remain stationary during the test, or dynamic, in which the forces generated by muscle contraction produce movement. The latter condition is the most common manner in which muscles work; they most often produce forces through dynamic contractions in which they are either shortening (known as a **concentric** activation, as happens to the thigh's quadriceps muscles when rising up out of a chair) or lengthening (an **eccentric** contraction against an external load, as happens when the quadriceps control body weight while sitting down in a chair). In an isometric activation, the length of the muscle remains constant during its activation (e.g., tests using a handgrip dynamometer, in which the handle stays at a preset, fixed position).

For dynamic tests, increasing the speed of movement significantly influences the ability of muscles to generate force; output is much reduced at high speed (flyswatters are very light weight to allow rapid swings). However, speed of movement has much less effect on eccentric test results (Enoka, 2001). A rule of thumb is that eccentric strength is usually higher than either isometric or concentric strength (which is the weakest of the three types of muscular effort). For example, a frail senior may be able to sit down in an armless chair successfully (eccentric muscle activity) but cannot get back up because of inadequate concentric leg muscle strength to lift the body weight out of the chair.

Although many different properties of muscle composition and neuromuscular performance that

Muscle strength can be measured under three different conditions:

Concentric contraction: Muscle shortens as it lifts a weight through a range of motion.

Isometric contraction: Muscle length remains constant during the contraction because of an immovable resistance (as in a handgrip test).

Eccentric contraction: An external load causes the muscle to lengthen while contracting (as when lowering a weight).

can be measured in a laboratory setting can provide considerable knowledge about an older person's muscular conditioning (Hunter, White, & Thompson, 1998), only the most common and practical tests are presented in this chapter. Brief mention is made of some advanced technology that may be encountered in a physical therapy setting.

A simple and very common assessment of muscle strength is to measure the heaviest weight that a person can move one time through a specified range of motion using correct form. This test is referred to as the **one-repetition maximum (1RM),** and the equipment used for the 1RM test can vary substantially, from simple barbells to more elaborate (and safer) weight-and-pulley machines. Tests of both upper-body and lower-body concentric muscle strength are recommended, such as the well-known seated chest press and leg press. The former is done in stable sitting position, pushing out with the arm and shoulder muscles against a handle connected to an external resistance such as a weight stack. From an initial position of bent elbows, the arms are extended outward from the chest until the elbow is fully extended. To get a stable baseline measure, these points are important: (1) allowing clients an initial practice session with the equipment, (2) standardizing the cadence or speed of the movement, (3) standardizing the angle of knees and elbows, (4) standardizing motivation such that all clients are encouraged to work at a similar rate, (5) ensuring that the same equipment and set-up are used for repeated tests, (6) administering at least two 1RM tests on separate days and using the best score.

The leg press test is performed in a similar manner, with the client seated in a stable position, hips flexed, knees bent, and feet on a large foot plate to push against. The client extends the legs outward until the knees are fully extended. Care must be taken to lower the weight stack in a controlled manner, without rapid acceleration of the leg joints in the reverse direction. If pneumatic equipment is used for these assessments, the air pressure needs to be carefully calibrated and checked prior to each test administration. Proper technique, as described in figure 7.5, is of great importance to avoid injury and obtain consistent test results.

When the goal of the testing is to make precise strength measurements, velocity of movement must be precisely controlled (because of the dramatic effect of muscle contraction speed on force production). Hence, rather elaborate and expensive machines (called **isokinetic** devices because they keep velocity constant) have been developed that regulate the speed of joint rotation closely while measuring strength. Isokinetic machines, which contain electric or hydraulic motors, also allow safe measurement of eccentric muscle strength (in effect, the powerful motor of the device moves a lever arm, and the person resists the motion as much as possible until a preset safe joint angle is reached). The most commonly tested movement is knee extension, but many other muscular actions (e.g., hip flexion and abduction, shoulder flexion) can be measured with this type of equipment.

Note the relationship between the percentage of maximal exertion that a given task represents and the ability to make repeated muscle contractions for that task. For example, a weight that represents 90 percent of 1RM can normally be lifted only four to five times in a row; however, activities requiring low contraction intensity, such as walking, use muscular forces that can be produced repeatedly for hours. This might explain why seemingly small gains in absolute muscle strength, even in the absence of measurable increases in muscle size, can dramatically improve an older person's ability to do submaximal, everyday tasks involving several minutes of effort (e.g., vacuuming, mowing the lawn).

Body Composition

The body consists of fat and nonfat components. The percentage of total body mass that is fat is generally called percentage body fat, while nonfat mass is called percentage lean body mass. Since one of the hallmarks of aging is loss of muscle mass

The 1RM test

- Objective is to find the maximum weight a person can lift once, without creating undue fatigue during the assessment.
- Only three to five cycles of adding weight are recommended.
- Clearly communicate the aim and nature of this *maximal* test to the client before and during the assessment.
- The weight lifted during the last successful attempt is recorded as the 1RM value.
- A spotter to control the weight is necessary when the person reaches a failure point.

Step 1. Instruct the client to warm up with light weights (about half the predicted maximum, determined through prior familiarization sessions with the test equipment).
- Good form (posture and stability) should be emphasized.
- Five to 10 repetitions at this weight are recommended.

Step 2. Allow a one-minute rest period, and then lead the client in some light stretching.

Instruct the client to complete three to five repetitions with a higher weight (60 percent to 80 percent of perceived maximum).

Step 3. Allow a one-minute rest period, followed by some light stretching. The exertion observed in step 2 should have appeared close to maximum capacity.

If so, a small amount of additional weight (2.5-5 pounds, or 1.1-2.3 kilograms) is added, and a lift is attempted. If the lift is judged successful—a complete movement with no need for assistance—an additional 2.5 to 5 pounds (1.1-2.3 kilograms) is added, and the lift is repeated after a rest period of three to five minutes. This process is continued until the client can complete no more than one repetition with good form.

Submaximal alternative to the 1RM test

This alternative is used if there is concern about pushing inexperienced or frail clients to their limit. The aim of this test is to determine the amount of weight that can be lifted several times before failure.

The following values, extrapolated from Sale & MacDougall (1981), can be used to set training intensity and to track progress (as participants get stronger, they can lift a given weight more times before failure).

Number of repetitions	Percentage of 1RM
10	76
8	78
6	86
4	90
2	96

FIGURE 7.5   Recommended procedure for the 1RM test.

and strength, considerable attention has been paid to quantifying this aspect of body composition and to the related health concern of increasing obesity (Franklin et al., 2000).

There are a variety of ways to measure body composition in both the field and the laboratory, and these approaches have different levels of accuracy. Advanced laboratory methods can obtain precise body composition values but have the drawback of requiring expensive equipment and a less convenient location (usually resulting in extra costs in money and time to the person being tested).

Although it is unlikely that you will conduct any of these tests, you should at least be familiar with the different types of laboratory methods available, which fall into two basic categories:

- **Hydrostatic** (underwater) **weighing, bioelectrical impedance analysis (BIA),** and assessment of air displacement (as measured by the well-known Bod Pod device), which are based on differences in the densities of muscle and fat tissue
- Imaging techniques such as dual-energy X-ray absorptiometry (DEXA) and the latest generation of magnetic resonance imaging (MRI) scanners, which provide cross-sectional areas or even volume estimates of the various tissue types

Underwater weighing can be inconvenient and difficult because the person to be tested must be fully submersed in a water tank. This method is therefore seldom used to assess older adults. The remaining tests all involve only passive participation by the person tested, but they vary in accuracy and cost. DEXA equipment is commonly available in hospitals, medical clinics, and university physiology research laboratories and is currently considered the gold standard for the measurement of bone mineral density.

Balance

The final laboratory assessment to be described in this chapter is the measurement of balance, a skill-related component of physical fitness. Over the past 10 years, a number of sophisticated instruments have been developed to test multiple dimensions of balance. Some of the dimensions of balance that can now be accurately measured using specialized equipment include static and dynamic balance, sensory organization and integration skills, and reactive postural control. Force plate technology is used to make both **kinematic** (quality of the body's motion) and **kinetic** (quantity of force produced) measurements.

Balance is defined as the ability to control the body's center of mass (COM) relative to the base of support (BOS), whether that base is stationary or moving (Rose, 2003). When standing quietly in space, the goal is to maintain the COM directly above the BOS, whereas during dynamic activities

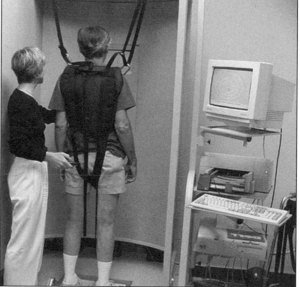

Specialized equipment can be used to measure multiple dimensions of balance, including static and dynamic balance, sensory organization and integration skills, and reactive postural control.

such as leaning or walking, the goal becomes controlling the COM as it moves through or beyond the BOS. The maximal distance an individual can move beyond a centered position without altering the BOS is referred to as the **limits of stability (LOS).** Field-based measures of balance are described in chapter 6, and methods to improve balance and mobility are described in chapter 14.

There are four measures of balance that should be considered when making a complete assessment:

1. *Static balance.* On average, older adults exhibit a greater amount of **postural sway** (movement over their BOS) than younger adults. To assess static balance, the older adult is instructed to stand quietly for a designated period of time (20-30 seconds) on a stabilometer or static force plate that can be used to measure both the magnitude and the velocity of the postural sway exhibited. When you test healthy older adults, it is recommended that you measure static balance with the clients' eyes open and closed and their feet in a more challenging position such as a tandem (heel-to-toe) or one-legged stance (Patla, Winter, Frank, Walt, & Prasad, 1990).

2. *Dynamic balance.* Simple daily activities (e.g., leaning into cupboards, walking, making beds,

mopping floors) require dynamic balance, the ability to control the COM while leaning through or moving beyond the LOS. Dynamic balance abilities are usually measured by instructing the individual to lean toward visual targets on a computer screen as quickly and accurately as possible after a visual signal to go is displayed. These tests determine the overall distance that a person can lean forward, backward, laterally, and diagonally; how quickly she or he reacts to the signal to move; and how quickly and accurately the body leans toward the target.

3. *Reactive postural control.* **Reactive postural control** (the ability to respond automatically to a loss of balance) can be accurately measured using a specialized technique called **computerized dynamic posturography (CDP).** Unlike static force plates, the platform used for CDP can be tilted up or down or moved forward or backward at different speeds and distances. Tests of reactive postural control provide information about the individual's ability to respond rapidly to an unexpected loss of balance caused by the sudden movement of the force plate. A person with good balance is able to respond quickly with a countermovement in the direction opposite the direction of plate movement. Adaptation tests (force plate tilts) and motor control tests (force plate slides forward or backward) provide valuable information about a person's ability to respond quickly and appropriately to an unexpected loss of balance and to repeated movements of the support surface.

4. *Sensory integration and organization.* An additional test of balance that can be conducted using CDP equipment is known as the sensory organization test. This test measures a person's ability to integrate and organize sensory information provided by the visual, somatosensory, and vestibular systems. By systematically exposing the person being tested to different sensory conditions (e.g., eyes closed, moving surface, moving visual surroundings), the tester determines how well each individual sensory system is functioning and how well the person can maintain upright balance when the information provided by the three systems is not in agreement. The results from this test also indicate whether an older adult is at higher risk of falls in certain sensory conditions (e.g., low lighting, compliant surfaces such as thick grass or sand, crowded or busy visual environments).

> There are two types of balance:
> Static balance is the ability to maintain the COM directly over the BOS.
> Dynamic balance is the ability to control the COM while leaning through or moving beyond the LOS.

Summary

Individual levels of physical fitness can be accurately assessed in the laboratory. An assessment of cardiorespiratory function provides valuable information regarding an individual's functional status (ability to maintain an independent lifestyle) and establishes heart rate limits for prescribing the appropriate intensity for safe and effective aerobic exercise. Similarly, laboratory assessment of muscular strength offers important information regarding the exercise workloads required to strengthen muscle effectively. Improved muscular strength directly influences older adults' functional independence. The assessment of body composition adds valuable information on overall physical fitness. New, sophisticated methods of measuring body composition (e.g., DEXA, MRI) offer very precise measurements of muscle and bone tissue density, which are important in detecting age-associated diseases (e.g., osteoporosis). Finally, the assessment of balance skills provides valuable information regarding an older adult's potential risk of falling. Appropriate exercise programs can be prescribed to address any deficits in physical fitness detected by these assessments.

Laboratory-based physiological assessments provide essential information that can be used to develop safe and effective exercise programming for older adults. For older adults just starting an exercise regimen, laboratory assessment provides valuable baseline measurements and sets appropriate limits for exercise. Older adults already involved in exercise programs can use the laboratory assessment to chart their fitness progress. In either case, fitness instructors of older adults can use this information to individually tailor the exercise program to meet the specific needs of the older adult client.

Key Terms

Recommended Readings

ACSM's Guidelines for Exercise Testing and Prescription (6th ed.). (2000). Philadelphia: Lippincott, Williams & Wilkins.

Heyward, V.H. (1998). *Advanced fitness assessment and exercise prescription* (3rd ed.). Champaign, IL: Human Kinetics.

Study Questions

1. Direct measurement of maximal oxygen consumption ($\dot{V}O_2$max)
   a. is less accurate than indirect measurement
   b. requires very basic equipment
   c. is appropriate for older adults
   d. is associated with a higher incidence of adverse effects

2. Indirect measurement of oxygen consumption ($\dot{V}O_2$)
   a. is more accurate than direct measurement
   b. requires sophisticated laboratory equipment
   c. should not be used to predict $\dot{V}O_2$max
   d. can be used only with younger clients

3. Compared with treadmills, leg cycle ergometers
   a. are more appropriate for testing people with balance problems
   b. provide more accurate measures of work rate
   c. are more difficult to move around
   d. are more expensive

4. The one-repetition maximum (1RM) test of muscle strength involves lifting a weight under ___ conditions.
   a. eccentric
   b. dynamic concentric
   c. isometric
   d. isokinetic

5. When conducting a one-repetition maximum (1RM) test, it is important to allow adequate rest periods so that the client does not experience
   a. muscle fatigue
   b. stress
   c. muscle hypertrophy
   d. both a and b

(continued)

6. Which of the following laboratory assessment techniques is not used to measure body composition in older adults?
    a. dual X-ray absorptiometry (DEXA)
    b. hydrostatic weighing
    c. graded exercise test (GXT)
    d. bioelectrical impedance analysis (BIA)

7. Which of the following tests can be performed using computerized dynamic posturography?
    a. adaptation test
    b. motor control test
    c. sensory organization test
    d. all of the above

Application Activities

1. Calculate oxygen consumption ($\dot{V}O_2$) for a client who is 75 years old and weighs 154 pounds (70 kilograms). During an Astrand-Ryhming cycle ergometer test on a Monark bike, your client reached a steady-state HR near 75 percent of predicted HRmax at a speed of 50 revolutions per minute and a bike resistance setting of 1.5.

2. Calculate oxygen consumption ($\dot{V}O_2$) for a client who, on a treadmill test, reached 75 percent of predicted maximal HR at a speed of two miles (3.2 kilometers) per hour at a treadmill grade of 12 percent.

Goal Setting and Behavioral Management

Sara Wilcox
Abby C. King

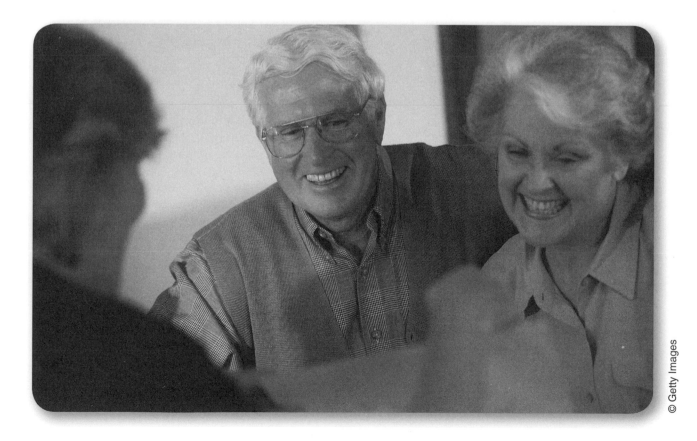

It is as important to understand the psychosocial factors that increase or decrease older adults' likelihood of adopting and maintaining an exercise program as it is to understand their health, fitness, and mobility status. One third of the population age 50 years and older is estimated to be sedentary, and one half of women age 75 years and older are sedentary (Robert Wood Johnson Foundation, 2001). In addition, dropout rates from exercise programs are high. The purpose of this chapter, therefore, is to provide the physical activity instructor with strategies to maximize exercise **adoption** (i.e., beginning a program) and **adherence** (i.e., maintaining a program) by older adults. Specifically, we discuss the factors that influence the adoption and maintenance of exercise in older adults, strategies for promoting behavior change and adherence, and implications of these issues for program design and management.

Factors Influencing Older Adults' Exercise Participation

No single factor can predict whether or not an older adult will initiate and maintain an exercise program. Rather, exercise behaviors are determined by multiple interacting factors. These factors can be grouped into three general categories: personal characteristics, program-related factors, and environmental factors (see reviews by King, 2001, and Wilcox, Tudor-Locke, & Ainsworth, 2002).

Personal Characteristics

The most consistent demographic factors that are negatively associated with exercise participation by older adults include being female, being in an ethnic minority group, older age (especially those 85 years old or older), rural residence, and low socioeconomic status. While exercise programs obviously cannot modify any of these factors, awareness of them can help you guide and tailor programs to address the unique barriers faced by these subgroups of older adults.

Health-related factors also affect exercise participation. Older adults in poor physical condition and poor health are less active than their healthy counterparts, and illness has been shown to be a strong predictor of poor adherence to exercise programs. Arthritic pain is a significant barrier to exercise by older adults, despite the benefits of exercise for people with arthritis. Pain or discomfort was one of the top five barriers to exercise identified in a recent study of older adults (Brittain, Jones, & Rikli, 2002). Older adults who smoke and those who are overweight also tend to be less active than their nonsmoking, average-weight peers.

Attitudes, knowledge, and beliefs as well as psychological factors also influence exercise behaviors of older adults. An individual's willingness to make changes in his or her physical activity level is typically a necessary but not sufficient factor for exercise adoption. Older adults who perceive greater benefits of exercise, as opposed to fewer barriers to exercise, are more likely to be active. A number of motivations for physical activity (perceived benefits) have been reported by older adults. The desires to improve health, prevent disease and disability, manage chronic illness, and improve mobility are commonly reported health-related motivations for exercise by older adults. Another motivation is the desire to improve mental health or mood, for example, by decreasing stress, depression, and anxiety and by improving energy and engagement in life. Older adults, like younger adults, cite appearance-related benefits as another motivation for exercise. Exercise enjoyment has also been associated with higher levels of physical activity and may be especially important for older adults. Exercise **self-efficacy,** or confidence in one's ability to undertake regular exercise successfully even when faced with obstacles, is a strong predictor of exercise adoption in older age. Finally, previous experience with exercise is associated with current exercise participation.

It is important to remember that older adults, especially older women, may hold more negative attitudes and beliefs about physical activity than younger adults because of inexperience, misconceptions, and stereotypes (O'Brien & Vertinsky, 1991). Commonly cited barriers to physical activity by older adults, especially older women, include the fear of falling or suffering an exercise-related injury such as a heart attack, lack of self-motivation or willpower, psychological distress (e.g., depression and anxiety), low exercise self-efficacy, and lack of knowledge or experience with the activity. Lack of time is the most frequently cited barrier to physical activity by adults in general (Sallis & Owen, 1999). Lack of time appears to be less important among older individuals; Brittain and colleagues (2002) found that lack of time was the second most frequently cited barrier to exercise in a large sample of older adults (lack of self-motivation was the most frequently cited barrier in this study).

Program Factors

Program-related factors include the structure, format, complexity, intensity, convenience, and financial and psychological costs associated with the activity. Most older adults prefer moderate-intensity activities instead of more vigorous ones. Physical activities that are convenient, inexpensive, and noncompetitive also tend to be preferred. For example, walking and gardening are cited most often by older adults as preferred physical activi-

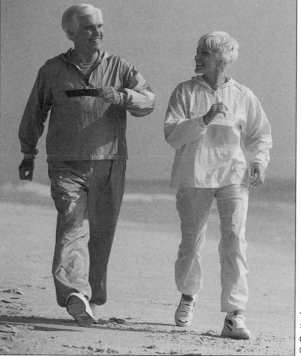

Many older adults prefer informal physical activity rather than a formal exercise class.

ties. Approximately two thirds of older women and men, regardless of current physical activity levels and race or ethnicity, prefer physical activities that can be undertaken outside of a formal class or group setting (King, Castro, et al., 2000; Wilcox, King, Brassington, & Ahn, 1999). Furthermore, adherence to supervised home-based programs is typically higher than adherence to class or group programs (King, Haskell, Young, Oka, & Stefanick, 1995; King, Pruitt, et al., 2000). Of the one third of older adults who do prefer group exercise, the social aspect of this form of activity is often a motivating factor.

Environmental Factors

Social and physical environmental factors also influence exercise participation. **Social support** (defined as assistance received through social relationships) from friends, family, and health professionals is positively associated with exercise adoption and maintenance. Social support appears to be more important to older women than men, yet many older women do not perceive that they receive support from their physicians and families to be physically active. Physical environmental factors such as the travel distance required for exercise, climate and weather, neighborhood safety, and availability of facilities for physical activity (e.g., parks, walking and jogging paths) could also affect physical activity by older adults, but these factors have received little systematic investigation. A recent study found that poor weather and the lack of social support were among the top five barriers to exercise identified by older adults (Brittain, Jones, & Rikli, 2002).

Potential personal, program-related, and environmental barriers to exercise and motivations for exercise by older adults are summarized in figure 8.1. By better understanding how these factors affect older adults in general and your clients in particular, you can more effectively select strategies

to help your clients overcome or minimize their barriers and enhance their motivations for exercise. We now turn to a description of strategies to promote exercise in older adults.

Strategies for Behavior Change

Changing a behavior such as physical activity can be difficult for adults of any age. The transtheoretical model is useful for understanding people's readiness and motivation for change (Prochaska, DiClemente, & Norcross, 1992; Prochaska & Marcus, 1994). The model states that behavior change is a process that comprises five stages (see

Barriers to exercise	Motivations for exercise
Health and medical • Illness or injury • Pain or discomfort • Lack of strength or stamina *Knowledge* • Lack of knowledge or ability *Motivational or psychological* • Lack of time • Lack of self-motivation (feeling lazy or unmotivated) • Not a priority • No enjoyment • Fear of injury • Low self-efficacy or confidence • Exercise perceived as inappropriate or unnecessary for older adults • Poor body image • Depression or anxiety *Program-related* • Lack of age-appropriate classes • Intensity too high • Inconvenient class times or hours of operation • Program cost *Environmental* • Lack of transportation • Unsafe environment (crime, traffic, etc.) • Poor weather • Lack of support from family, friends, health care providers	*Health and medical* • To feel good physically • To improve overall health • To reduce risk of disease • For rehabilitation • To maintain or improve mobility • To maintain or improve ability to do activities of daily living • To reduce risk of falls • To improve fitness • To improve strength • To reduce or manage body weight *Mental health* • To have more energy • To reduce stress and anxiety • To reduce depression • To enjoy life more fully • To feel good mentally *Appearance-related* • To maintain or improve appearance • To reduce or manage body weight *Social* • For social contact and interaction • Encouragement by family or friends • Recommendation of health care provider *Other* • For enjoyment of activity • For competition or personal challenge

FIGURE 8.1 Exercise barriers and motivations for older adults.
Data from E.L Brittain, C.J. Jones and R.E. Rikli 2002.

figure 8.2). In the precontemplation stage, people have no intention to adopt or change a behavior because they may not be aware of the problem, they may be in denial about the problem, or they may be unwilling or uninterested in changing. In the contemplation stage, people are thinking about adopting or changing a behavior in the near future. They are aware of the benefits of the behavior but are also acutely aware of the difficulties of changing. In the preparation stage, people intend to take action to change their behavior in the immediate future and have generally taken initial steps toward change. For example, they may have purchased walking shoes, joined a gym, or begun to take short walks in the neighborhood. In the action stage, people have made consistent changes in their behavior but have not yet maintained the behavior for a long period of time. Finally, people in the maintenance stage have been participating in the desired behavior for at least six months. Most clients seen by physical activity instructors are in the preparation, action,

or maintenance stage because they have begun to take action toward change. Keep in mind that your clients may not always move forward from one stage to the next. For example, a person who is in the action or maintenance stage of change may relapse to an earlier stage of change when faced with a health or personal crisis.

Perhaps one of the most important lessons from the transtheoretical model is that interventions are most successful when they are tailored to the client's stage of readiness for change. For example, setting specific exercise goals would not be useful for a client who is in the precontemplation stage, because the client is not ready to change his or her behavior. It would be more helpful to provide your client with information about exercise. Marcus and Forsyth (2003) described practical ways to apply the transtheoretical model to physical activity promotion.

In addition to assessing your client's readiness for change, it is also important to assess his or her self-efficacy. Self-efficacy is a construct that originated

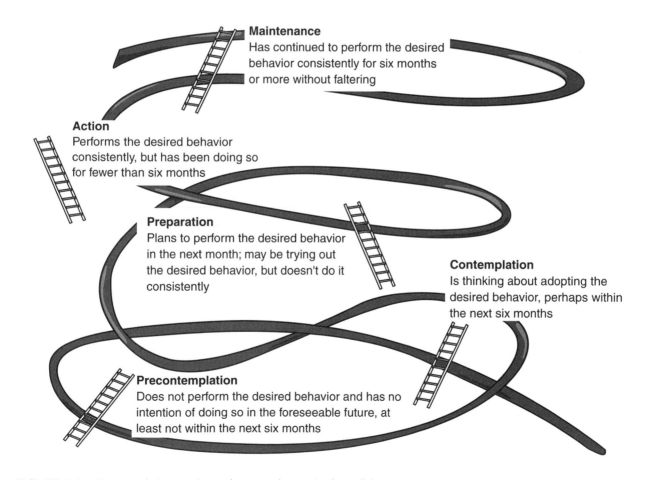

FIGURE 8.2 Stages of change from the transtheoretical model.
Reprinted from the Centers of Disease Control, 1999, *Promoting physical activity: A guide for community action* (Champaign, IL: Human Kinetics), 59.

in social cognitive theory (Bandura, 1977, 1982). It refers to a person's confidence in his or her ability to engage in a behavior even when faced with barriers. Self-efficacy is strongly related to exercise and other health behaviors in older adults. For clients who have low self-efficacy, there are four ways in which self-efficacy can be learned and enhanced. The most potent way is through *performance accomplishments;* self-efficacy increases when a person successfully executes a behavior. By encouraging clients to set realistic goals that they can meet, physical activity instructors can increase their clients' self-efficacy.

Another way in which self-efficacy can be positively influenced is through *persuasion.* We have all probably accomplished something we initially thought was very difficult because someone encouraged us to try. Physical activity instructors can encourage clients and express confidence in their abilities. Of course, it is important that this expressed confidence be genuine. Self-efficacy is also enhanced through *observational learning.* That is, we often learn by observing another person's behavior and its outcomes and then modeling that behavior. People tend to be most persuaded when the individual they are watching is perceived as like themselves, when the individual initially struggles with the behavior but ultimately succeeds, and when the individual is rewarded for his or her behavior. Using other seniors as models can be very motivating. A woman who has never exercised could be introduced to a woman who had a similar history but is now regularly active. Finally, *emotional arousal* that is too high tends to decrease self-efficacy. Our confidence is lowered when we feel nervous or negative about a task or situation. Older adults may have concerns about injuring

themselves through exercise, and basic education about the risks and benefits of exercise and reassurance might be useful. Similarly, instruction and supervision in the use of exercise equipment can reduce feelings of anxiety and self-consciousness that an older adult may feel. Enhancing self-efficacy appears to be particularly useful in the adoption stage of exercise.

Step 1: Explore Expectations and Exercise Objectives

Clients enter an exercise program with vastly different expectations about exercise and what it will do for them (i.e., outcome expectations or perceived benefits). It is important for these initial expectations to be explicitly discussed for at least two reasons. First, these expectations should dictate the type of exercise program that is recommended. Clearly, different programs should be recommended to an overweight older adult who wants to lose weight, to a frail older adult who wants to improve balance and reduce the risk of falls, and to a healthy but less active older adult who wants to run a 10K race. Second, a discussion of expectations can indicate how realistic these goals are. A client who expects to lose 20 pounds (9 kilograms) in two months through a walking program is likely to be very disappointed after two months of hard work and little weight loss. You can correct clients' misconceptions that are revealed during your initial screening and assessment and thus prevent later disappointments that could cause them to drop out of the program.

Step 2: Set Goals

The next step is to assist the client in setting goals for achieving his or her overall objectives. In goal setting, your role is to help direct the client toward appropriate goals. It is critical, however, that the client takes primary responsibility for setting his or her own goals. The role of the physical activity instructor is to ask questions ("How likely is it that you can meet that goal next week?"), request clarification ("What days will you exercise next week?" "What time of day works best for you?"), and make suggestions ("I've found that focusing only on weight loss can be frustrating for many people. I suggest that we work together to set goals around your actual walking—goals that you have more control over. We'll keep your longer-term

> These are four strategies to increase your clients' self-efficacy:
>
> 1. Encourage realistic goals, and provide proper instruction and demonstration of exercises (*performance accomplishments*).
> 2. Encourage clients, and express your confidence in their abilities (*persuasion*).
> 3. Use older adults as role models (*observational learning*).
> 4. Provide appropriate instruction, supervision, and reassurance (*reducing emotional arousal*).

objective in mind when setting these goals."). Ideally, exercise goals should not be prescribed or dictated by the instructor.

Characteristics of Good Goals

An important role of the physical activity instructor is to ensure that goals meet four requirements: They should be measurable, specific, realistic, and behavioral. First, ask yourself, "Will my client know when he or she has met his or her goal?" That is, can the goal be measured? An example of a measurable goal is, "I will attend an exercise class three days per week for the next month." An example of a goal that cannot be easily measured is, "I will exercise more." It is not clear how "more" is defined here. Goals must also be specific. A specific goal, such as, "I will attend the 10:00 A.M. exercise class on Mondays, Wednesdays, and Fridays," helps the client plan his or her behavior and increases the likelihood of meeting the goal.

Next, a goal must be realistic. People are likely to be very motivated when they first begin an exercise program and may set unrealistically high goals. Although you do not want to dampen clients' enthusiasm, you also want to be sure that their goals are realistic. In general, it is best for clients initially to set small goals that they are quite certain can be achieved. If goals are not met, clients are likely to feel that they have failed and to be at increased risk of dropping out of the exercise program. Overly ambitious goals can also lead to soreness or injury.

Finally, although clients often focus on physiological or performance-related outcomes, such as weight loss or improved strength and fitness, physical activity instructors should encourage clients to set behavioral outcome goals, such as

attending three aerobic exercise classes and two strength-training sessions per week. Physiological and performance-related outcome goals, such as weight loss, often take a long time to achieve, and the client may feel frustrated if progress is slow. In contrast, clients have much more control over their behavior than over the outcomes of their behavior. Encourage clients to view exercise as important in and of itself, with an array of benefits that go well beyond weight loss and similar outcomes.

Short-Term and Long-Term Goals

Both short-term and long-term exercise goals are important. Clients often focus on long-term goals. For example, they may want to increase strength by a certain percentage, lose 50 pounds (23 kilograms), be able to touch their toes, or run a 5K road race. However, when initiating a new behavior, the client must set short-term goals that are almost certain to be achieved. It is hard to stay motivated when your only goal is to lose 50 pounds because this goal takes time to achieve. Encourage clients to set daily and weekly exercise goals. Your clients will experience a sense of accomplishment and mastery when they achieve what they set out to do. Achieving these short-term goals is also the most potent way for your clients to increase their self-efficacy, an important determinant of future behavior. Monitor your clients' progress on longer-term goals and adjust short-term goals. Like short-term goals, long-term goals should have a behavioral focus. For example, one woman's short-term goal might be to attend two aerobic exercise classes per week for the next two weeks. Her long-term goal might be to increase her frequency to three aerobic exercise classes per week and to engage in upper- and lower-body resistance training two days per week by the sixth month of her program. Goals should be discussed, monitored, and adjusted regularly based on the client's progress, health status, and long-term objectives.

Step 3: Provide Feedback and Monitor Goals

Physical activity instructors often help their clients to set goals but then never review their progress toward these goals. Regularly review your clients' goals, their successes, and their struggles. Focusing on successes as well as struggles shows you what factors help clients meet their goals. You can then point out these helpful factors to your clients during

---

Your client's goals should have these characteristics:

1. Measurable – your client should be able to determine whether or not the goal was met
2. Specific – your client should specify when he or she will perform their exercise
3. Realistic – goals that your client is sure to achieve will enhance self-efficacy
4. Behavioral – your client has more direct control over goals that are behavioral (e.g., walking 3 times per week) than goals that are outcome-oriented (e.g., lose 10 pounds)

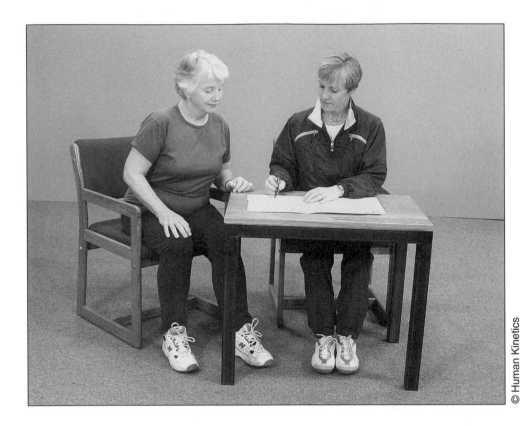

© Human Kinetics

Assist your clients in setting short- and long-term goals.

periods when they struggle. Goals should be frequently reviewed (every week or two) with your clients at the start of a program and less frequently (monthly or bimonthly) after they have succeeded in meeting some of their goals.

Encourage clients to use a log for self-monitoring (such as the exercise log shown in figure 8.3) where they can record the activity, its duration, its intensity, and any other information that may be relevant to the program (e.g., their mood or energy level). Pedometers, or step counters, are a low-cost and potentially effective way to self-monitor a walking program. Research has shown that clients who engage in more self-monitoring are more likely to change health behaviors (Boutelle & Kirschenbaum, 1998).

In addition to providing feedback and monitoring progress toward goals, conducting a behavioral analysis with your older adult clients can be useful. A **behavioral analysis** is a systematic way of examining the factors that increase or decrease the likelihood of exercising. An easy way to remember how to conduct a behavioral analysis is to focus on the "ABCs" of behavior change. *A* represents the antecedents to behavior. **Antecedents** are cues that set the stage for target (exercise) or nontarget (sedentary) behavior. They include thoughts, emo-

tions, perceived barriers and motivators, and factors in the physical and social environment that affect behavior. Some antecedents increase the likelihood of the target behavior. For example, leaving walking shoes by the bed serves as a reminder to walk the next morning and increases the likelihood of walking. Conversely, antecedents such as feeling stressed or tired decrease the likelihood of exercising. Encourage clients to use cues and prompts that increase the likelihood of exercise. *B* represents the behavior itself. The type, intensity, location, and purpose of the activity have differing antecedents and consequences that can, in turn, influence future behaviors. *C* represents the **consequences** of the behavior. These consequences can be reinforcing or punishing. Receiving praise for exercising or enjoying the social aspect of an exercise group are examples of reinforcing consequences that increase the likelihood of future exercise. Pulling a muscle during an exercise session or having a spouse complain that you are never around because of your new exercise program are examples of punishing consequences that decrease the likelihood of future exercise. The choice of the behavior itself can impact the types of consequences experienced. For example, vigorous exercise may cause muscle soreness or injury, which reduces the likelihood of

Day	Description of activity	Duration of activity (minutes)	Heart rate or RPE*	Other comments
Sunday				
Monday				
Tuesday				
Wednesday				
Thursday				
Friday				
Saturday				
My exercise goals for next week are to:				

* Rating of perceived exertion (using Borg's scale; see chapter 7, figure 7.4).

FIGURE 8.3 Sample exercise log.

When conducting a behavioral analysis, focus on the ABCs:

1. Identify *antecedents* to your client's behavior. Antecedents are thoughts, emotions, perceived barriers and motivators, and aspects of the environment that set the stage for target (exercise) or nontarget (sedentary) behavior.

2. Assess the *behavior* that results from the antecedents. For example, does your client skip his or her exercise session on days he or she finds stressful? What type of behavior does your client choose? Is the activity enjoyable to your client?

3. Examine whether the *consequences* of your client's behavior are reinforcing or punishing.

adhering to the program. Walking in a park, on the other hand, may be very pleasant, increasing the likelihood that older adults will continue this type of activity. Finally, walking that is done for transporta-

tion rather than exercise has different antecedents and consequences.

Your behavior as the instructor is also important in the ABC model. Providing appropriate warm-up and cool-down exercises, matching the exercise intensity to the abilities of the group, providing praise and encouragement, and displaying warmth to clients are examples of instructor-related antecedents, behaviors, and consequences that can affect your clients' exercise behaviors. Chapter 19 offers more in-depth discussion of the qualities associated with good leadership and instruction.

A behavioral analysis involves exploring with the client the events, feelings, and situations that tend to trigger exercise or sedentary behavior, aspects of the exercise itself that increase or decrease exercise (e.g., the type, intensity, and setting of the exercise), and the reinforcing or punishing consequences of exercise (see table 8.1). This can be done through a discussion with the client, a short questionnaire that asks about these issues, or the client's keeping a log or diary for a week that records the factors that facilitate or impede physical activity. Once these

TABLE 8.1   Behavioral Analysis

Antecedents	Behavior	Consequences
THE LIKELIHOOD OF EXERCISING DECREASES		
Spouse complains that client never spends time with him because she is always exercising.	Client misses exercise session.	Client receives attention and affection from spouse.
Client is in a hurry and does not do any warm-up exercises.	Client completes exercise session.	Client experiences muscle soreness the following day.
Client is busy during the holidays.	Client skips exercise sessions.	Client feels guilt and a sense of failure.
THE LIKELIHOOD OF EXERCISING INCREASES		
Client lays out exercise clothes for the next day at bedtime.	Client attends morning exercise class.	Client enjoys the social interaction of the class.
Client reminds himself or herself of the health benefits of exercise when not in the mood to exercise.	Client completes exercise session.	Client's children praise him or her for adhering to the exercise program.
Client's spouse offers to walk with him or her.	Client and spouse walk together.	Client enjoys the interaction and feels supported.

relationships are outlined, you can work with the client to modify the antecedents of the behavior, aspects of the behavior itself, and the consequences of the behavior in order to increase the likelihood of continuing to exercise. The reinforcing antecedents and consequences change over time, so it is important to reexamine this framework throughout the program.

Another way to help clients attain their exercise goals is to encourage them to seek out social support for exercise. Social support has consistently been found to be related to exercise participation; those who receive more social support for exercise have higher rates of adherence than those who receive less social support. Social support can come from the client's family, friends, coworkers, exercise classmates, or physical activity instructor. Social support provided by an exercise partner can be very useful to some individuals, but social support can take many other forms. As a physical activity instructor, you have valuable *informational support* to share with clients: advice, suggestions, and information regarding exercise. *Instrumental* or *tangible support* is another type of social support that is often practical in nature, for example, a spouse's help in preparing dinner to free up more time for walking

or a friend's offering a ride to attend an exercise program. *Emotional support* generally refers to expressions of love and empathy and can include encouragement for being active. Many people are reluctant to ask for help. It can be useful to discuss with clients the type of support they need and then brainstorm ways to get this support. You can also convey encouragement and genuine concern for your clients through your actions and by fostering a supportive program environment.

Once the client has identified his or her objectives, set short- and long-term goals, and developed a plan for modifying behavioral antecedents and consequences, it can be useful for the client to sign a written **behavioral contract** (Neale, 1991). This contract should explicitly outline the client's specific goals, how they will be measured, and the consequences of the client's behavior. How will the client be rewarded when the goals are met? What will happen if goals are not met? Both the instructor and client should receive a copy of the contract, and this contract should be referred to and updated regularly. Behavioral contracts increase a client's commitment to behavioral change and serve as a concrete reminder of the behavioral plan. Figure 8.4 is a sample behavioral contract.

Exercise is important to me because (list the benefits you hope to receive from exercising):

My specific exercise goals for the next two weeks are to (list your goals; be sure that they are measurable):

To reach these goals, I will exercise (list specific days and times):

To record my behavior, I will:

When I reach my goals, I will reward myself by:

If I don't reach my goals, I will:

My longer-term exercise goals (for the next three to six months) are to:

I agree to work hard toward reaching my exercise goals. I will contact my exercise instructor for assistance if I am having trouble reaching my goals.

Signed: _____ Date: _____

Witness: _____ Date: _____

FIGURE 8.4   Sample behavioral contract.

Step 4: Use Rewards and Incentives

Reinforcement has a greater impact on behavior than does **punishment.** Clients should be encouraged to reward themselves for meeting their behavioral goals. You can ask clients, "What will you do to reward yourself when you reach this goal?" It is important that the client choose his or her own rewards, since what is reinforcing for one person may not be reinforcing for another. Physical activity instructors can also build reinforcements into their programs, such as praising clients, offering incentives for class attendance, and providing formal recognition. When a person initiates a new behavior, reinforcements should be regular and consistent. Over time, however, reinforcements should be more occasional. As exercise becomes habitual, the client will ideally find exercise reinforcing in and of itself (intrinsic motivation) and will rely less on external reinforcements (extrinsic motivation).

Step 5: Use Problem Solving to Overcome Obstacles

Even when all these steps are followed, clients will inevitably encounter barriers to adhering to their exercise program. Many of the same techniques described for behavioral analysis can be used to engage the client in problem solving. For example, a client who is always too tired and unmotivated to exercise at the end of the day might consider exercising first thing in the morning. Again, solutions to barriers that clients generate themselves are most likely to be successful. It is often difficult for physical activity instructors to refrain from giving advice. However, not only are clients more likely to act on their own solutions, this approach also reduces the likelihood of the "yes but" struggle between the instructor and client, when the instructor provides a suggestion and the client responds with why it will not work. An example of how to facilitate problem solving with clients is provided in figure 8.5.

Step 6: Promote Long-Term Adherence

The choice of whether or not to exercise is a daily decision. Although a person's risk of dropping out of an exercise program is lower when he or she has maintained participation for six months or longer, **lapses** (i.e., missing several exercise sessions) and **relapses** (i.e., returning to a sedentary state) are the rule rather than the exception. Once your client has incorporated an exercise program into his or her lifestyle, it is a good time to introduce relapse prevention strategies. According to relapse prevention models (Marlatt & Gorden, 1985), lapses and relapses are often triggered by high-risk situations coupled with the absence of coping responses.

Problem

A 68-year-old retired client comes to your office frustrated that he has not been able to exercise all week because he has been baby-sitting for his grandchildren every night (he usually exercises at night). How should you approach this client?

Possible solutions

- You think of an easy solution to this barrier. Share your solution with the client.
- Ask your client if he has any ideas for overcoming the barrier.

Recommended approach

Your client can probably come up with a solution on his own, and he is more likely to act on a solution he generates. Try to elicit a solution from your client, and reflect back any emotions you perceive.

Sample script

Instructor: "It seems that before you started baby-sitting, you were exercising regularly. I can see why you are frustrated. Do you have ideas about how you can get back into your exercise program even though you have this new responsibility?"
Client: "Not really . . ."
Instructor: "So it seems that there is really no way around this barrier?"
Client: "Well, I'm not sure I'd go that far. My exercise program is important to me; it's just that I really like exercising at night, and now I can't."
Instructor: "So it's not an ideal situation, but it sounds as if you might have an idea for getting around it."
Client: "I guess I might be able to exercise in the morning."
Instructor: "OK, that's one option. How confident are you that you could exercise in the morning?"
Client: "I'd say probably 80 percent."
Instructor: "That's not bad. Are you willing to try to adjust your schedule this week and let me know how it goes next week?"
Client: "Yes, I can do that."

FIGURE 8.5   Client-generated problem solving.

Helping clients to view lapses and relapses as a normal part of behavior change can be useful. Encourage clients to identify situations when they are likely to experience lapses or relapses in their exercise program. The most common situations include travel, holidays, illness, stress, poor weather, and competing family obligations. When clients anticipate these high-risk situations and develop strategies (both cognitive and behavioral) to deal with them, they are better prepared in the actual situations and tend to have higher self-efficacy in coping with them. Illness and family obligations, particularly caregiving, are especially relevant for older adults. It can be difficult for anyone to restart an exercise program after recovering from a cold or flu, but it is particularly challenging for older adults, who tend to remain ill longer and may experience a greater loss of function during this period.

Many thoughts go through a person's mind when deciding whether or not to exercise. Thoughts such as "I'm too tired" and "I'm not in the mood" often precede (i.e., are antecedents to) the decision to not exercise. An important part of relapse prevention is helping people question their "all-or-nothing" thinking. After missing an exercise session or two, a person often feels as though he or she has completely failed. This person might decide to wait until the following week or the following month or even the following year to resume their program. In addition, it is common to feel discouraged when goals are not met and outcomes are not reached. These thoughts can lead to a brief lapse in an exercise program or to quitting the program altogether.

Clients can be taught to replace their negative thoughts with more realistic or positive ones. The first step is for the client to be aware of his or her thoughts and how thoughts lead to behaviors. Encourage clients to challenge their thoughts. A useful technique is to ask what the client would say to a friend with the same thought, and encourage the client to focus on similar thoughts. You can also model healthy thoughts by emphasizing that adherence is not an all-or-nothing phenomenon. For example, when a client says, "I had a stressful week and only exercised twice—I really blew it," you can respond, "I think it's great that you were still able to get in two sessions, despite your stressful week!" It is important that neither you nor the client forgets that engaging in *some* level of physical activity is better than engaging in *no* physical activity.

Although it is important to brainstorm ways to overcome barriers and high-risk situations, there will inevitably be times when it is nearly impossible for a person to exercise. One strategy that may initially seem counter to your natural instincts is to schedule a brief, planned lapse with your client. It is important that the time frame of the lapse be defined very specifically. Also, the client should have a very specific plan for resuming the exercise program after the lapse. Otherwise, it can be difficult to start up again after the scheduled time has passed. A planned lapse gives the client permission to stop exercising, and thus the client is less likely to feel guilty or to view himself or herself as a failure, which is a common trigger for a relapse.

Finally, an important aspect of relapse prevention is helping clients to differentiate between a lapse and a relapse. The all-or-nothing trap is powerful, and clients should be reminded to view exercise and adherence as a continuum. This more realistic view reduces negative thoughts and emotions associated with lapses and thus reduces the likelihood of a complete relapse. A summary of cognitive and behavioral strategies to increase exercise adherence is shown in table 8.2.

Physically Active Lifestyles

In addition to increasing participation in regularly scheduled, leisure-time physical activity, all participants should be encouraged to look for additional, more routine forms of physical activity to add to their day. Given that overall volume of physical activity is positively related to a range of positive health outcomes (U.S. Department of Health and Human Services, 1996), clients should be encouraged to find ways of increasing their energy expenditure outside their formal exercise group or personal training program. For instance, taking stairs rather than elevators, parking farther from stores to allow more walking, and other ways to increase walking during daily chores and routine activities should all be encouraged as part of a well-rounded physical activity program. This may be particularly important in light of some evidence indicating that older adults may actually compensate for energy expenditure in a formal exercise class or group by reducing their energy expenditure at other times in the day (Goran & Poehlman, 1992).

TABLE 8.2   Cognitive and Behavioral Strategies to Increase Exercise Adherence

Strategies	Explanation
Behavioral analysis	Conduct a behavioral analysis, and work with clients to determine ways to modify antecedents and consequences of their exercise behavior.
Behavioral contracts	Use behavioral contracts that specify exercise goals and the consequences of both reaching and not reaching goals.
Social support	Encourage clients to enlist social support for their exercise program from family, friends, exercise classmates, and fitness instructors. Provide support and encouragement to clients in your exercise program, and identify ways to promote support in exercise classes.
Self-efficacy	Aim to increase clients' self-efficacy by ensuring that their goals are realistic and can be met, providing peer role models, offering encouragement, and providing instruction to decrease anxiety and self-consciousness.
Cognitive strategies	Encourage clients to replace unhelpful thoughts (e.g., all-or-nothing views of adherence) with more productive thoughts.
Preparation for lapses and relapses	Prepare clients for lapses and relapses, develop strategies to reduce their occurrence, and consider scheduling planned lapses.
Reassessing and adjusting goals	Periodically reassess clients' exercise goals and help them adjust goals as needed.
Reassessing physical performance	Periodically reassess clients' physical performance and help them adjust exercise goals as needed.

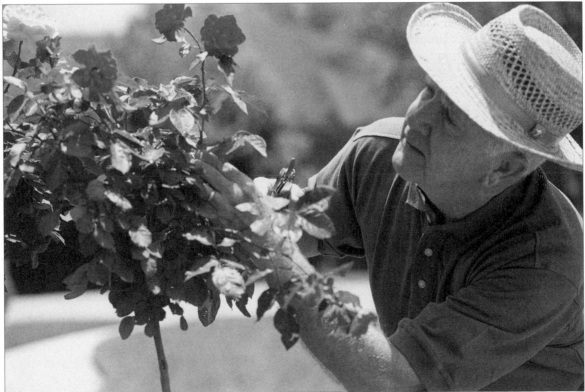

© Getty Images

Finding new ways to increase physical activity while doing daily chores and activities should be encouraged as part of a well-rounded physical activity program.

Implications for Program Design and Management

The cognitive and behavioral strategies described in this chapter can be applied in many different settings, to a variety of physical activities, and across a range of older adults' functional levels. For example, the strategies described in this chapter have been successfully applied in supervised home-based programs as well as in group programs; in resistance training, fall prevention, aerobic conditioning, and active lifestyle programs; and among populations ranging from frail older adults to high-functioning, healthy older adults (Brawley, Rejeski, & Lutes, 2000; Ettinger et al., 1997; Jette et al., 1999; King, 2001; King, Haskell, Taylor, Kraemer, & DeBusk, 1991; King, Pruitt, et al., 2000; King, Rejeski, & Buchner, 1998; Stewart et al., 1997, 2001).

These strategies have also taken different formats. For example, behavioral change strategies and action plan progress can be reviewed in person at the individual or group level, or via telephone or mail. Telephone or mail contact can be particularly useful for older adults, who may have more difficulty attending group programs due to transportation problems, scheduling conflicts, or family caregiving responsibilities.

A critical requirement in all these various situations is that you tailor the program and strategies to the client's needs, physical and cognitive abilities, interests, and preferences. These strategies cannot be applied in a "one-size-fits-all" manner. Therefore, you must possess the flexibility and creativity required to meet clients at their level. Most physical activity instructors enjoy working with older adults and are interested in helping people. These are two of the most important characteristics that you can possess, but they are not enough. Researchers have found a number of characteristics of helping professionals that predict positive behavioral outcomes, regardless of the type of intervention or treatment (Goldstein & Higginbotham, 1991). These characteristics include being a good listener and having empathy, flexibility, openness, genuineness, and competence. Important instructor characteristics are described in greater depth in chapter 19 of this book.

The specific ways in which strategies described in this chapter can be integrated into exercise programs depend on the nature and format of the program. In some, though not all, exercise programs, the instructor has an opportunity to meet with clients individually and focus on goal setting and behavioral analysis. Prepared worksheets, such as the behavioral contract and self-monitoring log shown in this chapter, help facilitate this process and make it more time efficient. These worksheets also provide the client with something to take home as a reminder of the goals and behavioral plan. In group exercise programs, self-monitoring logs and behavioral contracts can be distributed before or after class.

Exercise instructors can also focus on a different behavioral strategy at each session. For example, during the cool-down portion of an exercise class, the instructor might discuss social support and strategies to increase it. Topics can be presented in rotation. Praising clients, facilitating group cohesion by using clients' names, and arriving early to class to talk with clients are also good ways to incorporate reinforcement and social support into your program. For group or facility-based programs, the physical environment should reinforce cognitive and behavioral strategies. Bulletin boards can be used to highlight a "client of the month" and to present behavioral strategies. For telephone-based interventions, semistructured telephone scripts can be used to review progress toward goals. When clients are not meeting goals, you can encourage them to use problem-solving strategies, review antecedents to their behavior, and use positive reinforcement. Phone calls can also emphasize the importance of social support and relapse prevention strategies. For mail-based monitoring, tear-off reply forms or postcards can be used for the client to indicate progress toward goals, new goals, and barriers. Prepared mailings (e.g., tip sheets on common barriers) can then be sent to address the specific issues indicated by the client.

The effectiveness of your behavioral interventions should be monitored and evaluated. Relevant questions that your evaluation could address include, "Are clients' needs being met?" "Are clients improving their health and well-being?" and "What strategies do clients find most and least useful?" Evaluations do not need to be expensive or time-consuming to conduct. For example, client surveys, suggestion boxes, and monitoring attendance before and after implementing a behavioral modification strategy in your program are relatively simple ways to evaluate your program.

Summary

Despite the many benefits that can be achieved through regular physical activity, drop-out rates from exercise programs remain high. Factors that influence the adoption and maintenance of physical activity are multidimensional and include personal characteristics, program factors, and environmental characteristics (social and physical).

Cognitive and behavioral strategies, many of which are derived from theoretical models of behavior change, can enhance exercise adoption and maintenance. These strategies can be used in individual and group settings. A client's readiness for change and self-efficacy for change are characteristics that should be assessed very early in a program. The next step is to explore clients' initial expectations about exercise and their overall objectives and to use this information to guide the choice of activities and goals. Goals should be generated by clients rather than by instructors, although instructors can facilitate goal setting. Regularly reviewing progress and revising goals, encouraging the use of self-monitoring logs, helping clients assess the antecedents and consequences of their behavior (behavioral analysis), using behavioral contracts, and encouraging clients to enlist social support for change are techniques to enhance goal attainment. Finally, long-term maintenance of physical activity is critical. Relapse prevention strategies include helping clients to identify high-risk situations, to view lapses as a normal part of behavioral change, to reduce all-or-nothing thinking regarding adherence, and to schedule planned relapses in some circumstances.

The cognitive and behavioral strategies discussed in this chapter can be applied to different types of clients, settings, and physical activities. However, they must be tailored to the client's individual needs, abilities, and interests. Physical activity instructors can incorporate behavioral strategies into group exercise programs as well as individual programs by presenting behavioral strategies during the class (e.g., during warm-up or cool-down), distributing self-monitoring logs and behavioral contracts, creating a physical environment that emphasizes behavioral strategies, and creating a social environment that supports and encourages clients. Physical activity instructors are encouraged to use cognitive and behavioral strategies in their programs for older adults in a flexible and individualized manner.

Key Terms

Recommended Reading

Marcus, B.H., & Forsyth, L.H. (2003). *Motivating people to be physically active*. Champaign, IL: Human Kinetics.

Study Questions

1. Which factor or factors influence the initiation and maintenance of physical activity?
    a. personal characteristics
    b. program factors
    c. environmental characteristics
    d. all of the above

2. Which demographic factor or factors are associated with sedentary behaviors?
    a. female sex
    b. male sex
    c. low socioeconomic status
    d. both a and c

3. What is the barrier to physical activity most frequently cited by older adults?
    a. lack of time
    b. lack of self-motivation
    c. health problems
    d. pain

4. Your client sets a short-term behavioral goal to "exercise more." Which of the following characteristics does this goal lack?
    a. specific
    b. realistic
    c. measurable
    d. a and c

5. Which of the following is true about exercise goals?
    a. Short-term goals should focus on behavioral outcomes (e.g., exercise), whereas long-term goals should focus on physiological outcomes (e.g., weight loss).
    b. Short-term goals should focus on physiological outcomes, whereas long-term goals should focus on behavioral outcomes.
    c. Both short- and long-term goals should focus on behavioral outcomes.
    d. Both short- and long-term goals should focus on physiological outcomes.

6. Which of the following is the best description of behavioral analysis?
    a. examining the antecedents and consequences of a behavior
    b. examining ways to decrease undesirable behavior
    c. examining ways to increase desirable behavior
    d. developing a system of rewards and punishments for behaviors

7. Your client has never done strength-training exercises before and is convinced that she cannot do them. Which of the following strategies would be most likely to increase her self-efficacy for strength training?
    a. encouraging and persuading her to try
    b. having her lift very light weights so that she can experience success in strength training
    c. demonstrating how to do each of the exercises
    d. having her watch a peer do each of the exercises

Application Activities

1. Keep a self-monitoring log for two weeks to get a better sense of what this experience is like for your clients. What did you like and dislike about keeping the log? After you have completed the log, ask one of your clients to keep a log for two weeks. Review the completed log with your client and discuss his or her experiences with keeping the log.

2. Ask one of your new clients to complete a behavioral contract. Practice how you would assist your client in setting measurable, specific, realistic, and behavioral goals and choosing appropriate reinforcements.

3. How would you approach a client who tells you that she is going to drop out of your exercise group because she is not making the progress that she expected? Focus on your listening rather than advice-giving skills.

4. Choose four behavioral change strategies and develop brief descriptions that you can present during the cool-down portion of your exercise classes. Discuss one strategy per class.

Part III

Core Program Principles and Training Methods

TRAINING MODULE 1:
Overview of Aging and Physical Activity

TRAINING MODULE 2:
Psychological, Sociocultural, and Physiological Aspects of Physical Activity and Older Adults

TRAINING MODULE 9:
Ethics and Professional Conduct

TRAINING MODULE 8:
Client Safety and First Aid

TRAINING MODULE 3:
Screening, Assessment, and Goal Setting

International Curriculum Guidelines for Preparing Physical Activity Instructors of Older Adults

TRAINING MODULE 7:
Leadership, Communication, and Marketing Skills

TRAINING MODULE 4:
Program Design and Management

TRAINING MODULE 6:
Teaching Skills

TRAINING MODULE 5:
Program Design for Older Adults With Stable Medical Conditions

Now that you possess the knowledge and skills to screen and assess your clients and to incorporate cognitive and behavioral change strategies into your exercise programs, the next step in the successful design and implementation of effective physical activity programs for a heterogeneous older adult population is understanding the core exercise principles and training methods. These are presented in part III. Chapters 9 through 14 address content presented in training modules 4 and 5. Module 4 recommends areas of study that include information about how to use results from screening, assessment, and client goals to make appropriate decisions regarding individual and group physical activity and exercise program design and management. Module 5 recommends areas of study that include information on common medical conditions of older adults, signs and symptoms associated with medication-related negative interactions during physical activity, and how to adapt exercise for clients with different fitness levels and stable medical conditions to help prevent injury and other emergency situations.

• Chapter 9 discusses the relevance of the disability model to physical activity programming for older adults and the potential functional benefits of different types of physical activities that should be included in a well-rounded exercise program for older adults. You will learn how to apply basic exercise principles (e.g., specificity and overload) for effective program design. Some important exercise principles that are unique to the older adult population are also considered.

• Chapter 10 describes acute physiological changes in the neuromuscular, cardiopulmonary, and metabolic systems that occur during the warm-up and cool-down components of an exercise program. Examples of appropriate warm-up and cool-down activities for older adults that engage participants emotionally, socially, cognitively, and spiritually are also presented.

• Chapter 11 provides a discussion of age-associated changes in joint and muscle flexibility and how these changes affect older adults' ability to perform various activities of daily living. Critical ranges of joint flexibility required for these basic activities are also identified. The remainder of the chapter provides examples of dynamic and static flexibility exercises for all the major muscle groups and joints in the body. The dynamic flexibility exercises are recommended for inclusion in the warm-up, while the static flexibility exercises can be easily incorporated into the cool-down component of the class or performed as a stand-alone component.

• Chapter 12 introduces you to the resistance-training variables that govern the development of muscular strength, power, and endurance: resistance, exercise order, sets, number of repetitions, and rest periods. You will also learn how to design a safe and effective resistance-training component that meets the needs and personal goals of older adult clients.

• Chapter 13 provides an overview of the exercise principles and variables that must be considered when designing and implementing the aerobic endurance component of a physical activity program. Guidelines for accommodating older adults with different fitness levels and functional abilities are also presented in this chapter.

• Chapter 14 describes how age-associated changes in multiple body systems are likely to affect various dimensions of balance and mobility. This chapter identifies the four essential skills needed for good balance and mobility and then provides a set of progressive balance and mobility exercises that address each of these essential skills. You will learn how to adjust the challenge level of balance exercises to accommodate clients with different balance and mobility skills.

9

A New Approach to Designing Exercise Programs for Older Adults

Dawn E. Gillis
Anita L. Stewart

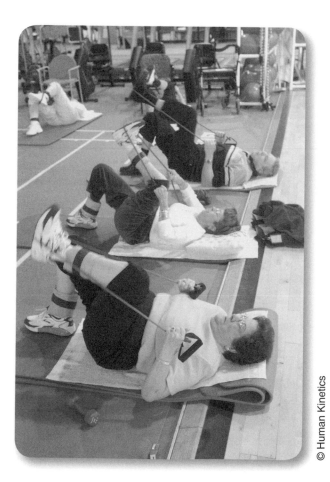

Designing and implementing exercise programs for older adults requires a unique approach, one that addresses individuals' needs and abilities. Traditional approaches to exercise programming for younger adults have generally focused on improving specific physiological parameters, such as cardiorespiratory endurance or muscular strength. These programs are often designed for people with specific goals in mind, such as athletic performance, fitness, body sculpting, or weight reduction. Although these goals may be appropriate for older adults as well, alternative goals may be helpful to accommodate the needs of many older adults, who are considerably more diverse in their level of health and physical function. Although many people remain relatively healthy and fit throughout their lives, others experience a decline in health, fitness, and functioning. Thus, an older adult population can range from those who compete as master athletes to those who have difficulty getting out of a chair. The unique approach presented in this book considers this variability by adding a focus on functional training and utilization of several principles to help develop safe and effective exercise programs for older adults.

This chapter begins by briefly describing the heterogeneity of the older adult population and a model for explaining how some older adults become disabled. We then discuss how this information, combined with screenings and assessments, can guide the planning of physical activity programs for older adults. We explain how different types of activities can affect various dimensions of physical functioning. Recently developed national guidelines and recommendations that address the specific needs of older adults are then summarized. Finally, important exercise principles specific to older adults and how to apply them in the development and implementation of physical activity programs for older adults are described.

Heterogeneity of Older Adults

Older adults are highly likely to have one or more chronic health conditions with arthritis, hypertension, coronary heart disease, stroke, and diabetes being the most common. Sixty-two percent of people 65 years of age and older have two or more chronic conditions; however, approximately 16 percent have no chronic conditions according to data from the 1996 Medical Expenditure Panel Study (Partnership for Solutions, 2002). See chapter 21 for further discussion of chronic medical conditions that are common among older adults.

In addition to having variation in number and types of medical conditions, older adults exhibit a wide range of physical functioning (Buchner, Beresford, Larson, LaCroix, & Wagner, 1992; Evans, 1995). **Physical functioning** refers to an individual's ability to do basic physical actions such as walking, climbing stairs, bending, and reaching. Even among those 80 years of age and older, many report no difficulty in physical functioning (Ostchega, Harris, Hirsch, Parsons, & Kington, 2000). Similar variation among older adults is found in performance tests of

> Most older adults have at least one chronic health condition and some limitation in physical functioning. However, some older adults have no chronic conditions and good functioning. This variation is found even among people 80 years of age and older.

physical functions such as walking or lifting heavy objects (Rikli & Jones, 1999; Simonsick et al., 2001). The major practical implication for physical activity instructors is that exercise programs need to be adapted to accommodate diverse health conditions and physical abilities of older adult clients.

Optimizing Physical Function Through Exercise

The disablement process model described by Verbrugge and Jette (1994; see figure 9.1) is the most recent adaptation of a model originated by Saad Nagi (1976, 1991). According to this model, pathology (chronic health conditions, injury) can lead to impairments in body systems (cardiovascular, musculoskeletal, cognitive, sensory, and motor). Aging can also lead to these types of impairments, even without pathology (Stewart, 2003). Eventually, the accumulated impairments can lead to limitations in physical functioning (e.g., walking, stair climbing), and ultimately to disability. **Disability** is usually defined as difficulty or inability to per-

form complex activities in domains of life such as work, recreation, household tasks, socializing, and self-care (Pope & Tarlov, 1991; Verbrugge & Jette, 1994). As a specific example of this process, loss of muscular strength (body system impairment) can lead to slower walking times (limitation in physical functioning; Buchner, 1997), and limitations in walking ability without intervention can lead to disability. However, early identification of emerging impairments and functional limitations, together with appropriately tailored physical activity, can delay or prevent subsequent decline (Stewart & Painter, 1998). In addition, research has shown that exercise can reverse functional decline (Cress et al., 1999; Schlicht, Camaione, & Owen, 2001).

A second theoretical perspective suggests that there is a threshold of physical or physiological fitness below which a person becomes dependent on others for help with daily tasks, that is, disabled (Shephard, 1993; Vita, Terry, Hubert, & Fries, 1998). According to this view, people gradually decline but accommodate or compensate for losses; however, below some critical point, they can no longer perform certain daily activities without assistance. According to Shephard (1993), sedentary people generally reach this threshold at about age 80 years, while active people often do not reach this threshold for 10 to 20 more years. Additional markers for physical fitness thresholds are described in chapter 6.

These two theoretical perspectives highlight the critical importance of optimizing physical functioning through exercise. Physical activity instructors can help clients maintain or improve their physical

The Main Pathway

Pathology	Impairments	Functional limitations	Disability
Diagnoses of disease, injury, congenital/developmental condition	Dysfunctions and structural abnormalities in specific body systems: musculoskeletal, cardiovascular, neurological, etc.	Restrictions in basic physical and mental actions: ambulate, reach, stoop, climb stairs, produce intelligible speech, see standard print, etc.	Difficulty doing activities of daily life: job, household management, personal care, hobbies, active recreation, clubs, socializing with friends and kin, childcare, errands, sleep, trips, etc.

FIGURE 9.1 Disablement process model: The main pathway of a larger model.
Verbrugge, L.M., and Jette, A.M. (1994). The disablement process. *Social Science and Medicine, 38*, p. 4.

functioning, regardless of where the clients are on the functional continuum. Comprehensive screenings and assessments (either in the field or in the laboratory, as described in chapters 5, 6, and 7) provide physical activity instructors with knowledge about each participant's physical impairments (e.g., reduced aerobic endurance or muscular strength), limitations in physical functioning (e.g., difficulty walking, climbing stairs, bending, or lifting), and disabilities (e.g., difficulty performing tasks such as personal care or shopping errands). Based on results obtained from the initial screening and assessment, physical activity instructors can begin to individualize and prioritize the most appropriate types of exercise for their clients.

Functional Benefits of Exercise

As mentioned earlier, the goals of exercise programs for older adults may differ from the goals for younger adults. One key difference is that many older adults can use exercise to improve or maintain their physical functioning and thus help them stay independent, or avoid disability. For instance, a certain level of lower-body strength is needed to get out of a bathtub or to climb stairs, and adequate levels of agility, power, and dynamic balance are needed to move out of the way of an approaching car (Rikli & Jones, 2001). Some functional tasks that may be made easier by performing different types of exercise are shown in table 9.1.

Exercise benefits can be made more salient to older adults if the benefits can be directly linked to the ability to remain independent. The physiological (fitness) benefits derived from exercise may be too abstract or uninteresting for some older adults. Many clients may be motivated more by self-identifying important tasks and activities of daily life and recreation and then having a physical activity instructor explain how various types of exercises can help them maintain or improve their ability to do these activities.

Exercise and Physical Activity Guidelines for Older Adults

In 1998, the American College of Sports Medicine (ACSM) published its first position stand on the importance of exercise and physical activity for older adults. The key message from the position stand is that regular exercise and physical activity can improve functional capacity and health and lead to greater independence and quality of life for older adults. Citing strong supportive evidence, the ACSM noted that older adults who participate in regular endurance exercise (such as walking, running, swimming, and cycling) and strength (resistance) training can gain many benefits related to healthy aging. Although the position stand reviewed experimental evidence of the benefits of exercise for older adults, it provided very little guidance for physical activity instructors on how best to set

TABLE 9.1 Functional Tasks That May Improve With Exercise Training

Type of exercise training	Functional tasks
Aerobic endurance training	Walk in order to complete errands or attend events, perform activities requiring stamina such as vacuuming and raking, climb stairs
Resistance training for upper body and trunk	Lift and hold a grandchild, place luggage in overhead storage during travel, carry groceries, open heavy doors, perform garden work such as pulling weeds, perform housework such as washing windows
Resistance training for lower body	Stand up from the floor, get into and out of a chair or bathtub, climb stairs, pick up a package from the floor, step onto a curb
Flexibility training for upper body	Turn head to look at traffic while driving or walking, fasten a zipper on the back of a dress, scratch an itch on the back, reach overhead to a cupboard, comb hair
Flexibility training for lower body and trunk	Put on socks and shoes, inspect feet, cut toenails
Balance and mobility training	Walk the dog safely; negotiate environmental hazards, curbs, and stairs; pull weeds in the garden; respond appropriately to unexpected losses of balance

exercise variables such as frequency and duration for older adults other than frail and very old individuals.

The ACSM (1998) position stand also included a discussion of the role of exercise in the maintenance of good postural stability and flexibility. Although more research was felt to be needed, the ACSM recommended a broad-based program including balance and strength training, walking, and weight transfers as part of a comprehensive fall prevention program. Although more research on flexibility training for older adults was felt to be needed, the ACSM's position was that individuals should include activities such as walking, aerobic dance, and stretching in their overall exercise program to improve joint range of motion.

More specific exercise guidelines for the elderly population have since been published in *ACSM's Guidelines for Exercise Testing and Prescription* (ACSM, 2000). (Only an overview is provided here since specific details related to exercise variables such as intensity are presented in chapters 11 – 14 of this book.) ACSM's book provides general exercise guidelines for a wide range of clients as well as specific sections addressing considerations in special populations such as cardiac patients, individuals with diabetes mellitus, and the elderly. Regarding exercise programming for the elderly, these guidelines emphasize the need for individualizing cardiorespiratory endurance and resistance-training programs. Whenever possible, the guidelines recommend that older adults accumulate at least 30 minutes of moderate-intensity exercise (such as brisk walking and yard work) on most, and preferably all, days of the week. The guidelines also state that additional benefits can be obtained with increased duration of moderate-intensity exercise or by performing higher-intensity exercise (after discussing this with a physician).

The guidelines recommend resistance training at least twice per week (with at least 48 hours of rest between sessions) for older adults to gain benefits related to muscular strength and muscular endurance. The guidelines also point out the importance of a well-rounded program of stretching at least two to three days per week for older adults to maintain flexibility and improve balance and agility. Tai chi and yoga may be useful ways of obtaining these benefits (see chapter 15 for a more in-depth discussion of these two forms of mind-body exercise).

Overall, the ACSM guidelines are an excellent resource for physical activity instructors to become knowledgeable about topics such as exercise prescription, health appraisal, and risk assessment. In general, a health screening is recommended before beginning an exercise program (see chapter 5 for a discussion of the specific components that should be included in such a screening). Guidelines are provided to determine when additional evaluation, including exercise testing, should be recommended. Even if not determined to be essential, additional exercise testing can provide the physical activity instructor with valuable information such as the clinical status and functional capacity of the client to consider in the development of a safe, effective exercise program.

The National Institute on Aging (NIA, 1998) published an exercise guide for older adults to help them better understand the benefits of exercise and how to incorporate it into their daily lives. The book provides guidance for individuals to determine when they should talk to their physicians before exercising and emphasizes the importance of gradually developing a well-rounded program of exercise that includes aerobic endurance, strength, flexibility, and balance exercises. The NIA guide recommends that, in general, older adults gradually progress to at least 30 minutes of moderate to vigorous endurance exercise on most or preferably all days of the week. The 30-minute goal can be accomplished by accumulating time in shorter sessions of at least 10 minutes each (see chapter 13 for more information on this exercise component). Older adults are advised to perform strengthening exercises for all of the major muscle groups at least two days per week, as long as the same muscle groups are not exercised on two consecutive days (see chapter 12 for a discussion of strength training). Some balance-training components should be added progressively as part of the lower-body strengthening routine, and additional balance exercises that can be done anytime, such as standing on one foot, can be performed (chapter 14 provides additional balance and mobility exercises). The NIA guide recommends stretching exercises after endurance and strength training, or three to seven days per week (after warming up) for those who are not performing other types of exercise. Diagrams and instructions for specific exercises are included in the guide. Specific examples of each type of exercise are also provided in chapters 11 to 14 of this book.

Becoming familiar with the exercise guidelines and recommendations established by ACSM (1998,

2000) and NIA (1998) can help you in at least three ways. The guidelines provide (1) evidence-based recommendations for exercise testing and prescription that you can use to design safe and effective exercise programs for older adults, (2) exercise options that can help you address the individual needs and interests of your clients, and (3) documentation of what constitutes safe practice according to experts in the field, which can help protect you from litigation when followed. Legal issues related to exercise programming are discussed in chapter 22.

Exercise Principles for Program Design

Two major principles of exercise, overload and specificity, need to be addressed when designing exercise programs. "The principle of **overload** states that for a tissue or organ to improve its function, it must be exposed to a load to which it is not normally accustomed. Repeated exposure is associated with an adaptation by the tissue or organ that leads to improved functional capacity." (ACSM, 2000). The load can be progressively increased by manipulating the type or mode of exercise selected, the position in which the exercise is performed, or other exercise variables such as the frequency, duration, or intensity of a particular exercise. For example, to improve the cardiovascular system, an older adult could gradually increase the number of days walks are taken, the walking distance, the walking speed, or the incline of the walking surface.

The principle of **specificity** states that the training effects derived from physical activity are specific to the type of exercise and muscles involved (ACSM, 2000). For example, a low-resistance and high-repetition exercise increases the oxidative capacity of the muscle but does little to strengthen the muscle. In contrast, a high-resistance, low-repetition exercise increases strength and muscle size but does little to increase muscular endurance.

Specific Exercise Principles for Older Adults

In addition to the traditional principles of exercise, overload and specificity, experts in gerokinesiology recommend applying three additional principles in programs for older adults: (1) functional relevance,

(2) challenge, and (3) accommodation (Jones, 2002; Rose, 2003). These principles exemplify the specialized knowledge and practical training needed to become an effective physical activity instructor of older adults.

Functional Relevance

The principle of **functional relevance** encourages selecting exercises that simulate the movements of everyday activities to be performed in environments that are similar to those regularly encountered by program participants (Jones, 2002; Rose, 2003). For instance, during balance and mobility training, participants can practice walking on a variety of surfaces that mimic everything from a thickly carpeted floor to a slick surface similar to an icy sidewalk. To make strengthening activities more functionally relevant, participants could practice picking up a weight such as a bag of groceries, carrying it across the room, and placing it on a shelf. Functional relevance is similar to the exercise principle of specificity, but its focus is on functional activities that simulate movements performed in daily life. The functional relevance principle makes older adults more aware of the connection between their exercise sessions and activities they perform in their daily lives.

Challenge

A second exercise principle related to the functional training of older adults is the **challenge** principle. Selected activities or exercises need to challenge, but not exceed, an individual's intrinsic capabilities (e.g., strength, cognition, sensorimotor ability), and the level of challenge can be altered by changing the task demands (seated, standing, or moving; single or multiple task) or the environmental demands (surface type, lighting, visual flow; Rose, 2003). Additional information about assessing an individual's intrinsic capabilities and matching them in an exercise program is presented in chapters 6, 7, and 14. For a client who has serious balance problems, for example, you should challenge his or her balance systems but at the same time provide a safe

> The principle of functional relevance emphasizes that exercises need to simulate functional tasks performed in environments of everyday life.

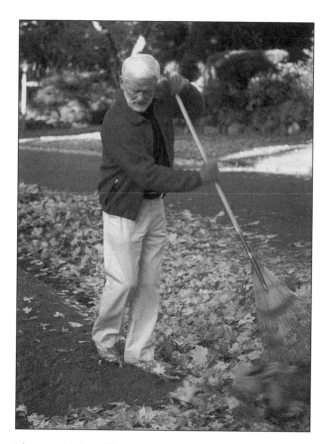

The principle of functional relevance focuses on exercises that simulate movements performed in daily life.

Source: *Health Canada website and Media Photo Gallery,* Health Canada, http://www.hc-sc.gc.ca. Reproduced with the permission of the Minister of Public Works and Government Services Canada, 2004

environment (a stable surface) so that he or she does not fall. This client could begin walking on a stable surface initially and then gradually progress to more challenging surfaces, for instance, or to reduced lighting conditions. The challenge could also be manipulated by adding a second task, such as counting while walking (Rose, 2003). In the resistance-training example of lifting, carrying, and putting away groceries, a participant might start with a light weight and place it on a low shelf and then progress to a heavier weight eventually placed on a higher level shelf.

There is a fine line between exercises that challenge a person enough to produce positive effects and those that place a client at risk of injury. The more information you have about your clients' medical conditions and physical status, the more effective you can be in providing the right amount of challenge safely. Clients' physicians should be involved as needed. While some of your clients

may want to take unnecessary risks, others may prefer comfort and be reluctant to increase the workload or challenge. It is important to remind the risk takers to progress more slowly, but it is equally important to gently prompt other clients to challenge themselves a little more (within a safe range). The challenge principle is discussed in more detail in chapter 14.

Accommodation

A third exercise principle important for older adults is **accommodation.** This principle states that participants should be encouraged to "perform exercises to the best of their abilities, but to never push themselves to a point of overexertion, pain, or beyond a level they consider to be safe" (Jones, 2002). Although the overload principle informs us that to cause a training effect, an exercise needs to challenge the system beyond what is usual, with older adults it is also important to apply the accommodation principle to ensure that they do not exceed their individual capabilities during exercise. The accommodation principle recognizes the fluctuating health and physical functioning of many older adults and encourages clients to perform to the best of their ability at that particular time.

For example, a person on cardiac medication may feel capable of walking two miles (3.2 kilometers) one day but the next day feel too weak to walk even 100 yards (91.4 meters). A client who may feel comfortably challenged by performing a low-impact aerobic dance sequence one day may experience very painful knee joints on another day. This fluctuating pain is common among people who have arthritis and other musculoskeletal disorders. To ensure that participants do not attempt to perform at the same level each time regardless of how they feel, they should be encouraged to become skilled at listening to their bodies and understanding the signs and symptoms of overexertion.

There are numerous practical implications of these exercise principles for physical activity instructors and personal trainers who wish to

> The challenge principle means that exercises need to challenge, but not exceed, an individual's intrinsic capabilities. The level of challenge of an exercise can be adjusted by changing the task demand or the environmental demand or both.

> According to the accommodation principle, participants should be encouraged to perform to the best of their ability, without pushing themselves to a point of overexertion or pain or beyond what feels safe to them at that particular time.

individualize programs for their clients. Teaching a group of older adults is generally more challenging because it requires accommodating a wide range of abilities and medical concerns, so the following chapters in this part of the book focus on group instruction. However, much of the material can also be applied to personal training.

Summary

Working with older adults provides unique rewards and challenges for physical activity instructors, stemming from the broad range of states of health and physical functioning of older adults and the focus on maintaining or improving all components of fitness and specific physical functions that affect day-to-day activities. Appropriate aerobic endurance, strengthening, flexibility, and balance and mobility exercises may help older adults maintain their independence well into their later years. By understanding the process of disablement and the role of physical activity in preventing or delaying disability, physical activity instructors can select particular types of exercise that meet their clients' goals and needs. By knowing each client's level of functioning, instructors can further tailor specific types of exercise to target the most essential functions (e.g., lower-body strength training to improve a person's ability to walk and get out of chairs). The ACSM and NIA exercise guidelines for older adults can help instructors become more

confident in designing and implementing well-rounded exercise programs with the input of their older adult clients.

Through the judicious application of the exercise principles of specificity, overload, functional relevance, challenge, and accommodation, instructors can better help their clients to achieve optimal outcomes safely. The chapters to follow encourage you to adopt this new approach that applies the exercise principles in the design of programs that include a focus on the functional benefits of exercise training. Functional training involves various physical activities that ultimately make the tasks and activities of daily living easier, safer, and more efficient.

Key Terms

accommodation 137
challenge 136
disability 133
functional relevance 136
overload 136
physical functioning 132
specificity 136

Recommended Readings

American College of Sports Medicine. (1998). ASCM position stand on exercise and physical activity for older adults. *Medicine and Science in Sports and Exercise, 30,* 992-1008.

American College of Sports Medicine. (2000). *ACSM's guidelines for exercise testing and prescription* (6th ed.). Philadelphia: Lippincott Williams & Wilkins.

National Institute on Aging. (1998). *Exercise: A guide from the National Institute on Aging* (Publication No. NIH 98-4258). Washington, DC: National Institutes of Health.

Study Questions

1. What percentage of people 65 years of age and over have no chronic health conditions?
    a. 5 percent
    b. 8 percent
    c. 16 percent
    d. 20 percent

2. The disablement process model defines disability as
    a. difficulty or inability to perform complex activities in various dimensions of life
    b. physical impairments of body systems
    c. functional limitations, such as limitations in walking or bending
    d. a common consequence of aging

3. The selection of exercises that simulate movements from everyday activities performed in practice environments that are similar to those regularly encountered by program participants embodies which exercise principle?
    a. challenge
    b. accommodation
    c. functional relevance
    d. specificity

4. In the challenge principle, examples of ways to alter the level of challenge are
    a. perform a task from a seated position versus a standing position
    b. dim the lighting in the room
    c. recite a poem while performing a walking task
    d. all of the above

5. According to the NIA guidelines, a balanced physical activity program for older adults includes
    a. flexibility, strength, and balance exercises
    b. aerobic endurance, stretching, and resistance-training exercises
    c. aerobic endurance, strength, balance, and flexibility exercises
    d. resistance-training and aerobic endurance exercises

6. Potential functional benefits of upper-body strengthening exercises include
    a. improved ability to lift and carry groceries
    b. improved upper-body strength
    c. improved ability to walk
    d. all of the above

Application Activities

1. You are working with an older woman who has just completed the chair stand functional fitness test. She did three chair stands in the 30 seconds, and she commented that it is difficult for her to get up from chairs and couches. Her physician told her that she could perform moderate-intensity exercise, and she has no medical conditions that would cause her difficulty getting up from the chair. Develop a list of discussion topics or questions that can determine (1) her interest in improving her ability to get down into and up from chairs, (2) whether she has difficulty in other activities that she does or would like to do, and (3) what types of activities or exercise training could lead to functional benefits that address these areas of concern. Also prepare an explanation that can help her link those types of training to the specific functional benefits, and include in your explanation at least one concept from either of the theoretical perspectives on how older adults become disabled.

2. Applying the principle of functional relevance, plan the activities for an exercise session for an independently living female client age 76. When asked how she spends her time each week, she said that she lives alone and spends a fair amount of time doing household tasks such as laundry and light housekeeping. She typically eats her meals at a nearby senior center, where she volunteers in the art studio. She would like to try a dance or tai chi class at the senior center but knows that some days her balance just isn't as good as it used to be. Her physician

(continued)

has encouraged her to stay active without any restrictions. How might you apply the challenge and principles when designing the balance and mobility component of her program?

3. An older man is interested in starting an exercise program and has asked you what types of exercise are recommended for older adults. He is going to talk to his doctor at an upcoming physical exam and wants some background information about appropriate exercises. Summarize the recommendations from the NIA and ACSM resources for him to give to his doctor.

10

Principles of the Warm-Up and Cool-Down

Kay Van Norman

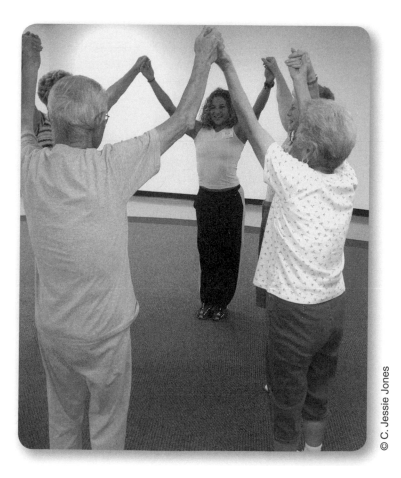

© C. Jessie Jones

Warm-up and cool-down exercises are designed to provide a safe transition to and an adequate recovery from more vigorous exercise. These elements of an exercise class are important for all age groups, but they are essential for older adults to prevent injury and facilitate the most efficient function possible. This chapter provides an overview of the acute physiological changes that occur while warming up and cooling down. Practical strategies for creating a safe and effective warm-up and cool-down for older adults are described. In addition, this chapter discusses the importance of using the warm-up and cool-down phases of an exercise class to engage your clients in other dimensions of wellness (physical, social, emotional, mental, and spiritual). A sample warm-up and cool-down are provided.

Physiological Changes Associated With Warm-Up

Warming up increases the internal body temperature, resulting in changes that prepare the cardiopulmonary, neuromuscular, and metabolic systems for higher-intensity exercise. A warm-up increases the efficiency of numerous body systems; for example, it increases lung circulation and improves delivery of oxygen to working muscles. It also affects nervous system function, improving coordination and reaction time. Warming up results in increased blood saturation of the muscles, tendons, and joints, thereby significantly reducing their susceptibility to injury. Figure 10.1 lists the physiological benefits of warming up.

Physiological change	Specific benefits
Increased release of oxygen from hemoglobin and myoglobin	Delivery of more oxygen to the working muscles More efficient use of oxygen
Decreased muscle viscosity	Improved mechanical efficiency and power
Increased blood saturation of muscles, tendons, and ligaments	Increased elasticity Decreased susceptibility to injury Increased delivery of necessary fuel
Increased speed of nervous impulses and sensitivity of nerve receptors	Improved coordination and reaction time
Reduced pulmonary resistance	Increased lung circulation More efficient aerobic metabolism
Improved cardiac blood flow	Decreased risk of myocardial ischemia
Increased metabolic rates	Improved efficiency

FIGURE 10.1 Physiological benefits of the warm-up.
Adapted from DeVries et al. 1994; Nieman 1999.

A physiological definition of warming up is increasing the temperature of muscles and blood for the body's transition from rest to activity (Nieman, 1999). This can be accomplished through **passive warm-up** (using external agents such as hot showers, saunas, or ultrasound) or **active warm-up** (using body movements). An active warm-up is generally preferred to a passive warm-up, regardless of the mode of exercise you are preparing for. However, passive heating in the form of a hot shower may be indicated for older adults with arthritis before they engage in fitness activities. Refer to chapter 21 for additional information on exercise adaptations for chronic medical conditions.

Warming up improves the efficiency of the cardiovascular response and may prevent a variety of cardiovascular irregularities that are commonly brought on by sudden strenuous exertion (American College of Sports Medicine [ACSM], 2000). Because the coronary blood flow adaptation is not immediate, a warm-up is needed as a transition period from rest to higher-intensity physical activity. In addition, warming up reduces the resistance of pulmonary blood flow, resulting in significantly improved blood circulation in the lungs (Nieman, 1999). Warming up properly also is an important safety precaution for managing older adults' risk of musculoskeletal injuries from aerobic and resistance training.

Increased body temperature acts as a mobilizing stimulus for the systems involved in oxygen transport, thereby increasing the efficiency of aerobic metabolism. There is evidence that a greater percentage of energy is derived from fat metabolism when a warm-up is done before aerobic exercise (DeVries & Housh, 1994). Not only does increased fat metabolism spare carbohydrates during exercise (important for endurance athletes), but it also can benefit individuals involved in weight loss programs.

The mechanical efficiency of the muscles is also improved by warming up, allowing them to relax and contract faster. Movements requiring strength, power, and coordination are enhanced as a result. In addition, warming up increases the blood saturation of the neuromuscular system, thereby improving delivery of fuel to the cells and facilitating the elasticity of muscles, tendons, and joints (Nieman, 1999). This improved elasticity is key to injury prevention for older adults.

Physiological Changes Associated With Cool-Down

In contrast to the warm-up, the purpose of **cooling down** is to slowly decrease body temperature, heart rate, and respiration to preactivity levels. For all practical purposes, the cool-down is a warm-up in reverse and may include many of the same low-intensity, continuous movements. The cool-down can decrease muscle soreness and help prevent potential exercise-related problems, such as dizziness and cardiac irregularities, that can occur in high-risk populations.

Mild, continuous activity following exercise keeps the leg muscles contracting, promoting venous return by the pumping of the contraction and relaxation cycle (Nieman, 1999). This prevents the blood from pooling in the extremities and reduces the fainting and dizziness that can occur when activity is abruptly halted. Less blood pooling also reduces delayed muscular stiffness after exercise. Continuous, low-intensity movement also helps reduce the level of lactic acid in the muscles and blood more rapidly than complete rest after exertion, thereby promoting faster recovery from fatigue (Nieman, 1999).

Finally, a cool-down helps to slowly decrease the level of **catecholamines** (epinephrine and norepinephrine) in the blood, which is raised by high-intensity aerobic exercise. High levels of catecholamines can cause cardiac irregularities among high-risk individuals, most often after rather than during exercise (Nieman, 1999). Although such exercise-related irregularities of the heart are relatively rare, a carefully constructed cool-down is an important safety precaution for all aerobic classes for older adults. Figure 10.2 summarizes the benefits of a cool-down.

Decreased body temperature
Decreased heart rate and respiration
Decreased blood pooling in extremities
Decreased catecholamine levels in blood
Decreased muscle soreness and recovery time

FIGURE 10.2   Physiological benefits of the cool-down.
From DeVries et al. 1994; Nieman 1999.

Guiding Principles of the Warm-Up

The warm-up should increase body temperature to provide a gradual transition to more vigorous exercise. It should also set the stage for safe and effective exercise by establishing proper movement techniques and exercise intensity. Finally, the warm-up should engage class participants socially, emotionally, and cognitively.

Increasing Body Temperature

To increase the body's internal temperature, an active warm-up is preferred to a passive warm-up. Lead your class participants in 10 to 20 minutes of low-intensity, continuous movement and easy range-of-motion activities to increase internal body temperature by approximately one to two degrees Fahrenheit (one-half to one degree Celsius). Consider the health and fitness levels of participants and the type of activity to be performed when determining the length and intensity of the warm-up. A longer warm-up is recommended for a higher-intensity exercise program and for frailer or less-conditioned clients (Nieman, 1999).

Safe and Effective Warm-Up

Many different forms of activity can be used to increase the internal body temperature and safely prepare older adult clients of different functional abilities for higher-intensity exercise. Examples include walking (on land or in water), rhythmic movements performed while seated or standing, and using cardiovascular equipment such as stationary bikes and recumbent steppers. Whenever possible, incorporate in the warm-up large-muscle movements that are the same as or similar to, but at a lower intensity than, those you plan to introduce later in class. Mimic movements to be used during later exercise at a slower tempo and intensity to serve as both warm-up and practice. For example, if the arms will be pushed overhead during the aerobic conditioning component of the class, have your clients perform the same movement through a similar range of motion but more slowly during the warm-up.

The environment in which you conduct warm-up activities also determines the types of activity you select. Environmental considerations include the amount of space available relative to the number of participants, the characteristics of the flooring, and the availability of equipment. Room temperature must also be considered, as it significantly influences how rapidly the internal body temperature rises in response to exercise.

When you teach a warm-up to a new group of clients, it is important to explain the importance of warming up and to carefully monitor the participants for signs of overexertion. How well each client responds to the intensity of the warm-up indicates how well he or she will respond to higher-intensity exercises.

Engaging Participants

The warm-up period of an exercise class is the perfect time to establish important social and emotional connections with the group. It provides an opportunity to converse with clients and encourage interaction, learn their names, greet them as they enter class, and introduce new participants to the group. These behaviors demonstrate your genuine interest in each individual in the group. Be sure to structure the warm-up to provide numerous opportunities for feelings of accomplishment and success in movement. Try to create a noncompetitive and safe environment where participants are encouraged to work at their own level, and frequently demonstrate variations appropriate for different ability levels. Provide positive reinforcement for all accomplishments and efforts, and downplay the need to be on the "right" foot at the "right" time.

The warm-up is also a good time to teach new movement sequences that you plan to introduce later in the class. This allows your clients to practice the movement at a slower speed and gain confidence before attempting it at a faster speed later in the class. Preparing your clients both physically and mentally to be successful in movement should be a primary goal of the warm-up. Music also plays an important role in fostering feelings of belonging, success in movement, and overall enjoyment of the exercise experience. The type of music and how it is managed throughout the class are both important considerations. (More information about incorporating music in activity classes is presented in chapters 19 and 20.)

Developing the Warm-Up

This section provides examples of warm-ups that apply the exercise principles of challenge and accommodation first described in chapter 9. Remember that your goal during the warm-up is to match the activities to the physical abilities of the participants. Teaching class participants how to monitor exercise intensity is also important. This section also provides simple strategies you can use to engage your exercise participants socially, emotionally, and cognitively.

Ability Level

Allow at least 15 minutes of continuous, low-intensity movement for healthy older adults to warm up before aerobic conditioning or other vigorous, high-intensity activities. Activities that gradually elevate the clients' heart rates to the lower limit of their target exercise heart rate range will produce the desired increase in internal temperature (ACSM, 2000). Frailer older adults can benefit from a longer warm-up (20 minutes) of continuous, gentle movements of the arms and legs that are performed in a seated position. This activity raises body temperature and increases blood saturation levels in the muscles, tendons, and ligaments. Frailer participants may begin to perspire (a sign that internal temperature is rising) after very mild activity, so it is important to monitor their responses carefully. Monitoring participants' responses to exercise is described in more detail in chapter 13.

Type of Activity

Have your clients perform continuous movement through a normal joint range of motion to increase their internal temperature. Select arm and leg movements that progress from small through progressively larger ranges of motion, and then progressively increase the difficulty of the pattern and the coordination required. For example, begin with biceps curls, and then do arm swings front to back and side to side. Follow with single-arm presses in front, down, to the side, and across the body, and progress to double-arm presses to the front, to the sides, and overhead, first in unison and then in opposition with the legs. Avoid static stretches for increasing range of motion during the warm-up. Save these activities for the cool-down,

Guidelines for an Effective Warm-Up

- Ten to 20 minutes of progressive exercise, gradually building the challenge and intensity (e.g., increasing size or speed of movement, adding arm movements and sequences)
- Age-appropriate music (100-110 beats per minute) with a steady and easily distinguished beat
- Continuous, rhythmic endurance exercises (e.g., easy walking, light marching, toe and heel presses, low knee lifts, and small kicks)
- Rehearsal (step by step but slower tempo) of exercise sequences to come
- Specific joint mobility exercises (e.g., arms overhead then circles along with low-intensity endurance exercise)
- Monitoring intensity (on the 6-20 point scale, RPE between 9 and 10 for older adults or between 7 and 9 for frailer older adults)
- Activities should promote many dimensions of overall well-being: physical, social, emotional, mental, and spiritual.

when muscles are thoroughly warm. (Examples of dynamic and static flexibility exercises that are appropriate for both warm-up and cool-down are presented in chapter 11.) The warm-up is also the perfect time to emphasize good posture, proper body mechanics, and breathing techniques during exercise.

Start your warm-up session with simple footwork, such as marching in place and toe and heel presses to the front, and then incorporate small kicks and knee lifts to engage the hip more fully before progressing to toe and heel presses and small kicks to the side. Use stationary movement before traveling movement to ensure that participants are transferring weight from foot to foot without balance problems before traveling. Start with forward and backward movement, and then progress to step touches to the sides before traveling sideways.

When the warm-up precedes resistance training, it should include walking around the room, rhythmic movement sequences, or using cardiovascular equipment to increase body temperature. These activities should be followed by movements that mimic those to be performed in the resistance-training component of the class (e.g., standing chest presses, biceps curls, standing rows).

Environment

An exercise environment that lacks adequate cardiovascular equipment or space for a group warm-up requires you to be more creative in your approach. You can use adjoining hallways or incorporate more stationary movements, such as marching in place, while performing progressively higher knee lifts, small kicks, or similar movements. Before performing standing rhythmic movements, however, consider the safety of the flooring. Select movements that can be performed in a seated position if the flooring poses a safety risk for your clients (e.g., a slippery or concrete surface).

If the room temperature seems warmer than normal, it is important to closely monitor your participants' responses and watch for signs of overexertion such as a flushed face or unusually rapid breathing. (Refer to chapter 13 for additional signs of overexertion.) According to the ACSM (2000), an ambient temperature higher than 82 degrees Fahrenheit (28 degrees Celsius) for moderate exercise or 84 degrees Fahrenheit (29 degrees Celsius) for vigorous exercise is not safe. An exercise environment that is too hot places your clients (especially those with high blood pressure) at a greater risk of cardiac problems. If clients become flushed, perspire easily, or mention how hot the room feels during the warm-up, it is probably too hot for aerobics. Modify the class to include little or no aerobic conditioning and substitute coordination, balance, flexibility, and relaxation exercises until the conditions change or a more suitable exercise space is located.

Intensity

Teach your clients how to check their heart rates and use a standard **rating of perceived exertion (RPE,** a subjective rating of how hard they feel they are exercising) immediately after the warm-up so they can be aware of how their bodies are responding to exercise that day. Use the same verbal cues each time you have clients take a pulse rate or determine an RPE, and make sure that your cues are clear and direct. Borg's (1998) RPE scale is the most widely used scale. During the warm-up, healthy older adults should not exceed an RPE of 9 to 10 on the 6-to-20-point version of the Borg scale, or 7 to 9 for frailer older adults. Periodically, and whenever new clients join the class, take time during the warm-up to review the procedures for monitoring exercise intensity. Refer to chapter 13 for more detailed information on monitoring

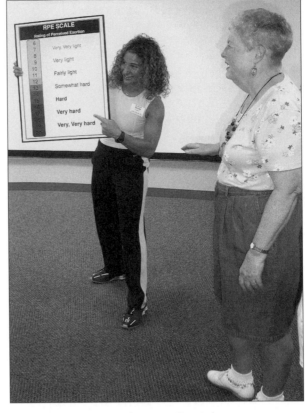

It is important to teach your clients how to rate their perceived exertion so that they can evaluate how hard they are working during the warm-up.

exercise intensity using Borg's RPE scale and on managing aerobic-training risks in general.

One way to evaluate clients' responses to the exercise intensity is to periodically use a circle formation during the warm-up and aerobic periods of the class. This allows you to watch closely for signs of overexertion. Ask your clients how they are doing or how the room temperature feels, and casually administer the **talk test** (a simple conversational assessment to guard against overexertion) to one or two clients during the warm-up. To pass the talk test, the client should be able to respond without gasping for air to a direct question that requires more than a one-word answer (e.g., "What are your plans after class today, Jane?").

Social Connection

The warm-up is a perfect time to establish an important social connection with your clients. Using a circle formation during parts of the warm-up allows close contact between participants and opportunities for friendly exchanges. Simple social mixer dances and activities also help participants learn one another's names and ensure that everyone is involved in the social interaction. Friendly conversation during the warm-up helps participants feel free to talk among themselves and contributes to feelings of belonging.

At the beginning of the warm-up, while performing a simple movement, take three to five minutes to establish mini-goals for that day's class. For example, set a goal to perform a simple coordination sequence that the clients already know well at a faster tempo, or perhaps add additional steps to the sequence. During the warm-up you can also engage your clients cognitively by having them identify the working muscle groups and their role in activities of daily living, and then invite them to think of an exercise goal for themselves. This approach at the beginning of class prompts participants to engage their minds as well as their bodies in the exercise. (See chapter 15 for more details on engaging mind and body in the exercise experience.)

Music

The music you select and how you manage it throughout a class can create feelings of belong-

ing, success in movement, and overall enjoyment of the experience. The proper tempo comfortably matches the speed of a movement sequence and sets the tone for the class. Music with a tempo in the range of 100 to 110 beats per minute with a steady and easy-to-distinguish beat works well for both the warm-up and the active cool-down segments of class. Faster music of a similar type, from 120 to 140 beats per minute, works well for the aerobic conditioning section of the class. Simple instrumentals without excessive embellishment and midrange vocals (medium pitch vocals that complement rather than overpower or compete with the melody) are good choices. Easy listening and relaxation music are good choices for flexibility and relaxation activities during the cool-down. Music popular when class participants were young adults can create a strong emotional connection, bring back memories, and have students singing along and enjoying their time in class. This connection helps participants feel that they belong and motivates them to continue attending the class. Some appropriate music selections are listed in figure 10.3.

Be sure to play music at a moderate volume, and turn the music down or off when explaining a new

Warm-up and cool-down music	Aerobics music
Max Bygraves Midrange vocals (110-120 beats per minute) Glenn Miller Big band selections (100-120 beats per minute) John Denver Midrange vocals (110-120 beats per minute) George Winston Instrumental piano for cool-down and relaxation (100 beats per minute or less) Mark Knopfler *Princess Bride* soundtrack, instrumental, for relaxation (100 beats per minute or less) Ray Lynch Instrumentals for warm-ups, especially "Celestial Soda Pop" on *Deep Breakfast* (110-120 beats per minute)	Max Bygraves Midrange vocals, many in medleys, such as "Won't You Come Home Bill Bailey?" and "Bye, Bye Blackbird" (120-130 beats per minute) Herb Alpert Many moderate-tempo instrumentals, such as "Spanish Flea" and "Sentimental Over You" (120-140 beats per minute) Glenn Miller Many moderate-tempo vocal and instrumental selections, such as "In the Mood," "Chattanooga Choo Choo," and "Chattanooga Shoe Shine Boy" (120-140 beats per minute) Roger Miller Midrange vocals, such as "Engine #9," "England Swings," and "King of the Road" (120-130 beats per minute) Royal Philharmonic Orchestra *Hooked on Classics* Vols. 1, 2, and 3 (130-140 beats per minute) Larry Elgart and His Manhattan Swing Orchestra *Hooked on Swing* Vols. 1, 2, and 3, instrumental medleys (130-140 beats per minute)

FIGURE 10.3 Music selections for the warm-up, the cool-down, and aerobics components.

exercise or changing to a lower-intensity portion of the warm-up. Straining to hear instructions over the music can be very frustrating for participants.

Success

To ensure your clients' success during the warm-up, avoid complex combinations and complicated steps. It is helpful to use simple movements and easy-to-follow, rhythmic patterns. Identify a simple "home" step, such as marching in place, that everyone can easily perform, and return to it frequently throughout the warm-up. When performing coordination sequences, begin with the leg movement alone, and then add the arm movement when participants have mastered the leg movement. Keep a careful watch on how the class is responding, and if they are having difficulty, return to the home step. Try a different approach if a number of your clients experience difficulties. This strategy ensures that each participant is successful a large percentage of the time, without drawing attention to anyone who may be having difficulty. Feeling at ease while

performing the movement patterns in time with the music can increase your clients' self-esteem and promote feelings of accomplishment.

Once your clients are able to successfully meet small challenges, their self-esteem and confidence in their abilities will be heightened (Wise & Trunnell, 2001). Gradually incorporate small challenges into your warm-up by adding more complex arm movements to simple, well-learned footwork. Practice coordination sequences that require the limbs to move in unison and opposition. Create short routines that can fit in various places in a song, and alternate them with the home step. Periodically add one or two new sets of steps lasting eight to sixteen counts to an established routine. These instructional strategies help to keep participants engaged cognitively by challenging their memory recall skills while still allowing success in movement. Research shows that successfully meeting challenges in one area of life often translates into increased confidence in one's ability to meet challenges in other areas of life (Bandura, 1997). Figure 10.4 provides a sample low-impact warm-up.

Music: Ray Lynch – "Celestial Soda Pop" and other songs from *Deep Breakfast*

Instructions: Perform these sequences and suitable variations for approximately 10 minutes. Begin with a front-facing formation; change to a circle holding hands; drop hands, resume arm movements, and move backward to widen the circle; and then move back to a front-facing formation. The absence of arm movement while in a tight circle holding hands allows the use of more intricate foot patterns. It also allows you to converse with participants, encourage social interaction, and identify a goal for the day. Avoid quick, jerky arm movements; keep them slow and fluid to safely warm up the shoulders. Use music that has a tempo of 110 to 120 beats per minute.

A March in place
   Continue marching while crossing arms in front and slowly opening over head in a large circle (two counts of 8)
   Shoulder rolls (forward for 8 counts, backward for 8 counts) while doing slow knee bends

B Alternating toe touches to the front (one count of 8)
   Alternating toe touches to the front with arms swinging (one arm forward, one arm back; 3 counts of 8)
   Repeat A

C Heel presses to the front (one count of 8)
   Heel presses to the front with arms swinging (one arm forward, one arm back; 3 counts of 8)
   Repeat A

D Alternating toe touches to the sides (one count of 8)
   Alternating toe touches to the sides with arms swinging side to side in unison
   Repeat A

E Alternating knee lifts to the front, touch hands to knees (one count of 8)
   Repeat A

FIGURE 10.4   Sample low-impact warm-up.

Repeat B, C, D, and E, but replace swinging arms with arm presses forward, down, and up. Use a variety of arm movements; in unison and opposition with legs, one arm at a time and both arms together.

F   March in place and with upper-back squeezes, arm circles, or arm stretches overhead or across the body (two counts of 8)

G   Step right, touch left, step left, touch right (two counts of 8)
Alternate step touches while moving forward (one count of 8)
Alternate step touches while moving backward (one count of 8)
Repeat moving forward and backward (two counts of 8) with arms swinging side to side in unison

---

FIGURE 10.4   *(continued)*

Developing the Cool-Down

The cool-down should reduce body temperature, heart rate, and respiration to preactivity levels, assist the return of blood flow to the heart, and facilitate the return of muscle and skin vasodilation to resting levels (Nieman, 1999). Reinforcing social connections, stretching, relaxation, and making a conscious transition to the rest of the day are also important aspects of a cool-down. It is important to allow enough time for a proper cool-down (at least 10 minutes) and to discourage participants from leaving class before it ends.

Before your clients leave class, instruct them either to monitor their pulse for at least 15 seconds or to rate their perceived exertion to ensure that they have fully recovered. If participants have to leave class early, make it a standard policy that they must complete the main activities 5 to 10 minutes early and walk around the space until their heart and respiration rates and body temperature have dropped. If someone leaves class unexpectedly, be sure to have an assistant or another class participant follow him or her to determine if he or she is experiencing a health problem.

After completing the aerobic endurance portion of the class, have your clients check the intensity of their workout by taking their heart rates for at least 15 seconds and rating their perceived exertion. Reduce the exercise intensity (slow walking or a similar activity) for one minute, then have them check their pulse and RPE again. Periodically ask each client how much his or her heart rate or RPE decreased during the one-minute recovery period. The rate of recovery varies, depending on how intense the exercise was for the individual. Refer to chapter 13 for more specific information on varying the intensity of aerobic endurance training. Chapter 16 describes the differences in heart rate your clients can expect to encounter in aquatic exercise classes.

Type of Activity

The cool-down is basically the warm-up in reverse, but with more static flexibility exercises and relaxation activities. Use low-intensity, continuous movement for 5 to 10 minutes to allow the body to adjust from exertion to rest. Use small steps from side to side and forward and backward, low marches in place, and heel presses and toe touches to the front and sides at progressively lower intensity to return the heart rate and respiration back to normal. Keep arm movements small and relaxed and predominantly below shoulder level. Mix gentle, dynamic stretches and coordination and balance activities with low-intensity, continuous movement.

The last stage of the cool-down (when the muscles and connective tissue are most pliable) should include static flexibility and relaxation activities. Healthy older adults benefit from stretches performed on the floor so that one muscle group can be isolated for stretching while the rest of the body is relaxed. In classes for physically frail older adults, gradually reduce continuous, seated movements and mix in gentle static stretches. While your clients are still seated, introduce activities that systematically stretch all areas of the body from the head down (i.e., neck, shoulders, arms, hands, back, hips, legs, and feet). Use relaxation strategies between stretches and at the end of class. Refer to chapter 11 for specific flexibility exercises and to chapter 15 for specific relaxation activities that you can use in the cool-down.

Guidelines for an Effective Cool-Down

- Continuous rhythmic exercises progressively decreasing in intensity for 5 to 10 minutes, depending on participants' fitness level

- A stretching phase that includes static stretching

- A variety of simple mind–body activities, such as yoga and tai chi

- Activities that reinforce social, emotional, and cognitive connections

- A relaxation phase to make the transition from exercise class to the rest of the day

Reinforcing the Wellness Connection

The cool-down is the perfect time for participants to reconnect with others in the class and for you to reinforce the relationship among the physical, social, emotional, cognitive, and spiritual domains of health. For example, holding hands in a circle while performing low-intensity cool-down activities is a great strategy for reconnecting socially. It provides an opportunity for participants to review goals achieved in the class and share jokes. These activities reinforce the positive nature of being part of a group, help end the class on a positive note, and help your clients begin to prepare for the rest of the day. Figure 10.5 offers a sample cool-down for healthy older adults.

Music: Max Bygraves "Somebody Loves Me Medley" (110 beats per minute)

A   In a circle holding hands, low-intensity march in place (two counts of 8)
Alternating step touches, moving forward and backward (two counts of 8)

Drop hands and walk backward for more space; stay in circle formation

B   Alternating toe touches front (two counts of 8)
Alternating heel presses front (two counts of 8)

Alternating toe touches side to side (two counts of 8)
Swing arms (very little) in opposition

C   March in place (two counts of 8)
Large circle of the arms up, over the head, and down (once)
Shoulder rolls (one count of 8 forward and one count of 8 backward)

D   Alternating toe touches side to side, arms in opposition (two counts of 8)
March in place (one count of 8)
Toe touches side to side, swinging arms in unison (two counts of 8)

Repeat, swinging arms in opposition and in unison

Move together to hold hands in circle; tap the right toe in front 8 to 16 times until everyone has the right foot free to move to the right.

E   Step sideways to the right, still in the circle (one count of 8)
Step to the left (one count of 8)
Repeat right and left (two counts of 8)
Step right (counts 1-4)
Step left (counts 5-8)
Repeat right and left (one count of 8)
Step right (counts 1-2)
Step left (counts 3-4)
Repeat right and left (counts 5-8 and again 1-8)
Repeat full sequence

FIGURE 10.5   Sample low-impact cool-down.

Note: Be sure to cue in advance for the changes in direction. If participants get confused, just march in place, then tap the right toe until everyone has the right foot free to move to the right, and begin again. Music should have a slow, distinct beat (110 beats per minute).

Repeat A-D

F   Holding hands in a circle, alternate marching in place with standing upper- and lower-body stretches like reaching arms overhead, Achilles tendon stretch (lunge), shoulder stretch (arm crossing in front and/or back), hamstring stretch (heel extended to front and flexing forward at hip). This is a great time to make personal contact with participants, visiting, asking about what they are going to do after class, sharing interesting news, and so on.

G   After 8 to 10 minutes of active cool-down, check pulse and RPE, and then progress to static flexibility exercises. Sitting on a mat or in a chair, perform flexibility exercises (see chapter 11).

H   End with relaxation breathing. Lie on your back, eyes closed, and take deep breaths. Quiet instrumental music and visualization of pleasant scenes can enhance relaxation. Refer to chapter 15 for instructions for relaxation breathing.

FIGURE 10.5   *(continued)*

It is important to set the right mood for the stretching and relaxation phase of the cool-down. Use a mat or pad to enhance comfort and relaxation when stretching on the floor. The music should be soothing and at a low volume, and lights can be dimmed to foster the right mood for visualization and active breathing, a simple technique to increase body awareness and lung capacity and promote relaxation (see figure 10.6). Refer to chapter 15 for other mind–body exercises and techniques for deep breathing and relaxation to use during the cool-down.

Transition to the Day

After the relaxation phase of the cool-down, the final minutes should be spent facilitating a thoughtful transition to the rest of the day and making any announcements. Review individual and group goals accomplished during class, and reflect on potential mini-goals for the day. Invite participants to identify a personal goal for the day, from accomplishing something in the garden, to relaxing with a good book or communicating something to a loved one. This approach reinforces identifying and achieving goals to improve self-efficacy. Highlighting social opportunities outside of class and inviting participants to share ideas and thoughts for the day also support social and emotional connections and foster group identity.

This time in the class can be a wonderful chance for participants to ask or offer advice on anything from gardening to personal relationships

A   Place the hands on the abdomen and become aware of how it moves while breathing.
Take a medium breath, allowing the abdomen to expand while inhaling and relax inward while exhaling.

B   Picture the lungs filling with air, pushing the diaphragm down and the abdomen out.

C   Practice slowly with medium breaths for one to two minutes. Then take several very deep breaths, inhaling and exhaling slowly.

D   Slowly raise the arms above the head while inhaling *through the nose,* and lower the arms to the sides while exhaling completely *through the mouth.*

E   When comfortable with active breathing, visualize something positive or pleasant throughout the breathing activity.

FIGURE 10.6   Active breathing.

and encourages interaction between participants outside the class. A group shoulder massage also brings participants together and is a fun way to bring the class to a close.

Summary

The warm-up and cool-down are essential components of an exercise class for older adults. The warm-up should be carefully designed to increase body temperature for optimal performance and reduced risk of injury. The cool-down is designed to return the body systems to their preactivity states. The warm-up and cool-down also provide the instructor with a perfect opportunity to engage participants socially, emotionally, cognitively, and spiritually in the exercise experience. Facilitating the psychosocial elements of physical activity improves clients' self-efficacy, both inside and outside class, and enhances their motivation to continue attending class.

Key Terms

Recommended Reading

Van Norman, K.A. (1995). *Exercise programming for older adults.* Champaign, IL: Human Kinetics.

Spiraduso, W.W. (1995). *Physical dimensions of aging.* Champaign, IL: Human Kinetics.

Study Questions

1. How does the body usually signal that it is physiologically warmed up?
   a. heavy perspiration
   b. slight increase in heart rate
   c. light perspiration
   d. dramatic increase in heart rate

2. The warm-up positively affects the neuromuscular system by
   a. increasing blood saturation
   b. increasing muscle elasticity
   c. making the muscle contraction–relaxation cycle more efficient
   d. all of the above

3. Warming up influences pulmonary blood flow by
   a. increasing the resistance to blood flow
   b. decreasing the resistance to blood flow
   c. creating a more constant resistance
   d. allowing wider variation in resistance

4. Passive warm-up refers to
   a. applying external heating agents to the body, such as hot showers or heating pads
   b. another person's moving the client's arms or legs through an easy range of motion to prepare the client for exercise
   c. engaging in whole-body movement to increase body temperature
   d. slowly moving the arms and legs through a limited range of motion

5. The purpose of the cool-down is to slowly decrease ___ to preactivity levels.
   a. respiration
   b. body temperature
   c. heart rate
   d. all of the above

6. Mild, continuous activity following exercise
   a. prevents blood from pooling in the extremities
   b. reduces levels of lactic acid in muscles
   c. increases levels of epinephrine
   d. a and b

Application Activities

1. Design a 15-minute warm-up suitable for a group of frail older adults who are beginning their first week of chair exercise classes. Indicate the music you plan to use and any other information that is relevant to the success of the warm-up.

2. Design a 15-minute warm-up for a group of independent-living older adults to prepare them for 20 minutes of strength training at 80 percent of their one-repetition maximum.

3. Design a cool-down for a low-impact aerobics class for independent older adults. Identify the sequence of activities and the music you would use.

11

Flexibility Training

Marybeth Brown
Debra J. Rose

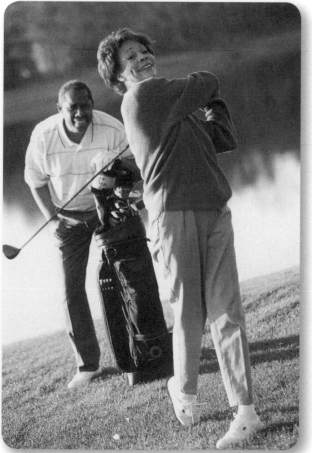

© Getty Images

Support for this work was provided to Marybeth Brown by the
National Institutes of Health (AG15796 and HD42272).

Flexibility, a term that describes the range of movement or motion possible at one or multiple joints, is important at all ages. When we were young, most of us enjoyed freedom of movement in all of our joints. Children have no difficulty breaking into a run spontaneously or picking up a stick and throwing it because their joints move freely. As we age, however, many factors contribute to a decline in flexibility (e.g., increased joint stiffness, changes in connective tissue, osteoarthritis). Indeed, for some older adults, the loss in joint flexibility can be so severe that the performance of daily functional activities becomes compromised. The good news is that exercises specifically designed to improve flexibility have been shown to be very effective for older adults. Although exercise alone is not likely to restore the movement potential that was present at a younger age, improvements in flexibility can lead to enhanced physical function. Improved flexibility also helps older adults feel better by reducing pain and stiffness, an additional benefit above and beyond the physiological benefits achieved.

The aim of this chapter is to clarify why people lose flexibility with age, the functional consequences of a loss in flexibility, and the minimal ranges of motion that should be maintained or restored at certain joints to improve older adults' performance of daily activities. In addition, a number of dynamic and static flexibility exercises designed to improve joint range of motion are presented.

Age-Associated Changes in Flexibility

Declines in joint **range of motion (ROM),** defined as the total excursion that is possible at a joint from the beginning of movement to the end of movement, are inevitable as a result of aging, but the rate of decline appears to be joint specific (Bell & Hoshizaki, 1981). For example, spinal extension declines, on average, by approximately 50 percent between the second and seventh decades (Einkauf, Gohdes, Jensen, & Jewell, 1987), while hip extension and knee flexion ROM decline on average by only 20 percent and 2 percent, respectively, over the same time period. The decline in joint ROM is also generally more evident in lower-body than in upper-body joints, consistent with the decline in muscle strength. Reduced flexibility in the lower-body joints has important implications for general mobility. Lower hamstring flexibility declines in both genders by approximately 14.5 percent, or one inch (2.5 centimeters) per decade (Golding & Lindsay, 1989), while losses of 15 percent (external rotation) and 11 percent (abduction) in ROM have been reported for the hip joints. Small but significant age-related changes have been reported in ankle dorsiflexion ROM. Small ROM changes independent of larger muscle strength losses have been observed (Nigg, Fisher, Allinger, Ronsky, & Engsberg, 1992), and ankle dorsiflexion strength has been shown to decrease by approximately 30 percent between the middle-age and the older adult years (Vandervoort et al., 1992). Any reduction in ankle ROM and strength increases the likelihood of trips and falls during the swing phase of gait.

With age, **stiffness** in all joints and muscle tissues also increases. Stiffness is defined as the force required to move a joint through a specified ROM (Holland, Tanaka, Shigematsu, & Nakagaichi, 2002). None of the tissues associated with mobility are impervious to old age, neither the tendons, ligaments, fascia, joint capsules, nor the fast- and slow-twitch muscles. Even muscles that are used routinely (e.g., calf muscles) show an increase in stiffness (James & Parker, 1989; Lung, Hartsell, & Vandervoort, 1996; Buckwalter et al., 1993). This increased stiffness is probably the most common complaint of older adults and results in a decline in ROM at most of the major joint complexes (Vandervoort et al., 1992; Svenningsen, Terjesen, Auflem, & Berg, 1989; Walker, Sue, Miles-Elkousy, Ford, & Trevelyan, 1984).

A number of biological factors appear to contribute to the increased muscle stiffness and reduced range of motion observed with age. These factors include an increase in the amount of inter- and intramuscular connective tissue, a change in the chemical composition of the connective tissue matrix and collagen, and breakdown of articular cartilage that increases arthritis in major joint complexes. In fact, it has been demonstrated by radiography that by the age of 75 years, 85 percent of older adults have osteoarthritic changes in the weight-bearing joints of the body (Moskowitz, 1989). As muscles age, they also lose mass as a result of the decline in the actual number of muscle fibers (Sjostrom, Lexell, & Downham, 1992). Subsequently, the connective tissue surrounding and within muscles increases as well (Eddinger, Cassens, & Moss, 1986).

Because connective tissues are composed primarily of collagen, they have much less give than skeletal muscle. Thus, more collagen within and around muscles results in reduced ROM. With age, collagen fibers also change such that there are more cross-links between fibers, making the collagen less extensible or more resistant to deformation (Cetta, Tenni, Zanaboni, & Maroudas, 1982). Connective tissues also contain a gelatinous material called matrix, which holds water and gives connective tissue its resilience. The collagen-associated matrix within all connective tissues also undergoes a change in chemical composition such that the material responsible for holding water (chondroitin sulfate) is lost with age. The loss of water

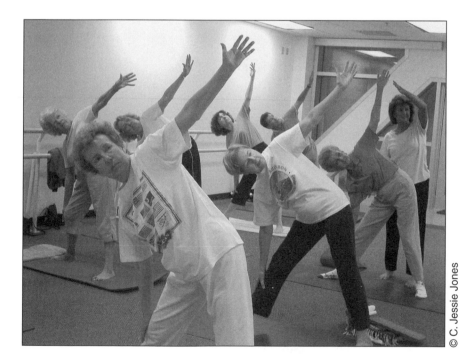

© C. Jessie Jones

Activities such as yoga can help to reduce the decline in joint mobility with age.

also contributes to making connective tissues less extensible and more resistant to being deformed (Buckwalter et al., 1993). These changes in connective tissue undoubtedly make it more difficult to move freely in old age.

A loss of muscle strength occurs concomitantly with the increase in stiffness. As a result, older adults have to use more muscle power to overcome their own inertia. For example, functional activities such as getting out of bed in the morning, getting dressed, bathing, and rising from low chairs become increasingly difficult with age. Because it is more challenging and, in some cases, painful to move, many older adults begin to operate within a smaller range of motion, thereby using less and less joint flexibility. As a result of this disuse, the joint becomes less capable of reaching what is considered to be a normal end range of motion. In fact, it is not uncommon to find a number of community-dwelling men and women who cannot perform essential daily activities, such as turning their heads far enough to see what is behind them as they back up a car, putting on clothes requiring an overhead motion, or rising from a low chair, because their range of motion is inadequate.

Although an age-related change in flexibility is inevitable, the magnitude of the decline is highly modifiable. Physical inactivity plays a particularly important role in the loss of flexibility with age and probably contributes more to the reduction in movement potential than normal age-related changes and pathological processes. Consequently, an important component of any well-rounded physical activity program for older adults should include flexibility training.

Flexibility and Function

The consequences of reduced flexibility are numerous. Activities of daily living most affected include those that require reaching overhead, getting into and out of a car (especially one with bucket seats), reaching into low cabinets, bending down to pick up an object from the floor, and stepping onto or down from a high step or curb. Other functional consequences of a limited range of motion include the inability to put on an article of clothing with zippers or fasteners in the back (e.g., a dress or bra) due to limited shoulder internal rotation. A reduction in shoulder elevation can restrict the ability

to put on sweatshirts, T-shirts, or any other item of clothing that requires more shoulder elevation than an older adult is capable of. Inadequate knee flexion coupled with limited trunk flexibility can make it more difficult, if not impossible, for older adults to put on shoes and socks.

As the number of functional limitations due to reduced flexibility increases, an older adult's functional independence becomes more and more compromised. Not as readily apparent are the consequences of limited flexibility for balance and strength. Both of these important domains are influenced by joint excursion. In addition, men and women with limited flexibility are more likely to sustain a muscle injury.

The association between muscle strength and flexibility in older adults has not been well defined. It is apparent, however, that when older adults gain flexibility, they typically experience an increase in strength also (Brown & Holloszy, 1991; Brown, Sinacore, Ehsani, Binder, & Holloszy, 2000). Perhaps the effort expended to gain range of motion is sufficient to challenge the surrounding musculature, thereby increasing muscle strength. Alternatively, increasing a joint's range of motion may release the muscles to such an extent that they can be used more readily. Regardless of the mechanism of change, improving your clients' flexibility will enable them to use skeletal muscle more efficiently.

For a variety of reasons, older adults are more susceptible to muscle injury than younger adults. Although direct evidence is lacking, one likely major factor is limited joint and muscle excursion (Lindsay, Horton, & Vandervoort, 2000; Ploutz-Snyder, Giamis, Formikell, & Rosenbaum, 2001). Ample evidence in the literature indicates that the muscles of young men and women with limited ranges of motion are more prone to injury than muscles of individuals who have normal ranges (McHugh et al., 1999; Noonan & Garrett, 1999). Hence, savvy athletes always warm up before athletic events to improve flexibility and decrease risk of injury. It should be noted that old muscle may not recover

> When older adults gain flexibility, they typically experience an increase in muscle strength.

from injury as quickly as young muscle (Brooks & Faulkner, 1996), although discussion of this topic is well beyond the scope of this chapter. It is consequently important for older adults to maintain full range of motion not just to prevent injury but to keep from losing strength or aerobic capacity unnecessarily if an injury should occur.

In addition to the functional benefits associated with improved flexibility, your clients will also feel better as a result of increasing their joint ROM. Improved flexibility can have a beneficial effect on posture that, in turn, can reduce pain, improve balance, heighten sense of well-being, and enhance self-efficacy. Improved spinal flexibility and the ability to stand more erectly also reduce breathlessness, as there is more room for chest expansion.

Critical Ranges of Flexibility

To date, few **critical ranges** (absolute minimum range of joint motion required to perform a certain activity) for flexibility have been published for daily activities. Ranges that have been reported for tasks such as walking, climbing stairs, getting onto and off a toilet, and getting dressed are presented in table 11.1. Critical ranges are important

to keep in mind when designing exercise programs to improve function. It is important as well to remember that some conditions do not permit reestablishing critical ranges. For example, older adults with total hip replacements are typically unable to bend the hip farther than 90 degrees. Knee joint replacements or prostheses rarely bend beyond 110 degrees.

The Benefits of Exercise and Flexibility Training

There is now sufficient evidence that older adults with range-of-motion deficits are very capable of improving their flexibility. It does not seem to matter what mode of exercise is used, as improvements in range of motion have been noted following traditional ROM exercises, dance, tai chi, and aquatic exercise (Raab, Agre, McAdam, & Smith, 1988; Brown et al., 2000; Munns, 1981; Frekany & Leslie, 1975; Misner, Massey, Bemben, Going, & Patrick, 1992). What matters most is stressing the **end range** of joint motion (i.e., the maximal distance a joint can be moved until a point of discomfort) using an activity that is fun and safe and feels good.

TABLE 11.1   Critical Ranges of Flexibility

Activity	Shoulder joint	Hip joint	Knee joint	Ankle joint
Putting on clothing overhead	90° elevation (including flexion, abduction) 45° external rotation			
Fastening or unfastening clothing in back	45° abduction, 70° internal rotation, 10° extension			
Walking at 3 mph (4.8 km/h)		30° flexion 10° extension	70° flexion	10° dorsiflexion
Ascending stairs		70° flexion	90° flexion	10° dorsiflexion
Getting on and off toilet		110° flexion	115° flexion	10° dorsiflexion
Getting down onto and up from floor, in and out of tub		120° flexion	135° flexion	10° dorsiflexion

Types of Stretching Techniques

Many different types of stretching techniques can be beneficial if applied correctly and at the right time during an exercise session. These different techniques can be divided into two main categories: **static** and **dynamic stretching.** Static stretching generally focuses on a particular muscle group and involves moving the joint through a single movement plane until a given end point is reached. The joint is then held in that position for a period of time (anywhere from 10 to 90 seconds). Static stretches are very safe to perform and present little likelihood of injury if performed correctly. In contrast, dynamic stretching moves a joint through a given range of motion but does not hold the joint in an end position for any period of time. Instead, the goal of this stretching technique is to progressively increase joint ROM with each subsequent movement repetition.

A certain joint or muscle group might be targeted for stretching through a single plane of motion (single-joint dynamic stretching), or multiple joints and muscles might be recruited and then moved through a single or multiple movement planes in task-specific patterns (multijoint dynamic stretching). This latter stretching technique constitutes a very functional approach to flexibility training and is beneficial for the performance of daily activities, which are usually dynamic and often require movement in multiple planes (e.g., reaching into the dishwasher to retrieve objects and then placing them on the counter, reaching into the back of a cupboard, cleaning windows, planting flowers). This approach to flexibility training nicely complements the functional resistance training described in chapter 12.

Well-controlled research studies have yet to be conducted to determine which type of flexibility training is most beneficial for older adults and when it should be done in an exercise class. However, there is general consensus among the experts that dynamic stretching is the more appropriate technique to use early in a class to facilitate warming up the body and muscles, while static stretching should be reserved until the body is at its warmest, when muscles and joints are most receptive to being stretched (Wolf, 2002). This might be at the end of

> It is recommended that dynamic stretches be performed early in the class to facilitate warming up the body and muscles and that static stretches be reserved for a later time when the body is at its warmest and the muscles and joints are more receptive to being stretched.

an extended warm-up, immediately following the aerobics section of the class and before resistance training, or during the cool-down.

Incorporating Flexibility Training Into the Exercise Program

Flexibility training can be incorporated into your physical activity program in many different ways. The warm-up provides a nice opportunity for dynamic stretching techniques, while a section of the cool-down can include static stretching techniques. A stand-alone flexibility component within your program is also an option. In addition to the more traditional flexibility exercises described in this chapter, there are other ways for your older adult clients to improve joint range of motion, such as certain types of dance, tai chi, Pilates, yoga, the Alexander technique, and the Feldenkrais Method. For more information about some of these techniques, please refer to chapter 15.

The Warm-Up

As indicated in the previous section, the best type of flexibility exercise to use in the early stages of the warm-up is dynamic. Dynamic stretching can often be achieved just by moving the limbs through a progressively larger ROM as the warm-up progresses. When the muscles are warmer (after approximately 10 to 20 minutes), you can perform specific dynamic stretches that involve the muscle groups that will be used in the movements planned for the next section of the class. Examples of single-joint and multijoint dynamic stretches that involve both the upper and lower body are presented in figure 11.1.

Seated activities	Standing activities
Floor reach: Sit on the edge of a straight-backed chair with no armrests or a chair with no backrest. Keep back upright. Arms are outstretched to 90°. Knees should be together and bent about 90°. Bend forward toward floor, reaching as far as possible toward the floor or touching the floor if ROM permits.	Reach and curl: From a standing position, reach arms overhead with palms facing up to ceiling; then tuck chin onto chest and curl down into a crouched position, hands touching floor. Repeat in a controlled manner slowly and continuously five times.
Seated trunk rotation: Sit on the edge of a chair with hands in front of the body holding an imaginary steering wheel. Slowly rotate trunk and head to the right until you can see an imaginary car in the right lane. Repeat rotation to the left side.	Picking apples: Reach up with single arm to pick imaginary fruit, and return to imaginary bag at hip level. Encourage clients to rise up onto balls of feet if their balance is good. Reach in a new direction with each repetition (e.g., same side of body, across body). Repeat with opposite limb after five repetitions.
Seated abduction: Sit on the edge of a chair with hands holding onto chair. Alternate abducting and adducting a single leg, increasing the range of motion on each repetition. Perform the same movement with both legs simultaneously to increase the challenge.	Climbing rope: Clients climb an imaginary rope. Emphasize good upward stretch with arms and trunk. Opposite leg lifts with each arm raise. Repeat five times. Encourage a larger ROM with each repetition.
	Knees up, Mother Brown: Exaggerated march in place. Arms and legs move in opposition. One arm is raised to 90° of flexion, while the opposite leg is brought up into as much hip, knee, and ankle flexion as possible.
Alternate knee to chest: Sit on the edge of a chair. Bring one knee up toward the chest. Grasp the knee and encircle it with both hands. Using both hands, bring the knee gently up toward the chest, touching the chest if possible. Repeat with opposite knee.	Side lunges with (a) spinal flexion, (b) arm reach across body, and (c) forward arm reach. Alternate movements on each subsequent repetition.
	Walking, with six to seven alternating bouts of long and short strides. Opposite arm should be raised with exaggerated, wooden-soldier-like movement. To make this activity more challenging, have clients walk with slightly flexed knees. Incorporate activities that simulate those to be performed later in class.

FIGURE 11.1 Single- and multijoint dynamic stretches for the warm-up.

The Cool-Down

In contrast to the warm-up, static flexibility exercises are preferred during the cool-down. At this point in the class your clients have thoroughly exercised their muscles and elevated their internal body temperature, so stretches that require longer holds will be more effective and safer to perform. You can use the time while clients hold a longer stretch to review aspects of the class, solicit feedback from your clients, and encourage them to do flexibility exercises even on the days they do not attend class.

General Precautions

Like any other program component, the flexibility exercises you select must be appropriate for your clients and performed correctly. Special precautions should be followed when selecting flexibility exercises for clients with certain medical conditions (e.g., osteoporosis, rheumatoid and osteoarthritis; refer to chapter 21). Because static and dynamic stretching techniques can improve flexibility, both can be employed in an exercise prescription. For example, a single static stretch is more comfortable than multiple repetitions of a dynamic stretch for a person who has significant joint disease and pain, at least in the early stages of an exercise program. On the other hand, for someone with poor body awareness, repeating limb movements multiple times seems to be helpful.

It is important that you encourage your older adult clients to move at their own pace to avoid injury. If any of the flexibility exercises presented in this chapter cause the client pain, an alternative exercise should be selected that stretches the target muscle or joint without discomfort. A client who has poor balance should perform exercises in a seated position or with the additional support of a chair or wall.

Flexibility Exercise Guidelines

Here is an appropriate set of guidelines for flexibility exercises:

- Select flexibility exercises on the basis of which joints have obvious range limitations and which muscles are stiff.
- Emphasize good body alignment.
- Perform dynamic stretches during the warm-up to facilitate warming up the body and muscles.
- Do not perform static stretches until the body is at its warmest and muscles and joints are receptive to stretch.
- Move slowly into a static stretch position.
- Stretch to a point of gentle tension, but not pain.
- Do not jerk, bounce, or force a stretch, because this could result in injury.
- Hold a static stretch for 10 to 90 seconds.
- Inhale before the start of the stretch, exhale during the stretch, and breathe evenly while holding the stretch at its end position.

Examples of Flexibility Exercises

Many of the flexibility exercises described in this section can be performed in a variety of different positions (e.g., sitting in a chair or on the floor, lying prone or supine, standing, kneeling with hands on the floor). You should choose flexibility exercises on the basis of information from preactivity screening and performance assessments. Each exercise has a simple name to facilitate recollection of the exercise. Your older adult clients can learn what exercise to perform by name. In addition, the muscle group or groups that are targeted by the exercise are identified.

It is important to emphasize appropriate breathing techniques as well as correct form. As a general rule, clients should inhale just before each stretch, exhale during the stretch, and breathe evenly while holding the end position in the case of static stretches. A focus on breathing during flexibility training is particularly important in light of older adults' tendency to hold their breath when exercising. Remember that flexibility exercises should be selected on the basis of which muscle groups are to be targeted later in the class. The selected flexibility exercises can also be performed one after the other with no need to rest after each exercise. Occasional rest periods may be incorporated if a client is debilitated, but there should be very little need for recovery. Above all, activities should be challenging, efficacious, and enjoyable. There is no pain for gain in this approach.

The following exercises are presented in top-to-bottom order: upper body, trunk, and lower body. You should present flexibility exercises systematically, starting with upper-body stretches, then trunk stretches, and finally lower-body stretches. The recommended readings at the end of the chapter offer additional flexibility exercises.

UPPER-BODY FLEXIBILITY EXERCISES

Exercises to improve older adults' upper-body flexibility are provided in this section, including exercises that can be done while seated or while standing. The dynamic flexibility exercises can be done in the warm-up, while the static stretches can be done during the cool-down. A stand-alone flexibility-training component can also be added to any exercise session.

Seated or Standing Position

Neck stretch

Target muscles: side of neck, upper back

Gently turn the head to the left and right, attempting to increase the range with each repetition. Encourage clients to perform each head turn slowly and to focus on a visual target at eye level to reduce the possibility of dizziness. Increase the time each turn is held if the client reports any dizziness or discomfort in the neck.

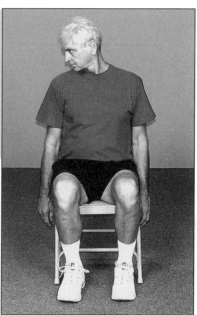
© Human Kinetics

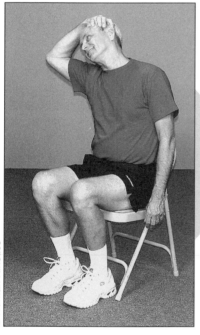
© Human Kinetics

Assisted side neck stretch

Target muscles: side of neck

Slowly bend the head to one side (ear toward the shoulder). At the same time, gently place the hand on the opposite side of the head so that the weight of the hand increases the stretch. Repeat to the other side.

Backward arm stretch

Target muscles: shoulder adductors, internal rotators

Raise the arms out to the sides of the body with the palms facing forward. Slowly move the extended arms directly backward as far as possible. Tell your clients to sit or stand tall with the ears directly above the shoulders and the eyes focused on a visual target at eye level.

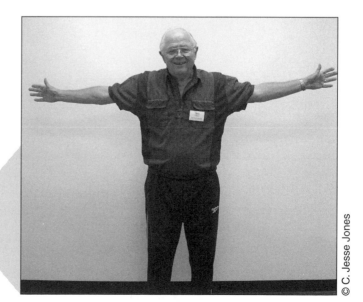
© C. Jesse Jones

Alternating arm swings

Target muscles: all scapular and shoulder muscles
Place the hands on the shoulders. Circle both arms in a wide arc, first backward and then forward.

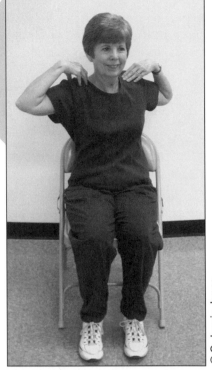

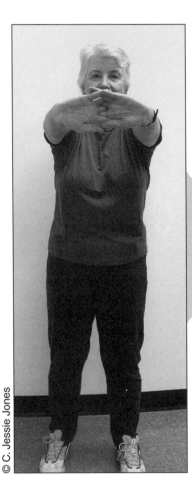

Upper-back stretch

Target muscles: upper back and shoulders

Sit upright in a chair or stand erect, and raise the arms forward to shoulder level. Clasp the hands together and turn the palms away from the body; tuck chin to the chest. Push the hands away from the body until a stretch is felt across the muscles of the upper back.

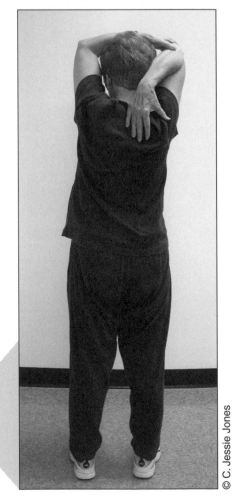

Triceps stretch

Target muscles: back of the upper arms, chest, and shoulders

Sit tall against the back of a chair or stand erect with relaxed shoulders and arms loosely hanging by the sides of the body. Position one hand behind the head with the upper arm close to the ear and the elbow pointed to the ceiling. Reach with the fingers of the bent arm down toward the middle of the back while gently pushing the upper arm back and down with the opposite hand. Keep the back straight during the stretch and the stomach and chin tucked in.

Side stretch

Target muscles: side of trunk and shoulders, also the outer thighs and hips when performed in a standing position

Sit tall against the back of a chair or stand erect. Gently lean the trunk to one side as the opposite arm reaches up above and then across the head to form an arc. Hold the position for 5 to 15 seconds, and then gently return to the starting position. Repeat on the opposite side.

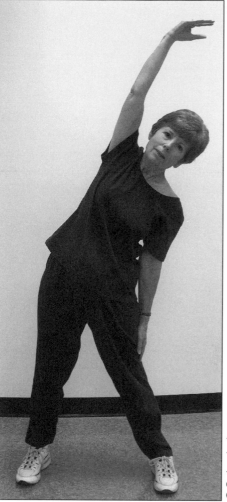

© C. Jessie Jones

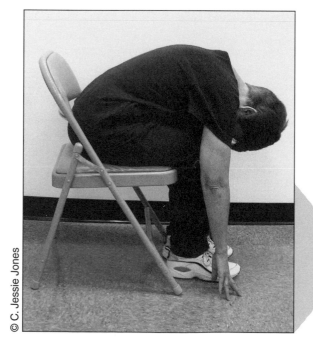

© C. Jessie Jones

Roll-down

Target muscles: lower back

Sit upright in a chair or stand with the feet hip-width apart. Slowly roll the upper body down toward the floor with the arms hanging loosely. Gently roll back up to the starting position.

Standing Position

Chest stretch

Target muscles: pectorals

Stand facing a corner or open doorway with one foot in front of the other. Raise the elbows to shoulder level and place the palms against the wall or door jam. Lean the body forward until the stretch is felt across the upper chest muscles.

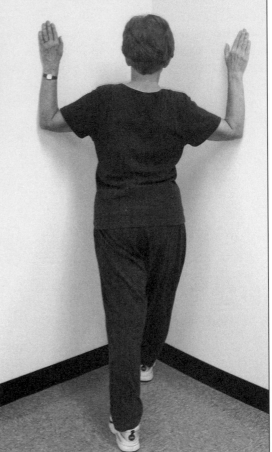

© C. Jessie Jones

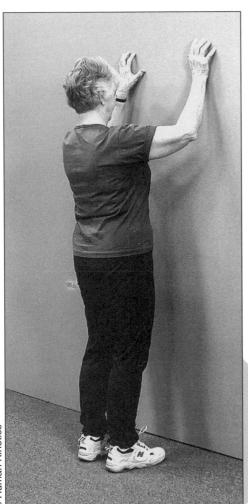

© Human Kinetics

Front wall crawl

Target muscles: scapular retractors and rotators, shoulder adductors and internal rotators

Stand facing a wall, approximately six inches (15 centimeters) away from the wall. Place both hands on the wall directly in front of the body. "Crawl" the fingers up the wall, bringing the arms up as high as possible with each repetition.

Side wall crawl

Target muscles: shoulders, oblique muscles of trunk

Stand with your side to the wall, feet approximately two feet (0.6 meter) away. Stand tall with the stomach tucked in, chest up, chin back, eyes directed forward. Walk the fingertips up the wall until a comfortable stretch is felt in the shoulder and along the side of the body. Move closer to the wall as the fingers move upward. Walk the fingers slowly back down to the starting position. Repeat on the opposite side.

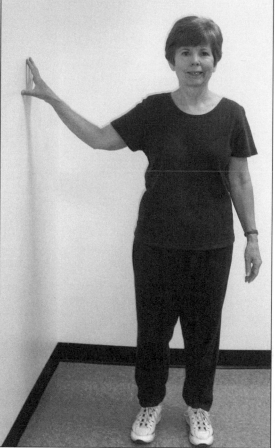

© C. Jessie Jones

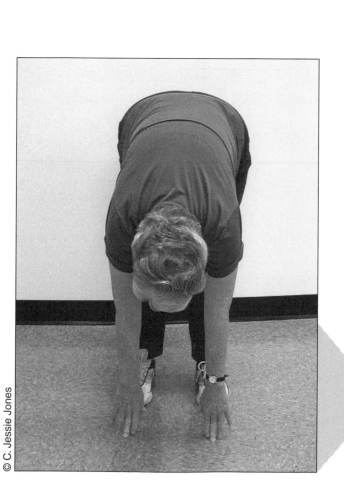

© C. Jessie Jones

Reach and curl

Target muscles: trunk extensors, flexors, shoulder adductors

Reach toward the ceiling with both arms, with back completely straight. Then tuck the chin to the chest and curl the body down into a ball with the hands touching the floor.

LOWER-BODY FLEXIBILITY EXERCISES

Many of the lower-body flexibility exercises described in this section can be performed in multiple positions for greater variety. Most of these activities can also be modified to make them easier or more complex and demanding, thus expanding the basic repertoire.

Lying or Kneeling Position

Side leg raises

Target muscles: hip adductors

Lie on your side on a mat, and place the palm of the uppermost hand on the floor at chest level to stabilize the body. Extend the lower arm above the head. Abduct the top leg up into the air, raising it higher and higher with each repetition. Point the toes away from the body as the leg is lifted.

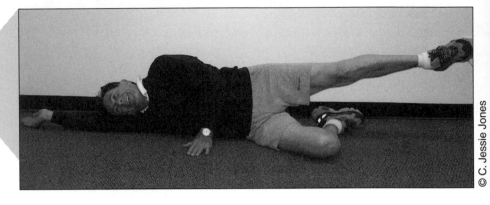

© C. Jessie Jones

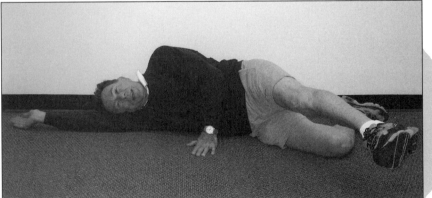

© C. Jessie Jones

Forward and backward kicks

Target muscles: hip flexors and extensors

Lie on your side on a mat, and place the palm of the uppermost hand on the floor at chest level to stabilize the body. Flex the ankle and slowly move the top leg as far forward as possible while maintaining a side-lying position. Point the toes and return the extended leg back to the starting position. Now move the top leg gently back behind the body while maintaining a side-lying position. Return the leg to the starting position. Roll onto the other side, and repeat with the opposite leg.

Hip rolls

Target muscles: gluteals, hips, trunk

Lie supine on the floor with the arms extended to each side and the knees flexed. Slowly lower both legs to the floor on the same side of the body while keeping the elbows, shoulders, and head flat against the floor. Return the legs to the starting position. Repeat to the opposite side.

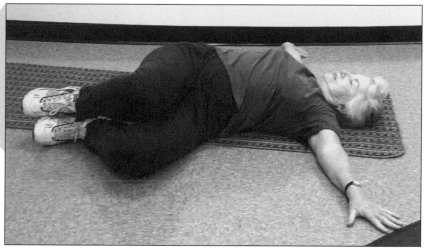

© C. Jessie Jones

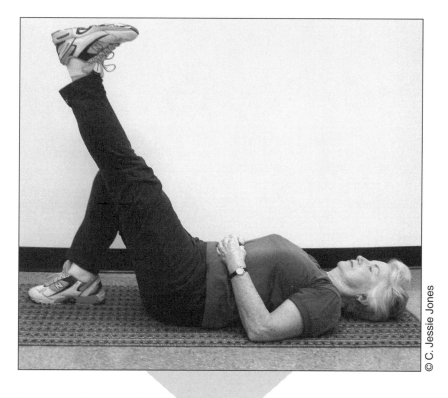

© C. Jessie Jones

Hamstring stretch, extended leg

Target muscles: buttocks, back of the upper thighs, calves

Lie on the back with knees bent and feet flat on the floor. The abdominal muscles should be contracted, and the lower back in contact with the floor. The neck is extended and the chin tucked in. The hands are placed on the lower abdomen. Lift and extend one leg up to the level of the opposite knee. Hold the leg in an extended position, flex the ankle, and point the toes toward the ceiling. Continue raising the extended leg, feeling the stretch in the back of the leg. Return the leg to the starting position, and repeat with the opposite leg. Note: This exercise can also be performed with a rolled towel looped under the foot of the extended leg to help guide it through the stretch if the hamstring muscles are tight.

Cat and camel

Target muscles: trunk flexors and extensors, hip flexors and extensors

Start in a kneeling position with the hands on the floor and directly below the shoulder. Knees are directly under the hips and the eyes are looking at the floor. Lower the stomach, arch the back, lift the head, and look forward, keeping both hands and knees in contact with the ground. Then reverse the movement: Round the back, and lower the head until it is between the arms. A floor mat under the knees increases comfort.

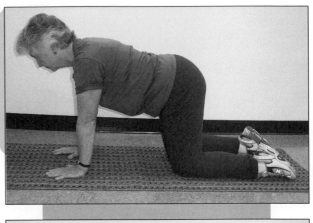

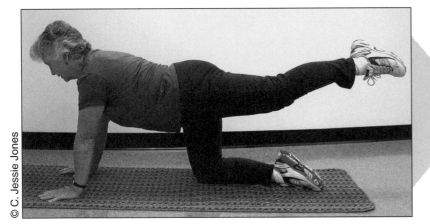

Alternating leg raises

Target muscles: hip flexors, trunk flexors

Kneel with the knees directly under the hips and the hands on the floor directly beneath the shoulders. Keep the head and eyes directed forward. Raise one leg off the ground; extend it and lift it toward the ceiling. Repeat with the opposite leg.

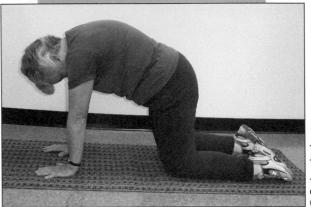

Spine stretch

Target muscles: upper and lower back, front of the ankles, lower legs

Kneel on all fours as in the previous exercise. Moving the buttocks backward, sink down so that the forehead touches the floor. Keep the hands on the floor with arms extended. Concentrate on lengthening the spine during the stretch. Return to the starting position.

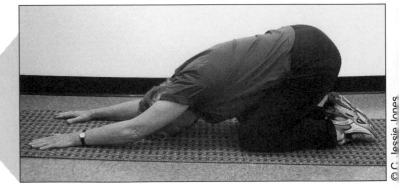

Seated Position

Sit-and-reach

Target muscles: hamstrings, hip flexors, ankle dorsiflexors

Place a chair against the wall. Sit at the edge of the chair with one leg extended and the toes of that foot pointed toward the ceiling. Place both hands on the hips. Slowly lean forward at the hips while keeping the trunk extended. The eyes are directed forward. A more advanced version of the sit-and-reach can be performed while seated on the floor with the legs extended.

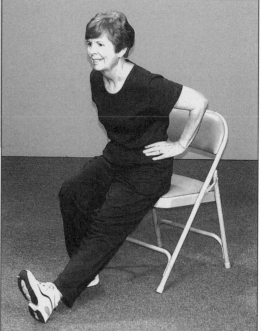

© Human Kinetics

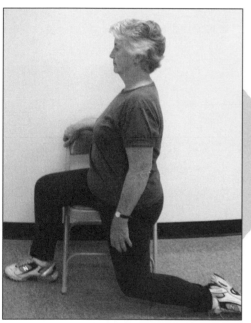

© C. Jessie Jones

Hip extensions

Target muscles: front of thigh and hips

Sit sideways on a chair close to the front edge. Hold onto the back of the chair with the closest hand for added support. Flex the knee of the opposite leg until it is pointing down to the floor and reach back with the foot while maintaining an upright posture.

Ankle circles

Target muscles: ankle and foot

Sit at the edge of a chair. Raise one leg off the floor and circle the foot at the ankle, first clockwise and then counterclockwise. Repeat with the other foot. This exercise can also be performed in a standing position, with or without support. Performing this exercise while standing unsupported adds a balance challenge.

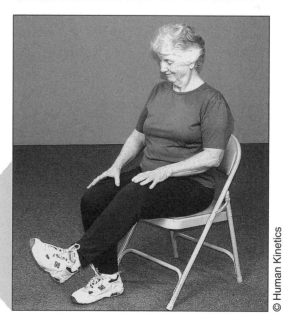

© Human Kinetics

Standing Position

Quad stretch

Target muscles: front of thigh

Stand upright with one hand against a supporting surface for balance. Flex one knee and raise the heel toward the buttocks. Slightly bend the knee of the stance leg. Reach behind and grasp the foot of the raised leg with one hand. Pull the heel gently toward the buttocks while keeping the thigh of the raised leg close to the stance leg. Relax and lower the leg to the floor. Repeat with the opposite leg.

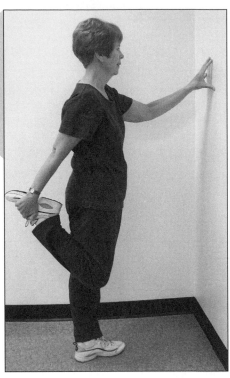

© C. Jessie Jones

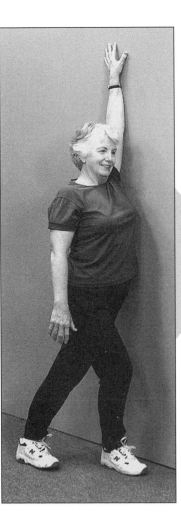

© Human Kinetics

Side wall stretch

Target muscles: hip abductors, oblique muscles of trunk

Stand upright close to a wall. Raise the arm closest to the wall above the head and rest it against the wall. Position the foot closest to the wall behind the ankle of the opposite leg. Slowly lean into the wall until a stretch can be felt along the outside of the thigh closest to the wall. Relax, and repeat on the opposite side.

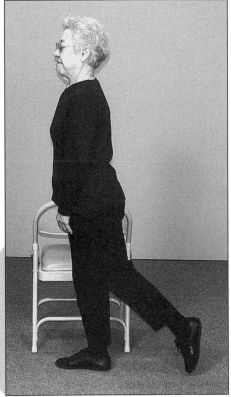

© Human Kinetics

Backward leg extension

Target muscles: hip and trunk flexors

With one hand on a wall or chair for support, extend one leg backward and away from the body while maintaining an upright trunk. Repeat with the opposite leg.

Summary

This chapter provided an overview of the age-associated changes in the joints and muscles that contribute to reduced flexibility. The critical ranges of joint motion needed for the successful performance of daily activities were identified. The functional consequences of reduced flexibility and the functional and psychological benefits of regular flexibility training were summarized. Age-associated changes in the joints and muscles that contribute to reduced flexibility include an increase in connective tissue, changes in connective tissue matrix and collagen, and breakdown of articular cartilage.

Two types of stretching techniques were then described. The first of these techniques, static stretching, involves moving the joint through a single movement plane and then holding it at an end position for a period of time. The other technique, dynamic stretching, involves moving the joint through single or multiple planes of motion without holding the end position for any length of time. Dynamic stretching techniques should be introduced during the warm-up section of the class, while static stretches should be used later (e.g., after the aerobics component or during the cool-down) when the body is at its warmest and the muscles and joints are more receptive to being stretched.

In the final section of the chapter, a number of upper- and lower-body flexibility exercises were described. These can be performed in a variety of different positions (e.g., seated in a chair or on the floor, standing, kneeling on all fours) and can be modified to accommodate different functional abilities and medical conditions that may limit available range of motion (e.g., osteoarthritis, joint replacement, chronic pain). Experiencing improved flexibility and understanding how flexibility can positively affect the performance of daily, recreational, and sporting activities can motivate older adults to make flexibility training a part of their daily routine.

Key Terms

Recommended Readings

Alter, M. (2004). *The science of flexibility* (3rd ed.). Champaign, IL: Human Kinetics.

Moffat, M., & Vickery, S. (1999). *The American Physical Therapy Association book of body maintenance and repair.* New York: Holt.

Robinson, L., Fisher, H., & Knox, J. (2001). *The official body control Pilates manual.* New York: Barnes and Noble Books.

Study Questions

1. The end range of motion refers to
   a. the minimum range of joint motion required to perform a certain activity
   b. the maximum distance a joint can be moved without any discomfort
   c. the maximum distance a joint can be moved in multiple planes of motion
   d. the maximum distance a joint can be moved to a point of discomfort

2. The greatest decline in range of motion with age is observed in
   a. hip extension
   b. spinal extension
   c. ankle dorsiflexion
   d. hip abduction

(continued)

3. Older adults with hip joint replacements are typically unable to bend the hip
   a. more than 110 degrees
   b. more than 70 degrees
   c. farther than 90 degrees
   d. beyond 60 degrees

4. The primary difference between static and dynamic stretching is that
   a. once the joint is moved to a given end point, the position is held without additional movement for a period of time during a static stretch
   b. the end position is held for a shorter period of time during dynamic stretching
   c. the joint is not moved at all during a static stretch
   d. static stretching is the more functionally relevant stretching technique

5. At what point should static stretching techniques be used in an exercise session?
   a. as soon as the class begins
   b. during the cool-down portion of the class only
   c. once the body and muscles are sufficiently warm
   d. at any point during an exercise session

6. Which of the following flexibility exercises would be best suited to improving the flexibility of the muscles in the lower back?
   a. seated upper-back stretch
   b. backward arm stretches
   c. seated roll-down
   d. sit-and-reach test

7. Which of the following flexibility exercises is most appropriate for an older adult who can no longer fasten a dress with a zipper in the back?
   a. alternating arm swings in a seated position
   b. seated upper-back stretch
   c. alternating arm swings in a standing position
   d. front wall crawl

Application Activities

1. Your client is a fairly typical community-dwelling 78-year-old woman who reports having some difficulty with bending and stooping. She cannot roll onto her stomach or get up from and down onto the floor. She cannot get her hands behind her back to fasten a bra or pull up a zipper. This woman also has difficulty getting up from low furniture. She has come to you for an activity program to make her feel better and enable her to perform basic activities of daily living more easily. Identify six flexibility exercises for this client to perform regularly.

2. Design a warm-up that includes a number of flexibility exercises to prepare a class of older adults to engage in (a) upper-body strength exercises or (b) step aerobics later in the class.

12

Resistance Training

William J. Kraemer
Duncan N. French

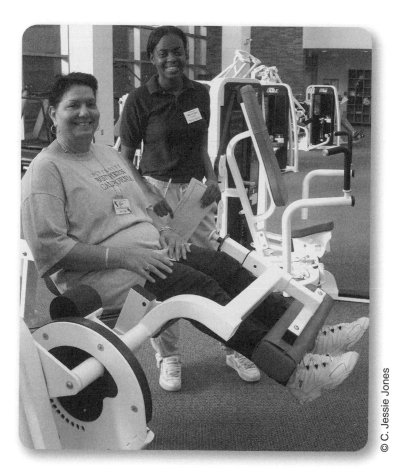

Advancing age is associated with a number of physiological changes that can be detrimental to both health and functional capacity. As a consequence of aging, individuals experience a well-documented loss of bone, muscle, and physical function that not only makes the activities of daily living (e.g., getting out of a chair, sweeping the floor, opening the window) more difficult but can also lead to injury and long-term disability (Baechle & Earle, 2000). The physiological consequences of aging are discussed in chapter 4, and an understanding of these changes is fundamental for developing strategies to counteract the physical decline associated with advancing age.

Today, **resistance training** is recognized for its significant impact on the quality of life and physical function of individuals of all ages, including older adults. Resistance training is an exercise intervention that can reverse much of the loss of muscle function and deterioration of muscle structure associated with aging and can improve physical health (Kraemer, Ratamess, & French, 2002). Through safe and correctly prescribed resistance training, older adults experience a variety of health and lifestyle benefits that include longevity and the maintenance of long-term independence (Evans, 1996; Feigenbaum & Pollock, 1999; Kelley & Kelley, 2000). The purpose of this chapter is to describe the health-related, physical fitness, and performance-related benefits of resistance training; how the exercise principles introduced in chapter 9 are applied to the resistance-training component of

a program; and how each of the acute resistance-training variables or training components can be manipulated in various ways to achieve successful training outcomes.

Benefits of Resistance Training

Traditionally, athletes seeking to improve strength, muscular hypertrophy, power, and sport-specific fitness have used resistance training. Today, because the benefits of resistance training are better understood, it is now looked upon as one of the most effective and least costly ways to preserve independent living and improve health in the aging population (Rogers & Evans, 1993). The following sections discuss the health- and performance-related benefits of resistance training.

Health-Related Benefits

The potential health-related benefits of resistance training have recently been elucidated, and resistance training is now recommended by national health organizations—including the American College of Sports Medicine (ACSM), American Heart Association, and the American Association for Cardiovascular and Pulmonary Rehabilitation—in conjunction with other exercise modalities (e.g., aerobic, flexibility, and balance exercise) for the maintenance and improvement of health and performance (Kraemer, Adams, et al., 2002). In a comprehensive health and fitness program, resistance training can reduce risk factors associated with many diseases and physical ailments and can preserve and improve functional capacity. Such benefits have been shown to improve the quality of life for a wide range of older adults and adults with health conditions, including those with low back pain, osteoarthritis, cardiovascular disease, neuromuscular disease, renal failure, and type 2 diabetes and those recovering from a stroke (Clyman, 2001; Hurley & Roth, 2000; Kraemer, Ratamess, and French 2002; Pollock et al., 2000). Regular resistance exercise results in a remarkable number of positive health changes in both elderly men and women. A number of these health benefits are described in table 12.1.

Physical Fitness and Performance-Related Benefits

As people become older, declines in strength, power, and muscular endurance decrease functional capacity and reduce quality of life (Gersten, 1991). A substantial proportion of this reduction is not a direct result of the aging process but rather a consequence of the sedentary lifestyle frequently associated with aging. Not only can resistance train-

ing improve many health-related components of physical fitness, it can also have significant effects on performance-related fitness, including speed, strength, agility, flexibility, power, balance, and muscular endurance. Such motor performance skills are required for a variety of recreational (e.g., walking, bowling, hiking, biking, gardening) and sport activities (e.g., softball, tennis, basketball, racquetball).

Numerous studies have demonstrated large increases in maximal loads lifted and an accompanying enlargement of whole-muscle and muscle fiber area in older adults after resistance training (Charette et al., 1991; Häkkinen et al., 1998; Sipila, Elorinne, Alen, Suominen, & Kovanen, 1997). From such studies it has been determined that high-intensity resistance training can induce large increases in muscle strength in frail men and women up to 96 years of age (Fiatarone et al., 1990). Gains in strength of between 32 and 227 percent have been reported following eight or more weeks of training; older adults respond to weight training in a manner relatively similar to younger adults.

The expression of muscular force is perhaps the most important aspect of both sport performance and an active lifestyle. All sporting and recreational activities involve some degree of power development (e.g., hitting, striking, carrying, kicking,

TABLE 12.1 Wellness and Health Benefits of Resistance Exercise

Physical characteristic	Benefit
Body composition	Increased lean tissue mass, metabolic rate, and daily energy expenditure result in body fat reductions of up to 9%.
Blood pressure	Small reductions in resting systolic and diastolic blood pressure reduce the risk of stroke and coronary heart disease.
Bone mass	The weight-bearing activity in resistance training improves bone health and reduces the risk of osteoporosis.
Glucose tolerance	Favorable changes in glucose tolerance and insulin resistance are observed after physical activity, including resistance training.
Lower-back pain	Increased strength and cross-sectional area of the vertebral muscles reduce lower-back pain by maintaining muscle balance.
Blood lipids	Resistance training has beneficial effects on blood lipid profiles, including lower total cholesterol and triglyceride concentrations.

cycling, throwing, lifting, running, jumping). In older men and women, walking speed relates positively with calf strength, hours spent in active leisure, height, and weight and negatively to age and the presence of health problems (Bassey et al., 1992; Bendall, Bassey, & Pearson, 1989). The increases in muscular strength, power, endurance, and hypertrophy (enlargement of muscle fibers) that accompany resistance training can therefore improve motor skills. For older adults who participate in regular sporting and recreational activities, resistance training is a means to improve many aspects of performance and thereby raise playing standards. Maintaining adequate levels of muscular strength, endurance, and power is also important for reducing older adults' risk of falls during the performance of their daily activities.

Principles of Resistance Training

The terms *strength training, weight training,* and *resistance training* all describe a type of exercise that requires the body's musculature to move (or attempt to move) against an opposing force or resistance (Fleck & Kraemer, 2004). Resistance exercises come in diverse forms; however, to maximize the benefits of resistance training, any form of resistance training must apply three basic principles: (1) overload, (2) variation, and (3) specificity.

Overload

Fundamental to all resistance training is the principle of **overload.** The overload principle states that for strength, muscular endurance, and power to improve, the demands placed on the muscles must increase over time to stress them beyond their accustomed loads. The adaptive processes of the human body respond only if continually called upon to exert a greater force to meet higher physiological demands (Kraemer, Adams, et al., 2002). The capacity of the muscle cells to exert force increases and decreases relative to the demands placed on the muscular system. When the demands on muscle decrease, as is the case with the sedentary lifestyle that often accompanies old age, the cells decrease in size (atrophy), and the muscles lose strength or the ability to exert mechanical force. However, if the muscle cells are overloaded beyond

normal daily use, as can occur in resistance-training programs, the cells increase in size (hypertrophy), which in turn increases strength, endurance, and muscular power.

Variation and Periodization

The systematic alteration of progressive overload over time creates **variation** in the physiological stresses placed on the body and optimizes the training stimulus. Variation in training volume and intensity is extremely important for optimal gains in strength, power, and endurance. A popular term for changing program variables is **periodization** (Fleck & Kraemer, 2004; Kraemer & Ratamess, 2000). Periodization is the planned cycling of training variables, including volume (number of sets) and intensity, to minimize the risk of injury and other symptoms of overtraining. For older individuals, precautionary measures to avoid overexertion and inappropriate stress should be taken. In the periodization of training for older adults, exercise intensity generally begins low and gradually increases, while volume starts high and slowly decreases as the individual becomes more accustomed to the exertions of exercise. These training variables can then be manipulated in future training sessions to constantly modify the training stimulus and promote optimal gains.

Specificity

Specificity refers to the body's responses and subsequent adaptations to particular program variables. The principle of specificity dictates that the nature of the adaptations observed with a resistance training program will be specific to the characteristics of load, velocity, movements, muscles exercised, and metabolic demands created by the exercise protocol (Kraemer & Ratamess, 2000). Several resistance exercise variables (e.g., load, volume, frequency, and rest periods) can be manipulated to alter the stimulus of progressive overload and overall adaptations to training. When developing suitable resistance-training programs for special populations (e.g., older adults), knowing how to adjust these acute variables is critical. The most effective resistance-training programs are individually designed to bring about specific adaptations while accommodating the needs and medical concerns of each individual. A number of these acute training variables are discussed next.

Training Components and Variables

A resistance-training program is designed using a variety of acute program variables, or training components. Altering one or several of these variables changes the training stimulus and ultimately affects the specific adaptations to the program (Kraemer & Ratamess, 2000). An almost infinite number of workout protocols can be created simply by manipulating the program variables; however, the choices for each variable determine the effectiveness and benefits of the training program.

Type of Resistance Training

A wide range of equipment has been used in resistance-training programs, including free weights, food cans of different sizes, resistance bands or tubing, fixed weights, and, more recently, functional devices such as medicine and stability balls (Fleck & Kraemer, 1997). With any of this equipment, the individual should be able to safely control the resistance throughout the full range of motion. On some fixed-weight machines, even minimal resistance is too great for older adults, who often experience difficulty producing the initial force to start the movement. Also, on some machines the increments in resistance, especially at the lighter resistances, are too large to allow a smooth progression. Modalities such as resistance bands overcome these problems, allowing easier initiation of the movement and the development of resistance throughout the ascending strength curve. Variation in exercise mode and the source of resistance is paramount in ensuring optimal training adaptations.

Training modalities should be specific to the abilities of an individual and his or her training goals. Exercises that accommodate the physical capabilities and functional capacity of older adults should be included; however, the choice of exercises can vary for older individuals, as for people of any age. In general, you should select exercises that stress all major muscle groups so that muscular balance can be maintained. The progression of exercises within the program should activate as much of the skeletal muscle mass as possible so that adaptation can take place. At least one exercise for each major muscle group should be performed per training session. It is important at some point in the program to use exercises that optimally stimulate the majority of the muscle tissue (e.g., total-body exercises such as squats).

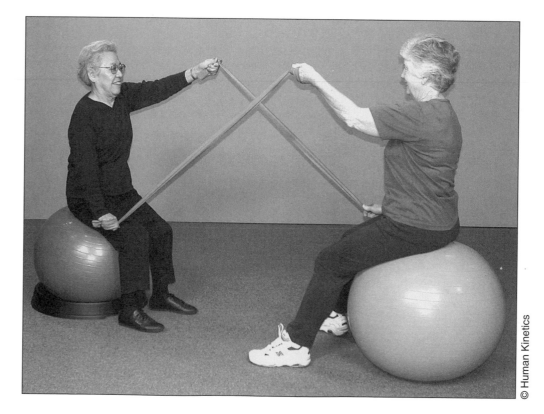

© Human Kinetics

Resistance bands can be effective for resistance training.

Single- and Multiple-Joint Exercises

Exercises can be divided into two basic types: single-joint and multiple-joint exercises. During **single-joint exercise,** one specific muscle group or joint action is targeted (e.g., biceps curl). Conversely, **multiple-joint exercises** target more than one muscle group or involve multiple joint actions or interactions (e.g., squat). It is recommended that both single- and multiple-joint exercises be included in a training regimen; both have been found to be effective for increasing muscular strength and hypertrophy.

Muscle Action

During resistance exercise, muscles can work in a variety of ways: concentrically, eccentrically, or isometrically. The nature of the muscle action influences the training adaptations. During **concentric contraction,** the muscle fibers and tendons shorten, whereas during **eccentric contractions,** the muscle fibers and tendons lengthen. For example, in the biceps curl, a concentric contraction raises the weight and an eccentric contraction lowers the weight.

The choice of isometric, dynamic concentric, dynamic eccentric, and isokinetic exercises is important when planning a resistance-training program. For example, eccentric muscle actions generate greater force (Komi, Kaneko, & Aura, 1987), are most conducive to **hypertrophy** (enlargement of the muscle cell; Hather, Tesch, Buchanan, & Dudley, 1991), and are less metabolically demanding. Eccentric muscle actions, however, are most likely to bring about delayed-onset muscle soreness (Ebbeling & Clarkson, 1989), particularly in individuals with little training history. **Isometric** (i.e., no change in muscle length as force is applied) muscle actions are more metabolically demanding than eccentric contractions yet less demanding than concentric muscle actions. Moreover, such contractions mostly increase strength at the specific joint angle at which they are performed. Whatever the train-

ing goals, a resistance-training program for the older adult should incorporate a variety of muscle actions. What matters is that the exercises be introduced progressively and that muscles be allowed sufficient time to recover following a particular muscle action, especially eccentric actions.

Resistance

Often referred to as the most critical aspect of a resistance-training program, **resistance,** or **load,** represents the amount of force exerted against working muscles and is expressed in absolute (i.e., weight in pounds or kilograms) or relative terms (i.e., as a percentage of maximal force; Kraemer & Ratamess, 2000). Generally, loads corresponding to 90 percent of a person's one-repetition maximum (1RM) are considered heavy; 70 percent to 90 percent of 1RM, moderate; and less than 70 percent, light. The resistance used depends on whether the goal is to develop muscular strength or muscular endurance, as altering the training load can affect the acute metabolic, hormonal, neural, and cardiovascular responses to training. **Muscle strength,** the strength of a muscle or muscle group, is the maximal force generated at a specified velocity, whereas **local muscular endurance** is the ability of a muscle or group of muscles to continue contracting repetitively for multiple repetitions.

A suitable load to stimulate strength development in a resistance-training program often depends on the individual's training status. This is particularly important for beginning lifters, where loads of at least 45 percent to 50 percent of 1RM are needed to increase dynamic muscular strength (Baechle & Earle, 2000). As an individual becomes more experienced, greater loads are required. To stimulate muscle cell hypertrophy and strength development, a resistance of approximately 80 percent of 1RM is recommended. When muscular endurance is the focus of the training, resistances of less than 80 percent maximum are required. The amount of resistance that frail elderly adults in their 90s can tolerate is at least 80 percent of 1RM (Fleck & Kraemer, 2004). Hunter and Treuth (1995), however, found that progression with lighter resistances (50-60 percent of 1RM) for older women may result in greater strength increases. The resistance needs to be carefully evaluated to avoid injury or increased pain from unsuitable overload.

> When designing resistance programs, make sure you're selecting exercises that stress all major muscle groups so that muscular balance can be maintained. To do this, use a mix of single joint and multi-joint exercises with both free weights and machines.

Exercise Order

The sequence in which exercises are performed during a training session can significantly affect performance and subsequent adaptation. The sequence of exercises depends on the goals of the training program and on energy metabolism and threshold of fatigue, particularly for older adults. Exercises that use larger muscle groups are typically placed at the beginning of a workout (Kraemer & Ratamess, 2000). Isolated muscle actions and single-joint movements should be used toward the end of the session. This order reduces muscular fatigue, allowing higher intensity or greater resistance in the large-muscle-group exercises. Optimal stimulation of the large muscle groups in the legs (e.g., leg press) and the upper body (e.g., bench press, seated row) should be a priority in a training program for older adults.

Sets

Resistance training is performed in **sets.** For example, lifting a weight eight times with no break between lifts constitutes one set of eight repetitions. As the number of sets increases, so does fatigue and the amount of recovery time required. The volume of exercise that can be tolerated is initially low, but tolerance increases as training continues. One-set (circuit-like) programs are the simplest starting point and are typically used in the early phases of a program to accommodate clients' low exercise tolerance. For progressive overload, the number of sets should be increased so that the muscles start to tolerate a greater volume of exercise. Resistance-training programs for older adults should not involve more than two to three sets of a given exercise. Many programs for older adults use a low-resistance warm-up set before the heavier sets. If the target muscle group needs more stimulation, another exercise for that muscle group can be added.

Number of Repetitions

The number of repetitions is closely related to load and also has an impact on training adaptations. Because of the high prevalence of cardiovascular problems and risk factors among older adults, repetition number must be carefully considered when designing resistance programs for this population. For example, when performing a set of repetitions to failure (or the maximal number of repetitions before

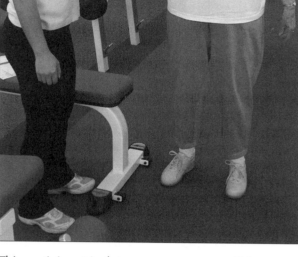

This participant is doing a warm-up set of biceps curls before increasing the resistance.

voluntary fatigue), blood pressure and heart rate can be significantly elevated compared to a shorter set. The highest blood pressures and heart rates normally occur in the last few repetitions of a set. In addition, joint compression during exercise to failure can cause subsequent joint soreness and pain. Therefore, for safety reasons older adults, especially those with cardiovascular problems, should not perform sets to failure. If muscular endurance is the particular focus, sets of 12 to 15 repetitions should be performed using lighter resistances. For strength development, a resistance high enough to permit 8 to 12 repetitions should be used initially.

Rest Periods

The **metabolic (energy) demand** of a workout is determined by the amount of rest taken between sets, exercises, or repetitions. Rest-period length depends on training intensity, goals, fitness level, and the targeted energy system (i.e., aerobic or anaerobic). Targeting energy systems is described

The Repetition Continuum

% 1RM	Repetitions
65%	14-15
70%	12-13
75%	10-11
80%	8-9
85%	6-7
90%	4-5
95%	2-3
100%	1 rep

in more detail in chapter 17 in the context of training of master athletes. Activation of muscle tissue is related to the resistance and the total amount of work performed, and so rest period lengths should be consistent with the program goals. The amount of rest will dictate the recovery between sets and impact the amount of resistance that can be used as well as the amount of work that can be tolerated in a particular workout. Short rest periods increase the contribution of energy from anaerobic sources. Short rest intervals are used to enhance local muscular endurance and improve **acid–base status,** (i.e., the pH and H^+ ion concentrations of a fluid or tissue), which is compromised with age. The increase in lactic acid with short rest resistance exercise protocols will demand a greater amount of inter- and intra-cellular buffering. Rest periods should be longer if heavier resistances are used. The amount of rest is also dictated by an individual's medical conditions. For some older adults with type 1 diabetes for whom gains in strength are the major goal, care must be taken to control the rest period between sets and exercises to avoid too great a metabolic stress.

Frequency

Training frequency refers to the number of training sessions completed in a given period of time, such as a week (Baechle & Earle, 2000). The frequency with which an individual performs resistance exercises needs to progressively increase as the body becomes more tolerant to exercise

stress. Resistance training can be performed as either a total-body workout or a split routine (e.g., upper body one day and lower body the next). Ultimately, the nature of the workout (total-body vs. split routine) determines the frequency with which each exercise is performed. Initially, total-body workouts two to three times per week are most appropriate for older adults. A split-routine that requires more frequent exercise sessions (three to five per week) can be used by individuals with more training experience. It is important that the training frequency allow sufficient recovery between exercise days. A general guideline is to schedule training sessions so that individuals with experience in resistance training have at least one recovery day between sessions that stress the same muscle group, and those just beginning training have two to three days.

Resistance Training for Older Adults

The principles of developing a resistance-training program are the same regardless of an individual's age. There are, however, a number of concerns that physical activity instructors should be aware of when working with older adults. First, it is very important to individualize the program, as older adults vary in their functional capacity and medical concerns. Existing medical ailments, exercise progression, and nutritional status should be evaluated before a client starts a resistance-training program (Baechle & Earle, 2000). Even though older adults retain the capacity to adapt to increased levels of physical activity (e.g., resistance training), guidelines for safe and effective exercise should be followed.

Proper breathing techniques, posture, and biomechanics during resistance training are critical to help prevent medical incidents. Another major concern is that the correct progression be used for older adults to avoid injury or acute overuse. Some data indicate that intensity must be carefully adjusted so as not to cause overtraining syndrome in older adults (Hunter & Treuth, 1995). It is possible that older adults take longer to recover from a training session, so varied intensities in a periodized format may allow better adaptation. The resistance-training programs used in many research studies involving older adults have been quite fundamental in design but have still yielded positive results. Therefore, early in training, advanced program design is not necessarily essential. Recommendations for progression were presented by the American College of Sports Medicine, the key points of which are presented in table 12.2 (Kraemer, Adams, et al., 2002).

When working with older adults, the physical activity instructor must appreciate that the frail elderly may initially possess minimal strength and be capable of producing a maximal force of only a few pounds. Therefore, in a progressive resistance-training program an older individual may lift only 0.5 pound (0.2 kilogram) during a set. Choosing the correct equipment capable of producing such low resistance increments calls for some care.

Design Considerations and Needs Analysis

The development of a resistance-training program for older adults consists of preactivity screening and assessment, setting individualized goals, designing a program, and developing evaluation methods. For older adults, resistance training should be part of their lifestyle, so continual reevaluation and assessment of program goals and program design are necessary for optimal results and adherence. As noted in chapter 5, the American College of Sports Medicine (2002) has advised that people who start an exercise program be classified into one of three risk categories to determine if a medical examination is recommended prior to participation.

TABLE 12.2 ACSM's Models of Progression for Resistance Training

Training component	Recommendation
Muscle action	For novice, intermediate, and advanced lifters, both concentric and eccentric muscle actions are recommended.
Loading	Novice to intermediate participants should train with loads corresponding to 60% to 70% of 1RM for 8 to 12 repetitions, and advanced lifters should use loads of 80% to 100% of 1RM in a periodized fashion. For progression, a 2% to 10% increase is recommended.
Volume	Novices should follow a general resistance-training program (consisting of either single or multiple sets). Multiple-set programs with systematic variation in training volume and intensity over time are best for intermediate and advanced participants.
Exercise selection	Both single- and multiple-joint exercises, with an emphasis on multiple-joint exercises, are recommended for novice, intermediate, and advanced lifters.
Free weights and machines	A novice to intermediate level training program should include both free-weight and machine exercises. An emphasis on free-weight exercises is recommended for advanced strength training.
Exercise order	Large muscle groups should be worked before small muscle groups, and multiple-joint exercises should come before single-joint exercises.
Rest periods	For novice, intermediate, and advanced training levels, rest periods of at least two to three minutes should be used between multiple-joint exercises using heavy loads. For other exercises, a rest period of one to two minutes may suffice.
Velocity of muscle action	Novices should use slow and moderate velocities initially. For intermediate strength training, moderate velocities should be used. For advanced strength training, a continuum of velocities from slow to fast is recommended.
Frequency	It is recommended that novices train the entire body two to three days per week. A similar frequency is recommended for intermediate participants, but those using a split routine should train three to four days per week so that each muscle group is trained one to two days per week. Advanced participants should work out four to six days per week.

Adapted from ACSM 2002.

After the individual's medical history and training status have been determined, a preprogram evaluation to document baseline measurements and evaluate responses to specific exercise modalities should be performed. Strength tests or exercise protocols are commonly used as an exercise test to evaluate EKG and clinical symptoms specific to resistance exercise modality. One-repetition maximum strength testing and resistance exercise workouts using as much as 75 percent of 1RM have been shown to cause fewer cardiopulmonary symptoms than graded treadmill exercise tests in cardiac patients with good left ventricular function (Faigenbaum, Skrinar, Cesare, Kraemer, & Thomas, 1990). One-repetition maximum testing is a safe and effective means of assessing older adults, provided that the client and the tester are adequately familiar with the test procedure and the appropriate testing guidelines are followed (Shaw, McCully, & Posner, 1995). Refer to Chapter 7 for the correct procedure for measuring 1RM.

Continual manipulation of acute program variables is recommended for long-term progression during resistance training by healthy, older adults. Caution must be taken with the rate of progression, as too much too soon can cause pain or injury. Older adults often have orthopedic problems that contraindicate the resistance training of affected joints. Recovery from a training session also takes longer for older adults, and care is needed not to exceed their physiological ability to repair tissues after a workout. Although higher resistances can be tolerated by some older men and women, the early phase of training should emphasize learning proper exercise techniques while minimizing the potential for injury and muscle soreness. Each individual responds differently to a given resistance-training program, based on his or her current training status, past training experience, and individual response to the training stress. A resistance-training program should aim to improve quality of life by enhancing muscular fitness, which includes muscle hypertrophy, strength, power, and local muscular endurance. Programs that include variation, gradual progressive overload, specificity, and careful attention to recovery are recommended (Kraemer, Adams, et al., 2002). Assessment of training progress should include testing strength (on the equipment used in training if possible), body composition, and functional abilities (e.g., getting out of a chair) and tracking existing medical conditions.

Once participants master basic exercises, standing exercises with **free weights** (e.g., barbells and dumbbells) and multidirectional medicine ball exercises can be incorporated into a program. Older adults should gradually progress from single-set workouts of 8 to 12 repetitions to higher training volumes with more sets of each exercise. Because recovery from training may take longer for older adults, an initial training frequency of twice per week is recommended during the adaptation period.

Strength and Hypertrophy Training

The basic resistance-training program recommended for health and fitness by the ACSM for healthy adults is an effective starting point for adults over 60. When the goal is increasing muscular strength and hypertrophy, evidence supports the use of variation in the resistance-training program. It is important that progression occur at a very gradual pace in programs for older adults. For improving muscular strength and hypertrophy in older adults, both multiple- and single-joint exercises are recommended. These exercises should be performed at a slow to moderate lifting velocity. One to three sets of each exercise should be completed, with one to two minutes of rest between sets and an intensity of 60 to 80 percent of 1RM for 8 to 12 repetitions per set.

Power Training

The available research evidence suggests that it is prudent to include high-velocity (nonballistic), low-intensity movements in the resistance-training program to maintain the structure and function of the neuromuscular system. Both single- and multiple-joint exercises are recommended for increasing power in healthy older adults. One to three sets per exercise using light to moderate loading (40-60 percent of 1RM) should be performed, and 6 to 10 repetitions at a high velocity promotes the development of muscular power.

Muscular Endurance Training

Local muscular endurance can be enhanced through circuit weight training, strength training, and high-repetition, moderate-load programs. Considering that local muscular endurance improvements are attained with low to moderate resistance loading, recommendations may apply to older individuals similar to those for younger individuals (Kraemer, Adams et al., 2002). Low to moderate loads should be used for a moderate to high number of repetitions (10 or more) with short rest intervals (less than one minute). Please refer to table 12.3 for suggested resistances and repetitions to achieve various training goals.

Resistance-Training Activities

As discussed earlier in this chapter, resistance-training programs for older adults should be individualized. Specificity of training is necessary to meet the particular needs of each individual. When designing a resistance-training program for older adults, you must consider which muscle groups

TABLE 12.3 Load and Repetition Recommendations Based on Training Goals

Training goal	Load (% 1RM)	Repetitions
Strength	60-80	≤8
Power	40-60	6-10
Hypertrophy	60-80	6-12
Muscular endurance	≤65	≥12

Reprinted, by permission, from T.R. Baechle and R.W. Earle, 2000, *Essentials of strength training and conditioning*, 2nd ed. (Champaign, IL: Human Kinetics), 414.

are most important for the functional activities of each individual and which are therefore the most important to target. For example, calf strength is significantly correlated with walking speed and mobility, power in the hip abductors and adductors can prevent lateral instability in gait, and muscular endurance in the biceps and triceps is important for many of the manual tasks performed each day (see table 12.4).

A variety of exercises can be used to stimulate muscular development, from body-weight-only exercises that require no equipment to machine-based circuit programs, free-weight exercises, and exercises that can be performed at home using food tins and other common, hefty objects. Examples of total-body workouts for older adults are described in figure 12.1.

Functional Training

The use of only linear movements does not address some of the more common functional movement patterns of everyday life (e.g., twisting, turning). **Functional training,** that is, exercises performed in an unstable environment, can improve muscle balance, strength, and functional capacity (Heitkamp, Horstmann, Mayer, Weller, & Dickhuth, 2001). Functional training means training in a manner that optimally carries over to real-life situations. Basically, this means training to improve

TABLE 12.4 Important Muscle Groups for Functional Activities

Muscle group	Relevance for functional activities
Dorsiflexors and plantar flexors	Important for walking and functional mobility (e.g., getting up from a chair)
Knee extensors and flexors	Required for all mobility activities Can prevent falls
Hip abductors and adductors	Required for lateral stability Increases stability when walking
Abdominals	Needed for the core stability vital to posture, balance, and mobility
Chest	Important for pushing and carrying Controls the upper body during gait
Back	Required for all pulling activities Controls posture in the spine
Biceps and triceps	Used for many activities of daily living (e.g., carrying groceries)
Shoulders	Needed for carrying Can help to reduce the impact of a fall

Beginner's home program

- For upper-body exercises, use food cans, wrist cuffs, or some other form of light resistance (2-5 lbs., 0.9-2.3 kg).
- Perform 1-3 sets of 8-10 repetitions.
- Rest 1-2 minutes between sets and exercises.
- Concentrate on full range of motion and balance. A wall or solid chair can be used for balance in the beginning.
- Appropriate exercises include front shoulder raises, wall push-aways, standing knee lifts, toe and heel raises, arm curls, good-morning exercise, side bends, standing knee curls, single-arm shoulder press, quarter squats, single-arm bent-over rows, side shoulder raises.

Program note: This is a light-resistance, callisthenic program to improve movement and range of motion. Progression to heavier resistances, especially for lower-body musculature, is vital for optimal improvement.

Beginner's program in the weight room

- Order of exercises: Large to small muscle groups
- Resistance: 60-75% of 1RM gradually adding resistance over time to 80% of 1RM, or the equivalent of 10RM-15RM range.
- Number of sets: One initially, progressing to three over a 12-week program
- Rest between sets and exercises: 2-3 minutes, or until recovered
- Appropriate exercises: leg presses, knee extensions, knee curls, calf raises, bench presses, seated rows, upright rows, arm curls, shoulder presses

Long-term periodized program in the weight room

Use a 12-week cycle, three days per week (e.g., Mon., Wed., Fri.), followed by an active rest of 2 weeks, and then repeat the cycle with appropriate variation in the program variables based on the training goals and needs of the individual.

- Order of exercises: Large to small muscle groups
- Resistance: 60-75% of 1RM (Mon.), 80-85% of 1RM (Wed.), 40-60% of 1RM (Fri.)
- Number of sets: One initially, progressing to three over a 12-week cycle
- Rest between sets and exercises: 2-3 minutes (Mon.), 3-4 minutes (Wed.), 1-2 minutes (Fri.)
- Appropriate exercises: leg presses or squats, knee extensions, knee curls, calf raises, bench presses, seated rows, upright rows, arm curls, shoulder presses
- Free weights (e.g., barbell, dumbbells)
- Fixed machine weights
- Resistance bands
- Stability balls
- Selected Pilates exercises
- Weighted cuffs (ankle, wrist)
- Medicine balls
- Manual resistance
- Body-weight resistance
- Aquatic exercises using water resistance

FIGURE 12.1   Sample resistance-training programs for older adults.

Adapted, by permission, from S.J. Fleck and W.J. Kraemer, 2004, *Designing resistance training programs*, 3rd ed. (Champaign, IL: Human Kinetics), 323.

strength in functional movement patterns rather than training simply to increase muscle strength or size. Functional movements are those that occur in all three planes of movement and involve acceleration, deceleration, and stabilization of the joint structures. Functional resistance-training exercises are executed in a variety of body positions, on a variety of surfaces, using a variety of resistance devices (e.g., resistance bands, weighted balls, specialized cable systems). The stabilizer muscles and not the mobilizing muscles limit functional strength. Development of the core muscles, which lie deep within the torso (i.e., the spine and pelvic muscles and muscles that support the scapula) and are used for stabilization, has a significant impact on the daily activities of older adults and reduces the incidence of injury as a result of falling.

Standard exercises

- Supine single-bent-leg raise
- Stability-ball single-leg raise
- Seated static contractions
- Supine pelvic tilts
- Pelvic tilts on all fours
- Abdominal curls (Progress from hands on thighs, to hands across chest, to fingers on temples.)

FIGURE 12.2   Functional training exercises suitable for older adults.

Though not as effective for developing strength and muscular hypertrophy as traditional weight-training methods, functional training promotes core stability and functional capacity, is simple to perform, and costs little. Figure 12.2 highlights some of the exercises suitable for functional training for older adults.

Functional training and core stability exercises can develop abdominal muscles (transversus abdominis, internal and external obliques, and rectus abdominis) and consequently help to protect the lower back (lumbar spine), stabilize the pelvis, and aid in performing exercises more efficiently and with less likelihood of injury. Functional training and core stability should be considered when designing a resistance-training program for older adults. Whether carried out using free weights, resistance bands, stability balls, or other forms of resistance, functional training should simulate muscle actions performed daily (twisting, bending, leaning). Most important for core stability are the stabilizing muscles of the trunk, and exercises to promote strength and muscle tone in this region should be included in the program. Figure 12.3 provides examples of abdominal exercises suitable for older adults.

Pilates is an exercise mode that focuses on improving balance, proprioception, and postural alignment by exercising the core postural muscles. Pilates promotes muscle recruitment and motor control by requiring stability to be maintained. Core stability can also be promoted through the

---

- Stability-ball chop-and-lift
- Supine heel slide
- Supine single-straight-leg raise
- Supine bent-knee fallout and return

Pilates exercises

- Roll-ups
- Hundreds exercise
- Oblique curl-ups

Abdominal movements should be performed through the full range of motion. Movements should be controlled, and steady breathing maintained. Progression is similar to other exercise modes (beginner: one set of 12RM-15RM; advanced: three sets of 15RM-20RM).

FIGURE 12.3   Sample abdominal exercises for older adults.

use of stability balls and appropriate exercises on an uneven base (e.g., wobble board, foam). For example, performing a shoulder press while sitting on a stability ball works not only the prime movers in the shoulder but also the stabilizers in the trunk (the abdominals) required to prevent loss of balance. Refer to chapter 14 for information about other types of balance activities that can be combined with the resistance-training component of a program.

Exercise performed in the water is an alternative mode of resistance training and provides well-balanced resistance over the entire body. Because of the effects of buoyancy and the limbs' and trunk's movement against the resistance of the water, all muscle actions in the water are concentric. The resistance can be increased by using hand and foot paddles, which increase the surface area against which the resistance is applied. Refer to chapter 16 for more information about the beneficial resistance properties of water and aquatic exercise in general.

Safety Precautions

Resistance training can be a safe and effective exercise modality for older adults if appropriate training guidelines are followed (Evans, 1999; Kraemer, Adams, et al., 2002). However, if program design is poor, resistance training can be potentially hazardous. Without the correct instruction and supervision, participants' risk of injury as a consequence of inappropriate resistance training increases. The risk of injury can be minimized with well-trained instructors, adequate recovery, and sound instruction (Baechle & Earle, 2000). As with any type of exercise or physical activity, resistance training requires that suitable safety precautions be employed. The risk of injury and infirmity must be minimized, particularly for older adults who are frail and may have special medical concerns. These are some safety recommendations that should be followed during resistance training for older adults: (1) Warm up muscles for at least 10 minutes before training. (2) Start with low resistance, and gradually add repetitions, intensity (resistance), and sets. (3) Conduct exercises through a full pain-free range of motion. (4) Discontinue any exercise that causes pain, or lower the resistance. (5) Never hold your breath; exhale during the exertion phase and inhale during the release phase. (6) Avoid hyperextend-

ing or locking joints. (7) Allow at least 48 hours between resistance-training sessions using the same muscle groups.

Summary

Research indicates that resistance training can be a safe and effective method of exercise for men and women of all ages and abilities. The benefits for older adults include increased strength, endurance, muscle capacity, flexibility, and energy and improved self-image and confidence. Endurance activities, which improve local muscular endurance, are performed at a significantly lower percentage of the maximal voluntary contraction. The enhancement of muscle and bone mass also has important benefits for an individual's health. Moreover, muscle strengthening enhances the performance of everyday activities, which in turn improves a person's overall health and well-being. Even for frailer older adults, research indicates that resistance training is beneficial. It is never too late to start a resistance-training program. Of course, the proper design and progression of a resistance-training program for older adults are vital to the optimization of its benefits.

Key Terms

Recommended Readings

Kraemer, W.J., Adams, K., Cafarelli, E., Dudley, G.A., Dooly, C., Feigenbaum, M.S., et al. (2002). American College of Sports Medicine position stand: Progression models in resistance training for healthy adults. *Medicine and Science in Sports and Exercise, 34,* 364-380.

Kraemer, W.J., & Ratamess, N.A. (2000). Physiology of resistance training: Current issues. *Orthopaedic Physical Therapy Clinics of North America: Exercise Technologies, 9,* 467-513.

Study Questions

1. To translate improvement in a weight-room task into improvement in a real-life task, what resistance-training principle is most important to consider?
   a. specificity
   b. intensity
   c. conversion
   d. periodization

2. A multiple-joint exercise
   a. stresses all muscles in the body
   b. uses muscles that cross more than one joint
   c. isolates the resistance to one muscle group
   d. can be done only with free weights

3. One of the most important physical capabilities needed for everyday lifting tasks is
   a. flexibility
   b. coordination
   c. power
   d. endurance

4. Which age group can benefit from resistance training?
   a. 40- to 50-year-old men
   b. 100-year-old women
   c. 70-year-old men
   d. all of the above

5. Periodization is best defined as
   a. planned rest cycles to minimize the risk of injury and other symptoms associated with overtraining
   b. the use of heavy weights with long rest periods to minimize the risk of injury and other symptoms associated with overtraining
   c. the planned cycling of training intensity to minimize the risk of injury and other symptoms associated with overtraining
   d. the planned cycling of training variables, including volume and intensity, to minimize the risk of injury and other symptoms associated with overtraining

Application Activities

1. Develop a one-minute talk to motivate a group of sedentary older adults to participate in resistance training.

2. Design a periodized training program for a group of healthy 70-year-old and older men and women, and delineate any gender differences you think are important in the program. Be sure to discuss various training variables.

3. You are training three clients. Your first client, an 85-year-old man, wants to be able to develop strength to climb stairs and get up from sitting down. Your second client, a 76-year-old woman, wants to improve her posture. Your third client, a 61-year-old woman, wants to improve her golf game. What resistance exercises would you recommend for each client?

13

Aerobic Endurance Training

Susie Dinan
Dawn Skelton
Katie Malbut

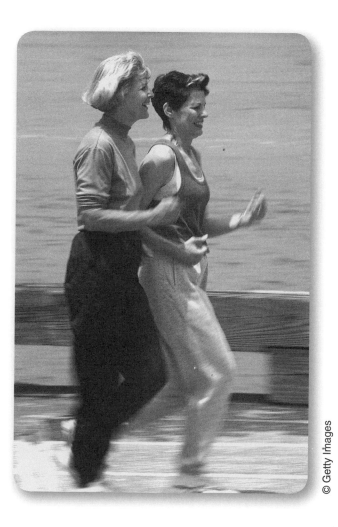

As discussed in chapter 4, the decline in maximal aerobic power ($\dot{V}O_2$max) with advancing age can have a devastating effect on the quality of life of the oldest-old. Everyday tasks and activities require a greater proportion of $\dot{V}O_2$max for older people, particularly those who are frail. For example, simple tasks such as dressing and undressing, with an energy cost of only two to three **metabolic equivalents (METs;** i.e., 7-10.5 milliliters of oxygen per kilogram per minute), requires as much as 50 to 75 percent of a frail 80-year-old woman's $\dot{V}O_2$max (Malbut-Shennan, Greig, & Young, 2000). The aerobic endurance component of your program not only can transform your clients' life but also provide you with a level of professional satisfaction that is hard to beat.

In this chapter the physiological and psychological benefits of aerobic training for older adults are described first, followed by a discussion of the important exercise principles and variables that need to be considered when developing the aerobic endurance component of any activity program for older adults. You will then learn how to manipulate each of these variables appropriately.

Benefits of Aerobic Endurance Training for Older Adults

Older adults maintain their ability to respond to aerobic endurance training even into their later years (Malbut-Shennan, Greig, & Young, 2000). Even women in their 80s and 90s can improve their $\dot{V}O_2$max by as much as 15 to 17 percent after 24 to 32 weeks of exercise training (Malbut, Dinan,

& Young, 2002; Puggaard, Larsen, Stovring, & Jeune, 2000). Aerobic endurance training also improves older adults' ability to sustain exercise at a fixed, submaximal level of energy expenditure. This can have a major impact on functional abil-

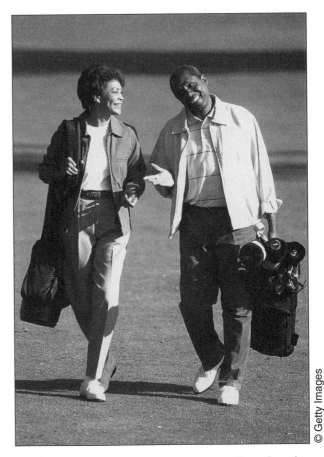

© Getty Images

Of all aerobic endurance activities, walking has the most natural relationship to activities of daily living and is easier to integrate into lifestyle and functional tasks.

192

ity, particularly for frailer older women, because everyday activities then represent a lower proportion of their $\dot{V}O_2$ and can therefore be performed for longer periods and with greater ease. There is also evidence that quality of life can be improved for older adults through aerobic endurance training (Hill, Storandt, & Malley, 1993; Lavie & Milani, 1995). It remains unclear, however, whether it is the exercise itself or the social contact that contributes more to improvements in mood and overall well-being (Hassmen & Koivula, 1997; Brown et al., 1995; Williams & Lord, 1995).

Most of the benefits of preventing coronary heart disease, stroke, hypertension, diabetes, and osteoporosis experienced by younger people can also be accrued by those who are physically active in later life (American College of Sports Medicine [ACSM], 1998; Young & Dinan, 2000). In frailer older people, however, aerobic endurance training takes on a role less of disease prevention and more of symptom alleviation. Aerobic endurance training counters some of the well-known age-related physiological changes, reverses disuse syndrome, helps to control chronic diseases, maximizes psychological health, and preserves the ability to perform activities of daily living (ACSM, 1998; Young & Dinan, 2000; Young 2001).

Principles and Considerations for Aerobic Endurance Training

This section describes how each of the exercise principles first introduced in chapter 9 (i.e., specificity, overload, functional relevance, challenge, and accommodation) is specifically applied to the aerobic endurance component of an activity program for older adults. It also discusses interindividual variability and rest and recovery, two programming considerations of particular importance for older adults.

Specificity and Interval Conditioning

Specificity is the foundation on which the successful application and manipulation of the other exercise principles and variables depend. Specific exercises elicit specific metabolic and physiological adaptations. For example, to improve a client's aerobic capacity, you must select physical activi-

ties that are aerobic in nature, such as walking on a treadmill at an intensity rated light to somewhat hard (11 to 13 on Borg's rating of perceived exertion [RPE] scale) (see p. 199). For maximum effectiveness, instructors should select exercises and exercise modes based on the results of pre-activity screening and assessment and then target the physical fitness parameters that need improvement. The exercises selected must also be specific to both the energy system being targeted (aerobic or anaerobic; Bompa, 1999) and to functional tasks performed in everyday life (Skelton, Young, Greig, & Malbut, 1995).

Everyday tasks such as hurrying to catch a bus or to avoid a downpour or climbing a hill during a walk to the store and leisure activities such as tennis, swimming, bicycling, and walking all demand intermittent bursts of energy over time.

This alternating effort–recovery pattern forms the basis of the **interval training** method. Classic interval training alternates periods of maximal or near-maximal effort with short periods of complete rest, while **interval conditioning,** an adapted interval training method, alternates short periods (one to six minutes) of higher-intensity exercise with an equal or longer recovery period (i.e., for a short time the effort expended is a little greater than is comfortable, and then the effort required returns to an easy, comfortable, and sustainable level [Brooks, 1997]). Interval conditioning is recommended for use with older participants, as it provides a flexible, systematic framework for progressing endurance training for older adults with a broad range of functional and fitness levels (Dinan, 2002). Before examining its use in greater detail, it is important to view interval-type training in relation to continuous training.

Research suggests that the physiological benefits of interval conditioning versus **continuous training** (six minutes or longer of uninterrupted activity, usually performed at a constant submaximal intensity) are similar (Haskell, 1997; Shephard, 1991). The main advantage of interval conditioning, for participants of all ages, is that the total volume of work is higher than when the submaximal intensity of exercise is constant. Alternating controlled fluctuations in intensity or duration with active recovery periods enables the older person to work harder for a longer time and with greater comfort. It also mirrors real-life energy demands more closely than continuous training. Therefore, it is recommended as the safest, most effective tool for improving both cardiorespiratory and functional aerobic fitness in the older person.

Brooks (1997) identifies three types of interval conditioning: spontaneous, fitness, and performance. When introduced sequentially, they form a logical progressive continuum of training. All three types of interval conditioning tap into aerobic and anaerobic energy sources during the higher-effort intervals and have **active,** aerobic, lower-effort recovery intervals. In each type of interval conditioning, the client periodically increases the intensity and then recovers actively before initiating another higher-intensity bout. Intervals can also vary in the durations of the effort and recovery phases; this allows physical activity instructors greater flexibility in prescribing exercise based on their observation of clients' performance and ratings of effort. An important feature of interval conditioning is that the client, armed with specific information about monitoring exercise, largely controls the intensity of the exercise. Specific guidelines for manipulating the different exercise variables for the three types of interval conditioning are provided in table 13.1. However, it is important to note that the performance end of the continuum is appropriate only for healthier, more fit older adult exercisers.

The ultimate goal is to design an aerobic endurance component that combines continuous- and

TABLE 13.1 Interval Conditioning Training Continuum for Older Adults

	Spontaneous conditioning		Fitness conditioning		Performance conditioning	
Goal	"Get me started"		"Train me"		"Challenge me!"	
	Getting skilled up: feeling fitter		Getting trained up: getting fitter; gaining the training gains		Getting even fitter: maintaining the training gains and beyond	
	Fitter moments		Fit for life		Fit for sport or performance	
	"I want to reduce breathlessness enough to get to the store and back without stopping and without feeling so exhausted that I have to rest for the whole day to recover."		"I want to be able to lengthen my walk to 30 minutes, increase my pace, and do uphill walking."		"I want to enter or improve my time in the super veteran category in my local triathlon."	
Fitness level	Deconditioned		Moderate to high (for anaerobic intervals)		High	
Intensity	Instructor programmed, participant controlled RPE guidelines 9-11		Instructor programmed, participant controlled RPE guidelines:		Set by instructor RPE guidelines:	
			Effort interval 11-13 progress to: 13-15	Recovery interval 9-11 remains: 9-11	Effort interval 13-15 progress to: 15-17	Recovery interval 9-11 remains: 9-11
	METS guidelines 2-4		METS guidelines 4-6 Progress to 6-8		METS guidelines 6-10 Progress to: 10-12	
TIME:						
* Work/ Rest: Effort/ Recovery ratio	Instructor programmed, participant controlled Aerobic Effort Recovery		Set by instructor Aerobic effort 1: recovery 1 Anaerobic effort 1: recovery 3		Set by instructor Aerobic effort 1: recovery 1 Anaerobic effort 1: recovery 3	

	Spontaneous conditioning	**Fitness conditioning**	**Performance conditioning**
*Duration	Instructor programmed, participant controlled Effort interval: 10 seconds to 5 minutes Recovery interval: 10 seconds to 5 minutes	Set by instructor Aerobic: 3-5 minutes Anaerobic: 80-90 and progress to 90-270 seconds Recovery: 3-5 minutes	Set by instructor Aerobic: 3-5 minutes Anaerobic: 80-90 and progress to 90-270 seconds Recovery: 3-5 minutes
Frequency	Participant controlled within fitness level and length of aerobic endurance component	Number of cycles depends on fitness level and type	Number of cycles depends on fitness level and length of aerobic endurance component
Type*	Walking, stationary cycling, and stair climbing and descending	Walking, jogging, cycling, rowing, swimming, exercise to music, circuit training	Timed or race walks, runs, swims, etc.; triathlons; mini-marathons
Approach	Individualized "easy-does-it" 'speed play'-Fartlek. No or minimal structure "Speed up a little until you reach the next tree and you are breathing a little harder but are not breathless, then ease off a little and recover."	Comfortably challenged More structured "Work a little harder than you usually do."	Improved sports performance, going beyond improved fitness; only for better-conditioned clients Highly structured

* Note: See Table 13.4 for appropriate activities and modalities. All interval conditioning programming must be tailored to the client's health needs, fitness levels, personal goals, and interests.

Adapted from Brooks 1995; Dinan and Skelton 2000.

> The key to interval conditioning is to alternate short periods of exercise in which the effort expended is just a little greater than is comfortable with equal or longer recovery periods of easy, comfortable, sustainable exercise.

interval-conditioning approaches. In the initial stages, however, interval conditioning is recommended because it is more flexible and it yields rapid and specific aerobic endurance gains that enhance the performance of everyday activities. After a period of interval conditioning (approximately 12-16 weeks), participants should be encouraged to progress by extending the duration of their workout to include continuous training using cardiovascular equipment (e.g., treadmill, stationary cycle, or stepper).

Overload

As first defined in chapter 9, the exercise principle of overload states that for continued improvement in fitness, the cardiopulmonary and musculoskeletal systems must be progressively overloaded by periodically increasing the frequency, intensity, time (duration), or challenge of an exercise (Heyward,

1998). Prevention of injury and overtraining is a priority at all ages. The instructor must strike a balance between ensuring sufficient progressive overload and preventing exhaustion and subsequent loss of coordination, muscle soreness, injury, and possible dropout. While it is true that cardiorespiratory overtraining is rarely a problem for noncompetitive older exercisers, maintaining this balance is even more critical for older adults because the safety margins are narrower, the consequences of overtraining are greater, and recovery takes longer. Manipulating the variable of intensity (speed, load) appears to be more stressful for the older adult exerciser than manipulating training volume (repetitions, time, frequency). In frailer older participants, whose bone strength, muscle force, and speed are already compromised, inappropriate programming can increase the risk of falls and injuries and overtraining.

These are some helpful guidelines for applying the overload principle to the aerobic endurance component of your activity program:

- Increase only one variable at a time.
- Increase duration before intensity.
- Increase duration in one-minute increments as tolerated (Fiatarone Singh, 2000).

- Increase intensity by using the arms in a more challenging way (e.g., arms above waist level) or by increasing resistance (e.g., carrying objects) before increasing the speed of the movement (Fiatarone Singh, 2000).
- Allow a minimum of two weeks for adaptation before considering increasing the overload (Dinan, 2002).

Functional Relevance

One of the unique principles for exercise programs for older adults, first described in chapter 9, is functional relevance. Examples of aerobic exercises that have functional relevance include activities such as stair climbing and descending, picking up objects and carrying them across the room, and certain line-dancing moves. Including specific functional tasks in your program can help your clients realize improvements in both muscle strength and functional ability (Skelton & McLaughlin, 1996; Skelton, Young, Greig, & Malbut, 1995). Although there is little evidence on specificity of aerobic training for older adults, it is likely that similar findings would apply. Therefore, it is best to select activities that are more functional in nature not only to improve physiological parameters but also to improve the performance of tasks and activities of daily living and to reduce the risk of falls.

Challenge

A second exercise principle critical to programs for older adults first introduced in chapter 9 is the challenge principle. This principle is similar to the overload principle, but it focuses on increasing the demands placed on multiple body systems rather than just manipulating the exercise variables (frequency, intensity, type, and time). The challenge of an aerobic exercise can be altered by increasing the complexity of the task, such as walking to music time, or by adding a second task, such as walking to music time in a particular direction and then walking to music time and using marching to turn and then walk in the opposite direction.

Accommodation

Another exercise principle specific to programs for older adults is accommodation. Because many of your clients may be taking multiple medications for various medical conditions, it is important to recognize that possible adverse side effects may influence

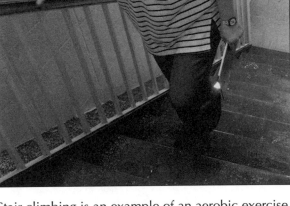

Stair climbing is an example of an aerobic exercise that has functional relevance.

> Accommodation through monitoring and adaptation is the key to meeting the greater fluctuations in health and functional capacity found in older adults.

their ability to exercise aerobically at the same intensity and for the same duration each week. Possible adverse effects of medications during exercise are discussed in chapter 21. It is not unusual for people with arthritic conditions to feel fine one day and then be in severe pain the next day. Assisting clients in learning to monitor their own exertion level, pain level, and personal safety limits and to adapt their exercise accordingly reduces musculoskeletal injury rates and risk of cardiac events.

Interindividual Variability

Some of your clients will progress very slowly and need a lot of encouragement because of their medical conditions, sedentary lifestyle, or personality. For your program to be effective, exercises must be individualized on the basis of the information derived from the preactivity screening, your assessment results, and the behavioral goals you have established in consultation with your client. It is also important to understand the unique personalities of your clients in order to communicate effectively with them. Refer to chapter 19 for a more detailed discussion of developing your skills for communicating with older adults.

When educating clients about cardiorespiratory fitness, you can boost their motivation by emphasizing the difference fitness can make in daily activities in which they report difficulty (e.g., breathlessness on hills, having to stop three times on the stairs). Engaging clients also means reassuring them that what they are experiencing is completely normal if they have not been active for a while; that progress will be slow; that they will receive individual attention; that there is no rush; that safety is the priority; that they will soon feel and see the difference; and that free-moving endurance exercise helps prevent falls, improves balance, makes for a healthier heart, and can also put a spring back in their step.

Rest and Recovery

It is crucial that you systematically plan for adequate rest and recovery periods in aerobic endurance training for older adult clients. Adequate rest and recovery help (1) prevent overuse fatigue injuries and falls, (2) enhance the functioning of the cardiorespiratory system, (3) improve aerobic and functional performance, and (4) promote exercise adherence. Residual fatigue or muscle soreness that interferes with a client's performance during the next exercise session or the next set of repetitions of a particular exercise is a good indicator that the recovery period was inadequate. Muscle acidosis is the primary performance-limiting factor in endurance exercise. Rest and recovery are essential preventive strategies and are most effectively achieved through careful program design and implementation.

Yessis (1987) identified three phases of recovery following aerobic exercise: ongoing recovery within a session, quick recovery immediately after a session (through removal of metabolic wastes), and deep recovery during and between sessions (through training adaptation that enhances the body's ability to recover quickly and efficiently). Effective aerobic endurance program design for all ages must therefore consider the recovery period required for each of the following: between effort intervals; between the cycles (sets) of effort and recovery intervals; between specific exercises;

> The key to older adults' recovery during endurance activities is best achieved through the active rest and recovery periods of interval conditioning.

between the components of a session; between consecutive aerobic endurance sessions performed on the same day (e.g., in circuit training and swimming); and between specific endurance sessions over days, weeks, and months. The amount of recovery between workouts depends on the ability and fitness level of the participant and the intensity, frequency, and duration of the activity. Deep recovery improves as cardiorespiratory fitness is achieved.

The key to older adults' recovery during endurance activities is ensuring active rest. Interval conditioning, with its lower-intensity active rest and recovery intervals, is most effective at clearing lactate and facilitating quick recovery phases for older adult exercisers. Advise your clients to come a little early to rest and refresh before the session and to allow 20 minutes to "relax and refresh" after the session in order to derive the greatest benefit from the exercise session.

Variables for Aerobic Endurance Training

In addition to skillfully and mindfully applying the exercise principles and exercise considerations discussed in the previous section, you must also understand how to manipulate each of the relevant exercise variables: frequency, intensity, time (duration), and type (mode). In this chapter we prefer the terms *time* rather than *duration* and *type* rather than *mode* because the acronym FITT (frequency, intensity, time, type) serves as a useful phrase for remembering these variables for the aerobic endurance component of the program.

Frequency and Time

The variables that have the most direct bearing on aerobic training volume are frequency and time. The older sedentary participant can gain substantial health benefits through 30 minutes of moderate exercise on most days of the week (U.S. Department of Health and Human Services, 1996).

> When designing your aerobic endurance com-
> ponent, use the acronym FITT as an easy way
> to remember the variables:
>
> **F**requency
> **I**ntensity
> **T**ime (duration)
> **T**ype

There is evidence that cardiorespiratory gains are similar whether the exercise occurs in several short sessions (e.g., three bouts of 10 minutes) or in one 30-minute period; however, it is not yet clear whether the health promotion and disease prevention benefits are as extensive for several shorter sessions (Fiatarone Singh, 2000; U.S. Department of Health and Human Services, 1996). For frailer participants, ACSM (1998) recommends a preparatory period of strength and balance training before aerobic training begins. Then aerobic training can be built up gradually, first by increasing the time and then by increasing the intensity. It may be necessary to start with as little as three minutes a day for frailer and/or less healthy and more deconditioned clients (Dinan, 2002).

Intensity

The intensity of physical activity determines the physiological and metabolic changes in the body. There are three common methods of measuring and monitoring the intensity of aerobic exercise: (1) heart rate, (2) Borg's RPE scale, and (3) metabolic equivalent (MET) values.

Heart Rate

The most common method of prescribing and monitoring exercise intensity is by targeting a training heart rate, which is established as a percentage of either **maximal heart rate (HRmax)** or **heart rate reserve (HRR,** maximal heart rate minus resting heart rate). Unfortunately, both of these methods have certain disadvantages. First, unless a true measure of HRmax has been obtained, it must be estimated. Such estimates are particularly unreliable in older people (Cooper, Purdy, White, & Pollock, 1977). Second, clients must slow down or stop exercising to take their heart rate. Third, heart rates that are self-measured by palpation have been shown to be inaccurate (Bell & Bassey,

1996). Finally, percentage of HRR may represent a higher than expected percentage of $\dot{V}O_2$max (Scharff-Olsen, Williford, & Smith, 1992), so using HRR percentage to prescribe exercise intensity may result in the older adult's working at an intensity that is higher than desired (Kohrt, Spina, Holloszy, & Ehsani, 1998; Panton et al., 1996).

Rating of Perceived Exertion

As first introduced in chapter 4, an alternative to using target heart rate to obtain the desired training intensity is using **Borg's rating of perceived exertion (RPE) scale.** This scale of self-perceived effort takes into account both central (e.g., heart rate and breathing) and local (e.g., muscle fatigue) sensations, so it does not rely on cardiovascular response alone to determine workload (Pandolf, 1982). It also does not require slowing down or stopping exercise to obtain a value, and it is effective for prescribing and monitoring exercise intensity for both younger and older adults (Malbut, Dinan, & Young, 2002; Koltyn & Morgan, 1992; Ceci & Hassmen, 1991).

A training intensity between 13 and 15 on the 6-to-20 RPE scale (see figure 13.1) is approximately equivalent to working at 70 to 80 percent of $\dot{V}O_2$max (Pollock, Wilmore, & Fox, 1984; ACSM, 1990; Malbut, Dinan, & Young, 2002), whereas an RPE of 11 to 13 approximates working at 49 to 70 percent of $\dot{V}O_2$max (ACSM, 1990). The relationship between RPE and percentage of $\dot{V}O_2$max has been reported to be independent of age (Sidney & Shephard, 1977). Figure 13.1 shows both Borg's RPE scale and his CR10 scale (ACSM, 2000).

According to the ACSM (1998) guidelines, starting with an exercise intensity of light to somewhat hard (11 to 13 on the RPE scale) and never exceeding an intensity of hard (15) appear to be most appropriate for previously sedentary older adults. For a frail older person, it is recommended that exercise intensity start at very light to light (9 to 11 on the RPE scale) and be increased slowly and cautiously.

However, whether you are using the 0-to-10 CR10 scale or the 6-to-20 RPE scale, Borg makes it clear that it is essential that the instructor and the participant understand what they are assessing and that the participant receives clear instructions on using the scale (Borg & Hassmen, 1999). The RPE scale instructions recommended by ACSM (2000) for clients during exercise testing are as follows:

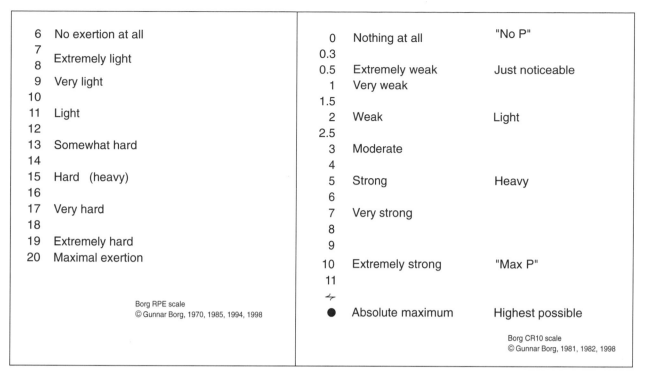

FIGURE 13.1   Borg's RPE (ratio) and CR10 (category-ratio) scales. Note: On the category-ratio scale, "P" represents intensity. For correct usage of the Borg scales, it is necessary to follow the administration and instructions given in ACSM, 2000. Additional valuable background information can be found in *Borg's Perceived Exertion and Pain Scales* (G. Borg, Champaign, IL: Human Kinetics, 1998).

Reprinted, by permission, form G. Borg, 1998, Borg's perceived exertion and pain scales (Champaign, IL: Human Kinetics), 47, 50.

During the exercise test we want you to pay close attention to how hard you feel the exercise work rate is. This feeling should reflect your total amount of exertion and fatigue, combining all sensations and feelings of physical stress, effort, and fatigue. Don't concern yourself with any one factor such as leg pain, shortness of breath, or exercise intensity, but try to concentrate on your total, inner feeling of exertion. Try not to underestimate or overestimate your feelings of exertion; be as accurate as you can. (ACSM, 2002, p. 79)

Metabolic Equivalent Values

The intensity of an exercise can also be regulated by selecting activities based on known metabolic equivalent (MET) values. Knowing the MET value of specific aerobic activities is important so that activities that may pose a risk to certain older individuals can be eliminated. Some activities have a wide range of MET values (e.g., ballroom dancing, 4-6 METs; aerobic dance, 6-9 METs; and skipping, 8-12 METs), while others vary little (e.g., walking at 3 miles per hour, 3-8 METs; cycling at 10 miles

per hour, 5-6 METs), because less-structured movements can be performed in a variety of ways. Ideally, for the first 8 to 10 weeks of any exercise program, endurance activities should be of a type that is easy to monitor and can be maintained at a constant intensity (e.g., speed of walking, wattage on a cycle, height of step, cadence of stepping, and tempo of exercise to music).

Type of Physical Activity

In addition to careful manipulation of the frequency, time, and intensity that will determine the cardiorespiratory overload, identifying the right type (mode) of physical activity is very important. Aerobic endurance exercise is defined as any activity that uses the large muscle groups, can be maintained for a prolonged period, and is rhythmic and continuous (Bell, 2001). When you select the type of aerobic endurance activity or exercise for your program, you should once again be guided by the results of the preactivity screening (chapter

5), physical and mobility assessments (chapters 6 and 7), and the behavioral goals (chapter 8) of your clients. Aerobic activities popular with older adults include walking, stationary cycling, treadmill walking or jogging, dancing, swimming, aquatic exercise, and exercise to music. A balanced combination of physical activities is as important as the selection of each individual activity in ensuring clients' safety, improved performance, and adherence.

The key recommendations for applying each of the exercise variables are as follows:

- Frequency: Exercise most days of the week; start with three days per week for frail and sedentary clients.
- Intensity: Intensity is most easily estimated by METs and most easily and effectively measured by RPE. Keep RPE between 11 and 13 (moderate to somewhat hard) for active, healthy older adults and between 9 and 11 (very light to light) for frail and sedentary older adults.
- Time: Exercise for 30 minutes most days; start with three periods of 3 to 5 minutes and build to three periods of 10 minutes per day for frail and sedentary older adults.
- Type: Choose activities that use the large muscle groups, can be maintained for a prolonged period, and are rhythmic and continuous. Walking is a great mainstay.

Types of Aerobic Exercises

Aerobic endurance exercise offers a wider range of potential modalities than any other fitness component and the largest number of activities that, with a little effort, can become part of your clients' everyday lives. Incorporating a variety of different aerobic endurance activities in a weekly exercise program minimizes overuse injuries, maximizes peripheral adaptation, and increases long-term motivation and adherence. This is particularly true of cross-training combinations that involve the large muscle groups of both the upper and lower body (e.g., recumbent stepper and circuit exercises). The dilemma of choosing the "best" type of endurance activity for a particular older adult client is assisted by evaluating each activity from three distinct yet related perspectives—health and training benefits,

risks, and programming advantages—and according to specific criteria or prompts.

First, the physical activity instructor needs to consider the health benefits and training effects specific to each exercise or mode of exercise in relation to his or her client's unique needs, goals, and preferences. For example, does the exercise preference reduce the risk of falls, preserve the client's functional ability, increase his or her opportunities for socializing, and so on (see table 13.2)?

Second, the instructor must analyze each exercise or exercise mode carefully to ensure that its risks never outweigh its potential benefits to the client. Using the prompts in the risk-to-benefit analysis tool (see table 13.3) will assist both the instructor and the client in deciding whether the exercise preference is an appropriate goal for the client or whether it needs to be permanently excluded for health and safety reasons, such as jumping jacks for a complete beginner or a cross-trainer for a client with knee problems.

Finally, the physical activity instructor should know what the specific programming advantages of different exercise modes are (see table 13.4). For example, knowing which activities score highest, not only on physiological and psychosocial criteria but also on cost–benefit and ease of integration into everyday life is important information to have at your fingertips. These programming advantages are highlighted in table 13.4.

As can be seen from table 13.4, walking quite simply has more programming advantages at any age than other forms of endurance activity. For this reason alone, walking should be the mainstay for any aerobic endurance program for seniors. As we age, participation drops in all types of physical activities except walking. Walking appeals to a wide range of people, is easily adapted to different fitness and functional levels and environments (indoors or out), and facilitates social interactions, particularly intergenerational ones. Of all endurance activities, walking is the most functionally relevant; it has the most natural relationship to and is the easiest to integrate into activities of daily living. By adding correct gait techniques and more complex skills and routes, this everyday activity becomes more interesting, challenging, and effective. It makes good programming sense, therefore, to promote walking as the foundation of aerobic endurance programs and active lifestyle approaches for older adults.

TABLE 13.2 Health Benefits and Training Effects of Different Modes of Exercise for Older Adults

	Walking	Aerobic dance	Circuit training	Step training/Stair climbing	CARDIO-VASCULAR EQUIPMENT		WATER TRAINING		Active lifestyle
					Cycle	Treadmill	Swimming	Aquatics	
HEALTH BENEFITS									
Prevents disease	++	++	++	++	++	++	+	+	—
Counteracts the effects of disease and reduces disability	+	++	++	+	+	+	+	++	+
Improves or maintains bone density	+	++	+	++	—	+	—	+	+
Reduces fall risk factors	+	++	+	—	—	—	—	+	+
Improves mental health or mood	++	+	+	+	+	+	+	++	+
Increases social opportunities	++	++	++	+	—	—	+	++	+
Preserves functional capacity in old age	++	++	++	+	+	+	+	+	+
TRAINING EFFECTS									
Improves submaximal $\dot{V}O_2$	++	++	++	++	++	++	++	++	+
Improves $\dot{V}O_2$max	+	++	++	++	++	++	++	++	+
Improves ability to perform specific functional ADL moves, e.g., sit to stand	+	++	++	++	—	+	+	+	++
Improves ability to sustain ADL endurance activities, e.g., walking and reduces fatigue	++	+	++	+	+	+	+	+	+
Improves reaction time	—	++	++	+	—	—	—	+	+
Improves balance and coordination	+	++	++	+	—	+	+	+	+
Improves (leg) strength	+	+	+	++	++	+	++	++	—
Improves flexibility	—	+	+	—	—	—	++	++	+
Improves posture and body control	+	++	++	+	—	+	+	+	+
Improves body and spatial awareness	+	++	++	—	—	—	++	++	+

Note the best exercise choices for each benefit are highlighted. All modes are assumed to be performed at a moderate (not elite or low) skill level with correct technique and alignment for a minimum of 30 minutes at a time. The "Active Lifestyle" mode assumes a combination of instrumental activities of daily living (IADLs), e.g., gardening, shopping, stairclimbing and recreational or sport activities. The social opportunities category is viewed with respect to its potential to increase opportunities to socialize both within and outside the activity. The aerobic dance, circuit training, and step training modes are assumed to be supervised groups. The status of each activity is graded on the bases of a combination of research evidence, consensus, recommendations and our opinion.

Key: Significant improvements ++; Noticeable improvements +; Little or no change —

TABLE 13.3 Exercise Risk-to-Benefit Analysis Prompt Tool

Effectiveness specific prompts. Ask yourself:	Safety specific prompts. Ask yourself:	Additional exercise prescription prompts. Ask yourself:	Personal considerations
• Is it health or performance related? Is it specific to everyday activities? • Will it accommodate an interval conditioning approach? • Will it allow small incremental progressions? • Does it improve bone density? • Does it prevent or reduce falls and injuries? • Does it protect joints? • Does it improve performance and posture? • Will it increase confidence, enjoyment, social opportunity? • Will it improve long-term commitment? • Does it suit the client's lifestyle?	• Is it biomechanically and ergonomically sound according to current best practices? (For example, short treadmills and drop-handle cycles are contraindicated for older adults.) • Is it biomechanically and energetically sound when performed by the individual? (For example, treadmill walking is contraindicated for a frail beginner.) • Is it stable and symmetrical? Do the muscles pull in the correct line of force? Does it allow a controlled, pain-free range of movement? (For example, step training with inappropriate step height and inadequate support could result in unbeneficial, unsafe exercise.) • Is the speed, resistance, body position, and length of levers appropriate, effective, and safe? (For example, exercise to music with too fast a tempo is inappropriate.) • Can it be done in a controlled manner, with a linear heart rate response, easily maintained work rate, and standardized progression in small increments?	• Is it adjustable? Can it be adapted to meet the needs of the individual? • Is it comfortable for this individual client? • Is a safe setting available (at home or in the community)? For example, does the space have adequate access and sufficient space? Is it in good repair and well maintained? Does it allow safe transitions from one area or piece of equipment to another? • Does it require special equipment (e.g., hip protectors, wall, chair, saddle padding) for this individual to perform it? • Can it be part of a balanced, varied, cross-training fitness program? • Does this mode require further consultation with a physician/therapist	• Will the client perceive it as a safe exercise mode? • Does it match the client's level of training or stage of behavioral change? • Does it match the client's perceived levels of skill and fitness? • Does it meet the client's perceived functional capacity and health needs? • Is it enjoyable? • Is it motivating? • Is it realistic?

TABLE 13.4 Specific Programming Advantages of Different Exercise Modes for Older Adults

	Walking	Aerobic dance	Circuit training	Step training/ Stair climbing	CARDIOVASCULAR EQUIPMENT		WATER TRAINING		Active lifestyle
					Cycle (station only)	Treadmill	Swimming	Aqua	
Advantages									
Low cardiac risk / high cardiorespiratory and functional endurance gains	✓✓	✓	✓✓	✓	✓✓	✓	✓✓	✓	✓
Accommodates interval conditioning approach	✓✓	✓	✓✓	✓	✓✓	✓	✓✓	✓	✗
Linear heart rate response	✓	✗	✗	✗	✓✓	✓✓	✓	✗	✗
Standardized progression increments, easily controlled	✓	✓	✓✓	✗	✓✓	✓✓	✓	✓	✗
Low to medium skill level	✓	✓	✓	✗	✓✓	✓	✗	✗	✓
Low impact	✓✓	✓	✓	✓	✓✓	✓✓	✓✓	✓✓	✓✓
Low injury risk	✓	✗	✗	✗	✓✓	✓	✓✓	✓	✓
Multi-level (i.e., a range of intensity levels to meet older individual's needs and goals)	✓✓	✓	✓	✗	✓✓	✗	✗	✗	✓✓
Mixes well with other modes	✓✓	✓	✓	✓	✓	✓	✓	✓	✓✓
Client's satisfaction with progress	✓✓	✓	✓✓	✓	✓✓	✓✓	✓✓	✓	✓
No or low cost (fees, equipment, clothing)	✓✓	✓	✓	✓	✗	✗	✗	✗	✓
Can be integrated into life safely	✓✓	✓	✓	✗	✗	✗	✓	✗	✓✓
Autonomous (unsupervised)	✓✓	✓	✓	✓	✓	✓	✓✓	✓	✓✓

The best exercise choices for each advantage are highlighted. The chart assumes that all modes are performed moderately (not elite or low) for a minimum of 30 minutes at a time, with correct technique and alignment. The active lifestyle mode assumes a combination of instrumental activities of daily living (IADLs) and recreational/sports activities. The aerobic dance, circuit training, and step training modes are assumed to be supervised groups.

Key: Very good ✓✓; Good ✓; Little or not at all ✗

Training Precautions

There are a range of programming precautions that must be applied to aerobic endurance training for older adults. While championing the exceptional potential of aerobic endurance training in even the oldest old, it is important to stress that the implementation of the training precautions by the physical activity instructor to the aerobic endurance component is crucial. This is because aerobic endurance training has potentially higher risks and involves a wider range of activities and environments than any other fitness component. It is important to revisit those risks briefly before moving on to their resolution through observing the training precautions. Table 13.5 summarizes the musculoskeletal, cardiovascular, and metabolic risks associated with inappropriate aerobic exercise by older people (Fiatarone Singh, 2000).

The number of injuries and medical emergencies can be reduced for older adults by following a few simple rules (Shephard, 1984). Table 13.6 summarizes the key precautions for optimizing the benefits of endurance training for older adults.

TABLE 13.5 Risks of Inappropriate Aerobic Endurance Exercise in the Older Adult

Musculoskeletal	Cardiovascular	Metabolic
Falls (excess fatigue, loss of coordination, unsafe exercises)	Arrhythmia	Dehydration
Fracture	Myocardial Infarction (MI)	Electrolyte imbalance
Joint or bursa inflammation, exacerbation of arthritis	Hypertension	Energy imbalance
Ligament or tendon strain	Hypotension	Hyperglycaemia
Muscle rupture or tear	Ischemia	Hypoglycaemia
Skin tears	Pulmonary embolism	Hypothermia (in cold weather)
Muscle soreness	Retinal haemorrhage or detachment, lens detachment (exercising too soon after surgery)	Heat stroke
Haemorrhoids	Ruptured cerebral or other aneurysm	Seizures
Hernia	Syncope or postural instability symptoms	
Stress incontinence		

Adapted, by permission, from M.A. Fiatarone Singh, 2002, The exercise prescription. In *Exercise, nutrition, and the older woman: Wellness for women over fifty*, edited by M.A. Fiatarone Singh (Boca Raton: CRC Press), 84.

TABLE 13.6 Training Precautions for Aerobic Endurance Training in Older Adults

General exercise guidelines for older participants	When exercise should not be done
• Outdoor exercise should be avoided in extremes of heat or cold or in icy conditions. • Prescribed exercise should progress slowly and cautiously. • Exercise should never leave the participant more than pleasantly tired the following day. • There should be an adequate warm-up and cool-down. • Sudden twisting movements and forms of exercise that adversely affect balance should be avoided (eg turns of more than 90⁰). • Activity should be halted temporarily for angina, premature ventricular contractions, or excessive breathlessness.	Contraindications to exercise are covered in chapter 5. These include acute and uncontrolled or unstable health conditions. Participants and instructors must strictly adhere to those criteria. Instructors and participants should also consider a number of additional intrinsic contraindications prior to aerobic endurance training. Older adults should not exercise if they • are feeling unwell or have a fever or acute systemic illness (e.g., bronchitis, respiratory infection, rheumatoid arthritis) • have new or worsened symptoms (e.g., pain, dizziness, breathlessness, unsteadiness)

General exercise guidelines for older participants	When exercise should not be done
• Vigorous exercise should be prohibited during acute viral infections. (Shephard, 1984) • Avoid exercising indoors where the air conditioning is inadequate. • Avoid unsupported exercise if balance problems are worse than usual. • Aerobic endurance activity should be eased off and halted temporarily if the legs or arms feel so tired and heavy that coordination or quality of movement is impaired (e.g., uncharacteristic clumsiness or slight tripping). • Ensure adequate hydration before, during, and after aerobic endurance exercise. • Toileting should occur before the activity to avoid interruption. (Dinan and Skelton, 2000)	• After a recent injurious fall without medical consultation The instructor must also consider extrinsic factors: • Paint or dust fumes • Damaged or slippery flooring • Unacceptable lighting, heating, or ventilation • Objects such as pillars in the middle of the working area • Unsafe footwear (high-heeled, open-toed, or sling-back shoes or untied laces, etc.) • Unsafe clothing (wide-legged trousers, tight belts, etc.) • A ratio of more than 25 participants to one instructor • A temporary or substitute instructor who is not a specialist in physical activity for older adults
When exercise should be stopped	**When exercise can be continued**
Once exercise is underway, it should be stopped if any of the following symptoms occur: • Severe dyspnea • Dizziness • Angina (chest pain) • Extra pulse beats or abnormal heart rhythms • Nausea • Confusion • Extreme fatigue • Near syncope • Intermittent calf pain (Shephard, 1990) • New joint or muscle pain or increased pain that is unresolved by adapting the exercise (Dinan and Skelton, 2000) • General or local muscle fatigue resulting in unresolved loss of coordination in the lower limbs, tripping over own feet, bumping into others or objects, or severe loss of concentration • Unresolved loss of concentration • Of particular concern, consistently refusing or being unable to follow instructions or perform exercises and thus putting him- or herself or others at risk Particular caution should be taken by participants with a history of arrhythmia, chest pain, congestive heart failure, hypertension, or a history of falls. Medical management must be sought and symptoms controlled before resuming participation.	• When breathlessness resolves by reducing the intensity of the exercise as gauged by the Borg RPE scale or by taking an active cardiorespiratory rest • When loss of coordination, loss of concentration, or aching or burning sensations in the muscle resolve by reducing the intensity, using a seated alternative activity, changing the task • When joint pain resolves on realigning the joint or improving exercise technique All the above physical signs are normal responses to exercise.

NOTE: Learning to listen to, interpret and respond skillfully to the body's messages is the key to safer, more effective exercise. The preactivity screening, physical performance assessment, individualized program planning induction and review, and the effective teaching of motor skills are all ideal and ongoing opportunities for the physical activity instructor to educate participants about the monitoring of the signs and symptoms of exercise.

The final precautionary strategies listed in table 13.6—preactivity screening, physical performance assessment, individualized program planning, effective teaching of motor skills, and the ongoing monitoring of signs and symptoms of overexertion—cannot be overemphasized in the ongoing safety responsibilities of the physical activity instructor when preparing, supervising, adapting, and evaluating aerobic exercise for older adults. (See chapter 18 for an in-depth discussion of important motor learning principles that can be applied to the teaching of motor skills.)

Observation of your clients is particularly important before beginning any session. Eye contact can help you better assess how a client is feeling, physically and psychologically, and help you decide how best to deliver the activities you have planned for each client. Advice to a client to "take it easy" should be explicit (e.g., "Do the exercises without the arm movements" or "Do the exercises sitting down today"). In an assisted-living setting, requesting a daily health update or additional assistance is a way of meeting the fluctuating health needs of your more frail clients. Staff training also helps to raise awareness and ensure that assistance to clients is administered safely. The risks and benefits of any type of exercise ultimately depend on many factors; following the precautionary training guidelines is a crucial 'best' practice first and must include how well the exercise is taught (Evans, 1999; Dinan, 2001) (see "Instruction" section on p. 207).

Implications for Program Design and Management

Whatever the exercise type, it is important to apply the principles and adjust the variables of training as recommended and to pay particular attention to progressive overload guidelines, progressing slowly and cautiously while accommodating individual functional limitations. Regular reevaluation of the aerobic endurance component of the program is necessary to respond to clients' changing needs and preferences.

For optimal benefits from the aerobic endurance phase of an exercise program, tailor the exercises to suit the individual needs of your clients. This is particularly important in group exercise settings, where clients are likely to have a wide range of fitness levels, pathologies and disabilities, and preferences. Designing a program for aerobic fitness involves the skillful application of each of the exercise principles (specificity, overload, functional relevance, challenge, accommodation, interindividual variability, progression, and rest and recovery) and the exercise variables (frequency, intensity, time,

and type) to meet the needs and goals of each client and, whenever appropriate, of each group.

Meeting Clients' Individual Needs and Goals

When deciding how best to adapt the exercise program to address the needs and personal goals of the client, it is important that you consider the question "Fitness for what?" For example, are your clients interested in improving their level of fitness so they can more easily perform the basic and instrumental activities of daily living, or is their aim to maintain their active lifestyles or even take part in athletic competitions? Once you have identified a client's interests, you can design a multilevel program (in which graded levels of intensity and graded exercise choice(s) are modeled by the instructor) to meet group goals as well as each participant's personal goals. These goals need to be SMART aerobic endurance goals (specific, measurable, agreed on, realistic and recorded, and timed); they need to be determined through negotiation and discussion and agreed on by the whole group. When promoting aerobic endurance training, the messages you convey must be adapted to address the benefits (and goals) that older participants find sufficiently motivating (see chapter 8). The more personal, functional, and for the majority, the more social the goal, the more motivating it will be for older clients (Health Education Authority, 1997; King, Rejeski, & Buchner, 1998).

Adapting Session Structure and Content

Adaptation is the key to safe, effective aerobic endurance program design. The changes are subtle but vital. The safety margins are narrower for *all* older participants, and without sufficient care some older people may suffer more falls. To be safe, particularly during free-moving group exercise, certain exercises need to be adapted or excluded.

Exercise Selection

Factors such as speed, the warm-up and cool-down, intensity, exercise selection, and the combination and repetition of exercises can independently or collectively render a potentially safe aerobic endurance exercise into a high-risk activity for a particular older individual. The risks of certain exercises outweigh the benefits for *all* older participants.

For example, these are activities and motions that should be avoided or adapted (Dinan, 2002; Skelton & Dinan, 1999):

- No turns of more than 90 degrees; even these may need to be altered to three- or even five-point turns for frailer individuals.
- No exercises involving lateral movement of one leg across the other, in front or behind (e.g., the grapevine). Although some controlled lateral movement is necessary to master compensatory stepping to regain balance (see chapter 14), this is very different from traveling across a room at a quicker pace and in a group. The client can simply bring the feet together rather than crossing them over to retain all the proprioceptive and aerobic endurance benefits while reducing the risks to a minimum.
- No sudden changes of step, speed, direction, or level. Many instructors working with older participants fail to invite, listen to, or accommodate their clients' feedback. As a consequence, some aerobic endurance components remain too difficult for clients to perform confidently: They move too quickly or involve too many complex step patterns. This makes for elite, high-risk aerobic endurance training. Instructors must recognize that even the fittest older adult is at greater risk on days when he or she is tired or has poor concentration.

Instruction

The importance of technical, administrative, communication, observation, mentoring, and negotiation skills cannot be overemphasized for ensuring safer, more comfortable, more enjoyable sessions and, more important, enhancing effectiveness and long-term commitment. Good exercise teaching of older adults is teaching done zealously! This sums up the specialized, constant, and exceptional level of attention and application you must provide when supervising aerobic endurance training for older adults.

To provide a safe and enjoyable activity environment, the following guidelines are recommended:

- Model each exercise and transition with correct technique and speed.
- Ensure that participants can hear and understand you by projecting your voice louder and

lower, making sure your lips can be seen and that your lips move normally, and adjusting the volume of music with participants' feedback. Use body language and exaggerated hand signals for ample warning of directional changes; this also improves clarity and safety for those with hearing or eyesight problems. Ensure that, if using circuit cards, lettering and numbers are in a thick, large, plain font on a light reflective color (yellow or white) and feature simple, accurate, single-line drawings or clear photographs of an older adult exercise model.

- Perform the least challenging option yourself rather than the most difficult alternative to validate working "at your own level."
- Avoid phrases that provoke competitiveness such as "Ready, steady, go" or "See how quickly you can get from here to the wall." Instead use phrases such as "When you're ready, off you go," "Walk briskly to the wall with as much energy and efficiency as you can," "Work at your own pace; avoid slowing down or speeding up to keep pace with your neighbor."
- Observation and correction require truly seeing, not just looking; analyzing movement needs; and providing a tailored solution discreetly and effectively.
- Emphasize body awareness skills. Regularly remind clients that "We all have different body sizes, leg lengths, and health and fitness levels, and we all have different amounts of energy on different days." and that listening to your body is an important exercise skill.
- Encourage clients to take active breathers and to adjust their pace to accommodate fluctuations in health and energy, for example, "If it's one of those days when you're feeling a bit sluggish, even after the warm-up, then today isn't the day for an endurance challenge." "Take it easy," "Stay comfortable," and "You can work harder next week" are all empathetic, encouraging, commonsense reminders.
- Encourage and motivate with specific praise and a gentle sense of humor.

Checklists also work well to keep your teaching standards high. The instructional techniques checklist provided here includes a number of important questions you should ask yourself regularly:

- Am I working hard enough on my teaching technique?

- How is my teaching position? Am I moving around and demonstrating from different angles?

- Are my coaching points effective? Are they precise, plentiful, accurate, and constantly reinforced?

- Am I using advanced cuing (visual and verbal) effectively?

- Am I constantly and consistently providing multilevel adaptations of the aerobic endurance exercises and then taking the lower level myself?

- Am I really seeing what my clients are doing so that I can analyze their movements and provide tailored solutions for each individual? Am I communicating these effectively and positively?

- Am I educating my clients about the purpose and benefits of different exercises and refining their use of the Borg RPE scale?

- Am I relating my feedback to their day-to-day performance, progress, and personal goals? Do I notice and praise improvement?

- Am I reviewing the program regularly, seeing where change or progression is needed for individual clients, and setting new goals?

- Am I encouraging and implementing client feedback about the content of my sessions, the exercise environment, or my teaching?

- Am I encouraging good posture and technique (the participants' and my own) on a regular basis?

- Am I patient, polished in my teaching approach, and punctual, and do I look like I am having fun when teaching?

- Am I making time before and after each exercise session to answer clients' questions and socialize and follow up on any absences?

Summary

Aerobic endurance training has a central role in maintaining health and function as we age, yet its potential is often underestimated and underutilized. Even the oldest old can improve their $\dot{V}O_2$max, functional ability, and quality of life with aerobic endurance training. For optimal benefits, the exercise prescription for older adults must tailor exercises to suit their individual needs. This is essential in older groups where there is a wider range of initial fitness levels, pathologies, disabilities, and preferences.

Exercise prescription involves the skillful, mindful application of exercise principles (i.e., specificity, overload, functional relevance, challenge, and accommodation) and variables (i.e., frequency, intensity, time, and type) according to the best practices for older adults. Older adults need multilevel, multiactivity, multipurpose aerobic endurance programs that use interval conditioning approaches to achieve life-related cardiorespiratory gains. Injury prevention must have the highest priority; structured, thoroughly adapted programs led by a skilled, empathetic, and committed physical activity instructor can greatly minimize the risks for the older participant.

The ultimate challenge for an instructor is to follow the aerobic endurance guidelines discussed in this chapter while accommodating the heterogeneity of your older adult clients. Your goal as a physical activity instructor is to encourage long-term participation in aerobic endurance activities by ensuring that all the important exercise principles are applied and creating a training atmosphere that is sociable and fun. Adaptation is the key to safer, more effective, and more enjoyable aerobic endurance exercise for older adults.

Key Terms

Recommended Readings

Brooks, D.S. (1997). *Program design for personal trainers*. Champaign, IL: Human Kinetics.

Dinan, S. (2001). Exercise for vulnerable older patients. In A. Young & M. Harries (Eds.), *Exercise prescription for patients*. London: Royal College of Physicians, pp. 53-70.

Study Questions

1. The appropriate training intensity for a *frail* older person starting an endurance training program is
   a. 8 to 12 METs
   b. an RPE of 11 to 13
   c. an RPE of 9 to 11
   d. 5 to 6 METs

2. Which of the following statements is accurate of An Activities of Daily Living (ADLS) based program?
   a. will give health benefits similar to those of a structured aerobic endurance training program
   b. is the preferred method of aerobic endurance training for older people
   c. will not ensure sufficient intensity, duration, and variety of aerobic endurance exercise
   d. will lead to training effects similar to those of a structured aerobic endurance training program

3. Which of the following statements is true?
   a. For older people, interval conditioning is not effective for achieving the energy gains needed for everyday activities.
   b. Interval conditioning is inappropriate for older people.
   c. The three types of interval conditioning are spontaneous, fitness, and performance.
   d. Interval training and interval conditioning are equally appropriate for older participants.

4. Manipulating which variable appears to be most stressful for older adult exercisers?
   a. intensity
   b. duration
   c. frequency
   d. type

5. Which of the following is not a recommended way to apply the principle of overload to aerobic endurance training?
   a. Increase only one element at a time.
   b. Increase duration before intensity.
   c. Increase intensity before duration.
   d. Allow a minimum of two weeks for adaptation before increasing the overload again.

6. Which exercise adaptation is not recommended?
   a. standardized, minimal, incremental progressions
   b. Instructor demonstrates all levels and then selects the most challenging level.
   c. alternatives for every exercise
   d. simpler, fewer moves

7. Which aerobic endurance exercise is contraindicated for older adult exercisers?
   a. stepping
   b. hill walking
   c. exercises involving lateral movement of one leg across the other such as the grapevine
   d. turns of less than 90 degrees

Application Activities

1. An older adult client asks for your assistance to improve her stamina so that she can play tennis at a more competitive level. Describe the types of aerobic endurance activities you would include during her first four weeks in your physical activity program.

2. Design a 30-minute aerobic endurance component that is suitable for a group of older adults who are generally healthy and have been regular participants in your class for at least 16 weeks. List the specific activities you would include, and identify exercises you would exclude and any adaptations you might consider to accommodate the different functional needs of your clients. Practice teaching this component to a group of older adults, and solicit their feedback.

3. If you are currently teaching a physical activity class for older adults, have someone videotape you teaching so that you can evaluate your performance. On the teaching techniques checklist provided in this chapter, check off each question you were able to answer in the affirmative. Make note of the questions you did not check, and think of ways to improve these teaching techniques and make an action plan to implement these in your next few physical activity classes.

14

Balance and Mobility Training

Debra J. Rose

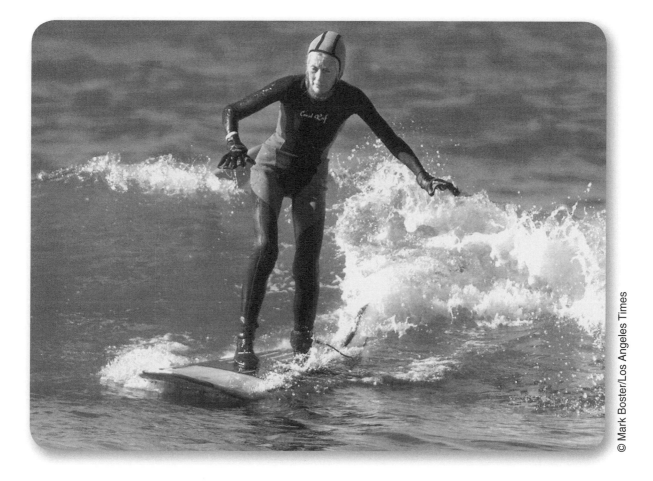

Good balance and mobility are essential to the successful performance of most activities of daily living as well as a number of recreational pursuits. In light of the fact that fall incidence rates among older adults currently pose a serious health problem in the United States and abroad, it is critical that any exercise program designed for older adults include activities specifically designed to improve older adults' balance and mobility. Both the incidence of falls and the severity of the injuries sustained increase steadily with advancing age. In the 65-and-over population, approximately 35 to 45 percent of generally healthy, community-dwelling older adults fall at least once a year, with the fall rate increasing after the age of 75 (Campbell, Spears, & Borrie, 1990; Rubenstein & Josephson, 2002). As a result of age-related declines in multiple physiological systems that lead to reduced muscle strength and flexibility, slower central processing of sensory information, and slowed motor responses, even a relatively mild fall could be potentially dangerous for an older adult (American Geriatrics Society, British Geriatrics Society, and American Academy of Orthopedic Surgeons Panel on Falls Prevention, 2001).

The good news is that in recent years, activities to improve balance and mobility have become increasingly evident in physical activity classes designed for older adults. What is less evident, however, is whether the chosen activities adequately target the multiple dimensions of balance and mobility in a systematic and progressive manner. Unlike other parameters of fitness such as strength, flexibility, and aerobic endurance, it is often not until the first fall that older adults realize that their balance system is significantly impaired.

The primary goals of this chapter are first to briefly describe the important age-associated changes in multiple body systems that affect balance and mobility and then to provide examples of the different types of balance activities that best address each of these age-related changes. The final section of the chapter presents instructional strategies for manipulating the challenge offered by a balance activity in a way that matches but does not exceed the intrinsic capabilities of the older adult client.

Before describing the age-associated changes in balance and mobility it is important to first define some terms in the context of this chapter. **Balance** can be defined as the process by which we control the body's **center of mass** (**COM;** i.e., the balance point or location about which all the segments of the body are evenly distributed) with respect to the base of support, whether it is stationary or moving (Rose, 2003). For example, when standing upright in space, our primary goal is to maintain the COM within the confines of the base of support. This aspect of balance is often referred to as **static balance.** Conversely, when we are walking, the COM is continuously moved beyond the base of support and a new support base reestablished with each step taken. Maintaining balance while leaning or moving through space is often referred to as **dynamic balance.**

Another term used frequently throughout this chapter is **mobility.** This term describes our ability to independently and safely move from one place to another (Patla & Shumway-Cook, 1999). Adequate mobility is required for many different activities we perform during our daily lives, including transfers, climbing or descending stairs, walking or running, and a variety of sport and recreational activities.

Age-Associated Changes in Balance and Mobility

Irrespective of how physically active we are throughout the course of our lives, certain inevitable age-associated changes occur in the multiple body systems that contribute to balance and mobility. While some of these changes have no observable effect on how well certain balance and mobility-related tasks are performed in different environments, other changes adversely affect dimensions of balance and mobility. For example, changes that affect multiple systems simultaneously (e.g., sensory, cognitive, and motor) or are compounded by existing medical conditions such as diabetes or

arthritis can be expected to affect not only the strategy older adults use to perform a certain balance task but whether they choose to perform it at all.

Although a number of age-associated physiological changes have been described in chapter 4, it is important that you understand how changes in the sensory, motor, and cognitive systems are likely to specifically affect the balance and mobility of your older adult clients. You will then be better able to decide what type of balance and mobility activities are most appropriate for your older adult clients. In general, age-associated changes in the peripheral and central components of the sensory and motor systems and changes in various cognitive functions, (i.e., attention, memory, and executive processing) have all been shown to alter the quality and speed with which tasks are performed, even by healthy older adults. The peripheral and central components of the sensory and motor systems are illustrated in figure 14.1.

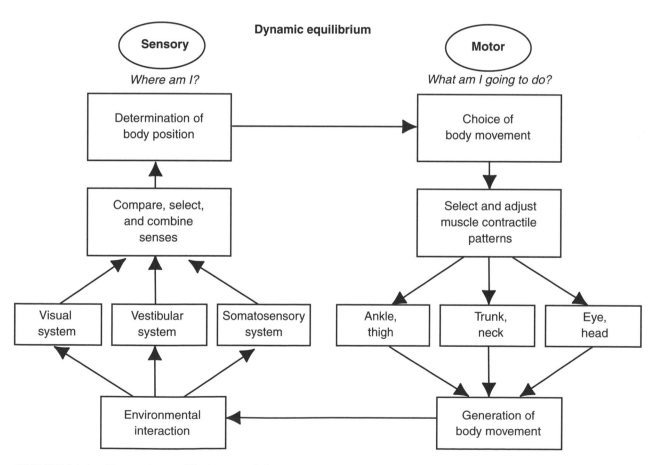

FIGURE 14.1   Dynamic equilibrium model.

Reprinted, by permission, from NeuroCom International Publications, 1990, "Illustration of Dynamic Equilibrium Model."

Sensory System Changes

The sensory systems that contribute to balance are the visual, somatosensory, and vestibular systems. Changes in the peripheral and central components of each of these systems affect balance and mobility to some degree. For example, the age-associated changes in the visual system that adversely affect an older adult's ability to perform a variety of balance and mobility activities include reduced visual acuity, narrowing of the field of vision, decreased depth perception, and loss of contrast sensitivity. Reduced visual acuity can also result from certain eye diseases, such as macular degeneration or cataracts. Any narrowing or blurring of the visual field makes it increasingly difficult to clearly discern the edges and shapes of objects in the environment. Any reduction in the peripheral visual field can also be expected to affect dynamic balance and mobility in particular because of the greater head and trunk rotation needed to see the missing information.

A decline in the ability to see depth affects an older adult's ability to safely negotiate obstacles, climb and descend stairs, and participate in sporting activities that require the accurate estimation of an object's position in space (e.g., tennis, golf, softball or baseball). Changes in contrast sensitivity make it more difficult to detect objects against a background or rapidly adjust to changes in lighting when moving from a brightly lit room into a dark corridor.

Age-associated changes in the somatosensory (i.e., touch and proprioception) system have a direct impact on postural stability and the ability to quickly restore upright control after an unexpected loss of balance. In addition, age-associated changes in **kinesthetic sensibility** (i.e., the conscious awareness of limb position and movement) also affect an older adult's ability to perform certain balance activities, particularly when vision is not available or is distorted (e.g., in busy or moving visual environments). A decline in the number of **cutaneous receptors** in the skin that detect pressure and vibratory sensations (i.e., Pacinian corpuscles) also affects both the speed and efficiency of different types of postural responses (Bruce, 1980). In addition to receptor loss, a decline of as much as 30 percent in the number of sensory fibers innervating the peripheral receptors has been observed with increasing age. These changes result in reduced somatosensation and greater reliance on the visual and vestibular systems for sensory information.

> Older adults can improve their ability to balance and move in altered sensory environments because the sensory systems are very adaptable, or amenable, to change.

Finally, age-associated reductions in the density of vestibular hair and nerve cells and a moderate reduction in the gain of the **vestibular-ocular reflex (VOR)** in the inner ear or vestibular system can also be expected to negatively affect postural control (Paige, 1991; Wolfson, 1997). Because the VOR helps stabilize vision when the head is moved quickly, any reduction in the gain of this reflex affects older adults' ability to accurately determine whether it is the world or they who are moving in certain situations. In addition to assisting with the correct positioning of the head and body with respect to gravity, the vestibular system becomes critical for balance when sensory information is not available from the other two sensory systems or when the information being provided by one or more of the other systems is not congruent (not in agreement) with the information coming from the vestibular system. This is called **sensory conflict** and can lead to a momentary loss of balance or even a fall in some cases. We often experience moments of sensory conflict during our daily lives when an object, usually moving through the peripheral visual field, leads us to believe that we are moving instead of the object. Sitting in a car at a traffic light and suddenly thinking that our car is rolling when it is the car next to us that is moving is an example of this type of sensory conflict.

Collectively, changes in each of the three sensory systems often result in slower processing and integration of sensory inputs and an inability to control the level of body sway when the amount of available sensory information is reduced. Among healthy older adults, the amount of body sway is most affected when somatosensory and visual inputs are distorted or absent (Woollacott, Shumway-Cook, & Nashner, 1986). The encouraging news is that the sensory systems are very adaptable, and if older adults are presented with progressively more challenging physical activities that involve these types of altered sensory conditions, they can learn to adapt their postural responses appropriately (Hu & Woollacott, 1994). One example of an appropriate activity is to have an older adult practice standing on a foam or moving surface with the eyes closed or while reading a poem. Standing on foam makes it more difficult to use somatosensory inputs, while engaging vision in the performance of a second task or removing it altogether effectively negates its use for maintaining upright balance. Additional balance and mobility activities that address this issue are presented in a later section of this chapter.

Motor System Changes

An increase in the time required to plan and then execute an appropriate motor response appears to be the greatest consequence of the age-associated changes in the motor system (Spirduso, 1995). Many older adults also begin to experience difficulty selecting the appropriate movement strategy to use in a given movement situation. Inappropriate **scaling** (i.e., adjustment of movement parameters, such as force, to match the action plan to the demands of the task or environment) of the selected response strategy is also evident in many cases. That is, older adults exhibit a tendency to over- or underrespond, particularly when their balance is unexpectedly perturbed or disrupted.

Electromyographic (EMG) studies have further shown significant age-related differences in the temporal sequencing of muscle activation patterns in response to unexpected losses of balance. Unlike the stereotypical and symmetrical patterns of muscle activation observed in younger adults, apparently healthy older adults exhibit considerably more variable activation patterns and a decline in their ability to inhibit inappropriate responses (Stelmach, Phillips, DiFabio, & Teasdale, 1989). Inappropriate postural responses are most evident when the functional base of support is reduced (e.g., standing sideways on a narrow beam), when the support surface is compliant or unstable (e.g., standing on a foam surface or rocker board), or when visual input is altered (e.g., visual environment moves so that vision no longer provides accurate information for balance; Alexander, 1994). Real-world equivalents of these experimental conditions include putting on a pair of trousers while standing on one leg (reduced base of support), walking across a grassy or slippery surface (standing on

foam or a rocker board), or walking along a busy city street (moving visual environment).

Age-associated changes in the anticipatory component of **adaptive postural control** have also been documented (Frank, Patla, & Brown, 1987; Inglin & Woollacott, 1988) and may be an important contributor to falls among older adults. Adaptive postural control describes our ability to modify the sensory and motor systems in response to changing task and environmental demands (Shumway-Cook & Woollacott, 2001). This type of control can be anticipatory (e.g., changing from one type of surface to another in good lighting, carrying objects while walking) or reactive (e.g., tripping over an undetected obstacle, being bumped in a crowd).

The research findings suggest that older adults are increasingly unable to activate the postural muscles required to stabilize the body before the muscles responsible for executing the movement are activated (e.g., activating the stabilizing muscle groups in the trunk and lower legs before pulling on the handle of a door). The reactive component of adaptive postural control is also affected with age. Specifically, healthy older adults are slower to execute a stepping response after an unpredictable loss of balance, even though their reaction to the loss of balance is not appreciably longer than that of young adults (Thelen, Wojcik, Schultz, Aston-Miller, & Alexander, 1997).

Other researchers have also demonstrated that healthy older adults are more likely to take multiple steps following a perturbation (Luchies, Alexander, Schultz, & Ashton-Miller, 1994; McIlroy & Maki, 1996). Coupled with the decline in absolute muscle strength and power described in chapter 4, these changes in the central and peripheral components of the motor system compromise an older adult's ability to make anticipatory and reactive postural adjustments quickly and efficiently. As is the case with the sensory systems, however, physical activities designed to challenge the motor system can significantly improve an older adult's ability to respond more quickly and appropriately when balance is compromised.

Changes in Cognition

One of the most noticeable cognitive changes observed with aging is an inability to perform multiple tasks simultaneously without compromising postural stability (Shumway-Cook, Woollacott, Baldwin, & Kerns, 1997). Recovering balance after

Older adults find it particularly challenging to perform multiple tasks at once because of age-associated changes in attention.

an unexpected perturbation also requires more attention for older adults than for young adults (Brown, Shumway-Cook, & Woollacott, 1999). These research findings suggest that older adults can find it particularly challenging to perform multiple tasks at once, particularly if one of those tasks involves the maintenance of postural stability. This knowledge is important for selecting balance exercises that require attention to be distributed across multiple tasks or that involve a high cognitive component.

Balance and Mobility Exercises

A wide variety of balance and mobility activities should be considered an essential component of any well-rounded physical activity program. At least 10 to 15 minutes during every class or personal training session should be allocated to balance and mobility activities. Balance and mobility activities can also be incorporated into the warm-up and cool-down sections (see chapter 10) in addition to the core component of the class. Another way for more advanced clients to incorporate balance activities is to perform selected strength and flexibility exercises in a balance-challenging environment. For example, clients can perform certain upper-body strength and flexibility exercises while sitting on a balance ball or standing on a foam pad. Remember that your primary goal when presenting balance and mobility activities to your older adult clients is to challenge but not exceed their intrinsic capabilities by systematically introducing increasingly complex balance and mobility tasks that can be performed in a variety of practice environments that simulate those encountered in daily life. A simple model of the factors that interact to affect mobility and balance is illustrated in figure 14.2.

You should vary either the task or environmental demands in a way that matches your client's individual capabilities. Two additional guiding

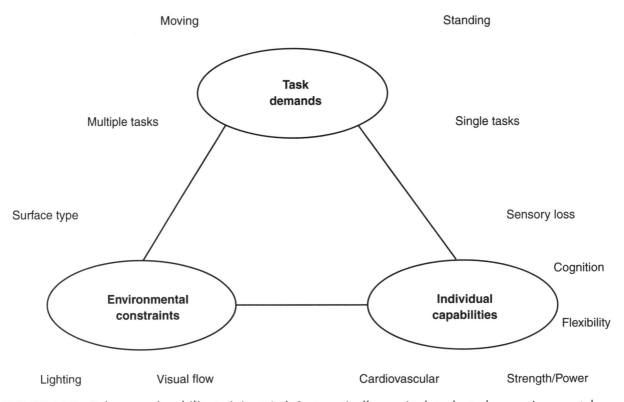

FIGURE 14.2   Balance and mobility training triad. Systematically manipulate the task or environmental demands of a balance activity to challenge but not exceed the individual capabilities of your clients.

Reprinted, by permission, from D.J. Rose, 2002, "Promoting functional independence in older adults at risk for falls: The need for a multidimensional programming approach" *Journal of Aging and Physical Activity* 10 (2): 207-225.

principles should be applied to determine which of the two variables to manipulate and when: First, if the goal is to tune up the motor system, it is most appropriate to alter the task demands of a particular balance and mobility activity. One easy way to manipulate the task demand is to perform a balance activity while standing or moving through space rather than sitting on a stability ball.

If the goal is to tune up each of the sensory systems that contribute to good balance and mobility, then your goal should be to manipulate the environment in which the task is performed. Our sensory systems are most receptive to changes in the environment. This manipulation can be done by having the client perform balance activities with reduced or no vision or while standing on a compliant or moving surface. Additional ways to manipulate the task or environmental demands and thereby alter the challenge of a particular balance or mobility activity are presented in table 14.1.

Four skills considered essential to good balance and mobility should be the focus of your efforts in this component of the program. These skills are (a) the voluntary and involuntary control of the center of mass (COM), (b) sensory integration and organization, (c) selection and scaling of postural strategies, and (d) development of a flexible and adaptable gait pattern. Let us now consider the

types of balance and mobility activities you can use to train each of these skills and how you can manipulate the practice environment or demands of the task for systematic progression.

Voluntary and Involuntary Control of the Center of Mass

The balance and mobility activities presented here are designed to improve the ability to maintain a more upright and steady position in space (static balance activities) or to move the body through space with greater control, speed, and confidence (dynamic balance). In addition, these exercises are also designed to improve adaptive postural control abilities (anticipatory and reactive) through manipulation of the task and environmental demands. Calling these the "belly button control" exercises readily conjures up an image in clients' minds of the body part that must be manipulated to maintain postural control. A few examples of seated, standing, and moving activities suitable for this type of balance training are shown in figure 14.3. Many more balance and mobility activities appropriate for training each of the four essential skills at multiple functional levels are presented in *FallProof: A Comprehensive Balance and Mobility Program* (Rose, 2003).

TABLE 14.1 Manipulating Task and Environmental Demands

	Easy	More difficult	Most difficult
TASK DEMAND			
Arm position	In contact with seat surface	Resting on thigh	Folded across chest
Base of support	Feet together	Feet in tandem stance	Single-leg stance
Pacing of exercise	Self-paced (own speed)		Externally paced
Length of movement sequence	Single activity	3 to 4 sequential movements	6 to 8 sequential movements
Additional task	Cognitive (e.g., counting backward)	Self-paced manual task (e.g., reaching)	Externally paced manual task (e.g., catching)
ENVIRONMENTAL DEMAND			
Lighting	Dim room lights	Dark glasses	Closed eyes
Support surface (seated)	Balance disk on chair	Stability ball (with holder)	Stability ball (no holder)
Support surface (standing)	Thin foam (0.25 inch, 0.6 cm)	Dense foam (2-4 inches, 5-10 cm)	Balance disk(s)

Balance challenge can be further increased by combining two or more task or environmental demands.

Seated balance activities (with eyes open and closed)

Equipment needed: Chair with or without backrest and arms, balance disks, stability balls

1. Sitting upright in space, first with eyes focused on a target and then with eyes closed, visualizing same target
2. Voluntary arm movements through space (single arm or both arms moving horizontally, vertically, and diagonally)
3. Voluntary trunk movements through space (leaning forward, backward, and diagonally from hips, rotating trunk to right and left)
4. Voluntary leg movements (heel and toe raises, marching, single-leg raises)
5. Dynamic weight shifts through space (shifting COM away from and back to midline in multiple directions, shifting to multiple positions in space without pausing at midline)
6. Dynamic body movements against gravity (bouncing up and down, front to back, and side to side)
7. Perturbations (push or pull at hips or at hips and shoulders) applied with varying force, with altered support surface to increase balance challenge

Standing balance activities

Equipment needed: Foam squares of different thicknesses, balls, benches of different heights, colored spots

1. Standing upright with changing base of support (feet together, tandem stance, single-leg stance), first with eyes open then with eyes closed
2. Dynamic weight shifts through space (leaning away from midline in multiple directions; shifting weight from side to side, forward and back, and diagonally)
3. Dynamic weight transfers through space (marching in place and while turning, forward and backward stepping, lunging in multiple directions, stepping up onto and off benches of different heights)
4. Kicking stationary and moving balls toward a target
5. Perturbations (push or pull at hips or at hips and shoulders) applied with varying force, with altered support surface to increase balance challenge

Moving activities

Equipment needed: Masking tape, colored spots, balance disks, small objects, various pieces of equipment to create obstacle courses, resistance bands

1. Walking with altered base of support: Tandem walking on a line or narrow beam, toe walking, heel walking
2. "Crossing the river." Lunge across an area marked by two lines that are moved increasingly farther apart, then return to starting position. Alternatively, attempt to step or jump across area.
3. "Rock hopping." Place colored spots at different distances apart within same area as in previous activity. Each client moves "down the creek" stepping only on spots. To increase challenge, (a) replace spots with balance disks for more instability, or (b) place small objects on floor within the area that clients must retrieve as they progress along the creek.
4. Design obstacle courses that require participants to control the COM during static activities (e.g., stepping up onto foam and standing with feet together for 10 seconds before moving to next obstacle) and dynamic activities (e.g., do tandem walking on a narrow beam in the obstacle course). To increase the balance challenge, you can place objects on the floor or at other levels that clients must place in a basket that they carry through the course.
5. Resistance-band walking. While client walks, partner or instructor increases and releases tension on a band wrapped around the hips.

FIGURE 14.3   Seated, standing, and moving balance activities.

Involuntary control of the COM can also be practiced in a seated, standing, or moving environment. Either you or a trusted assistant can deliver small, quick perturbations (pushes or pulls) to the individual seated on a ball or standing. These can be applied at the level of the hips, shoulders, or hips and shoulders simultaneously to prompt a small amount of trunk rotation during the perturbation. Quickly pushing the ball on which the client is seated is also an effective method of causing perturbation. To force clients to involuntarily or reactively control the COM, it is important that they be unaware that the perturbation is about to occur. Applying different amounts of force to the body or ball also keeps the client guessing.

Resistance bands can also be used to perturb balance in a moving environment. As the client attempts to walk around the room, the instructor or a partner first applies tension to a resistance band that is wrapped around the client's waist and then unexpectedly releases the tension, forcing the client to make a rapid postural adjustment. Because these activities pose a great challenge to older adults' balance abilities, it is very important to pay careful attention to creating a safe practice environment. Spotting less balanced clients during each activity and positioning clients close to a wall or sturdy chair for additional support are effective ways to promote safety.

Be sure to observe how quickly and efficiently the client is able to respond to unexpected perturbations. A client with good reactive balance control will respond quickly to the unexpected loss of balance in a direction opposite the direction of the push or pull. Unfortunately, this type of activity can be performed only once or twice before the client begins to change his or her postural set to one that is prepared for the perturbation. Once this happens, your client demonstrates the ability to anticipate rather than to react to an unexpected perturbation. While this is also an important aspect of balance to practice, recognize that their postural control has shifted from reactive to anticipatory. Teaching clients how to respond to an unexpected or even an expected perturbation better prepares them for being jostled in crowds, opening doors, or tripping on uneven sidewalks.

Sensory Integration and Organization Activities

The instructional ideas presented in this section are designed to optimize the use of each of the three sensory systems that contribute to balance. If there is no indication in the client's medical history of impairment of the sensory system that you want to challenge, then the primary goal for this set of balance activities is to construct a practice environment that encourages the older adult to use one particular sensory system more than another to maintain balance. Medical conditions that indicate impairment in a specific sensory system include macular degeneration and cataracts (vision), peripheral sensory neuropathy (somatosensory system), and Ménière's disease (vestibular system). If there is evidence of impairment in a particular sensory system, your goal is helping the client to compensate for that loss.

For example, eye diseases such as macular degeneration or glaucoma seriously impair an older adult's use of vision to control balance. In this case, your goal would be to help the client learn how to better use somatosensory and vestibular inputs to compensate for the losses in the visual system. As another example, if an older adult client has a history of diabetes that has adversely affected his or her ability to sense touch and pressure beneath the feet (i.e., peripheral neuropathy), you would have that client practice balance activities to teach them how to better use the unimpaired visual and vestibular systems.

When working on improving your older adult clients' sensory organization and integration skills, you should follow the second guiding principle presented earlier in the chapter: manipulate the environment rather than the task demands initially. Most of the seated, standing, and moving balance activities presented in figure 14.3 can be used to improve your clients' sensory organization and integration skills.

In addition to reviewing each client's health and activity questionnaire and the results of any balance testing you conducted at the outset of the program (see chapter 6 for a discussion of appropriate balance tests), you are well advised to observe your clients' behavior while they stand on a firm surface with their eyes closed and then on a foam surface with eyes open and closed. Of course, if the functional level of your clients made it possible for you to administer the Fullerton Advanced Balance Scale described in chapter 6, you will already have a good idea of your client's performance in each of these different sensory conditions. Being able to stand steady on a firm surface with the eyes closed requires good use of somatosensory inputs, while standing on foam with eyes open and then closed requires the effective use of vision when the eyes are open and the vestibular system when the eyes are closed. If any of your clients perform any of these activities poorly, you should make sure that they begin multisensory activities in a seated position or with additional manual support (assistant, wall, or sturdy chair). Although the most effective way to evaluate impairments in each of the three sensory systems that contribute to good balance is by using computerized dynamic posturography (see chapter 7), the required equipment is usually available only in clinical rehabilitation settings.

Somatosensory System Activities

If your goal is to increase clients' reliance on somatosensory inputs for controlling balance, you should have them practice progressive balance activities both on a firm, broad surface *and* with reduced or absent vision. These exercises can be performed while seated, standing, or moving, depending on each individual's intrinsic capabilities. While some clients find it challenging enough to perform certain seated exercises with vision reduced (e.g., wearing sunglasses), others have no difficulty performing standing or moving balance activities with their eyes closed. The important thing is that the surface be firm so that they can derive as much sensory information from the surface as possible. Teaching clients to better use the somatosensory system for controlling balance can measurably increase their safety when performing activities in dark or poorly lit environments (e.g., going to the bathroom in the middle of the night, entering movie theaters after the lights have been lowered, walking outside at night).

Visual System Activities

Although it is a commonly held belief that adults rely on vision more than any other sensory system, many older adults do not use it very efficiently for controlling their balance and mobility. To help your older adult clients better use vision for balance, it is important to teach them how to fixate their eyes on specific targets in space. While they are performing a balance activity in a seated or standing position, they should be verbally cued to fixate on a target directly in front of them and at eye level. A vertical target, such as a door jam or line on the wall, is a particularly good target to choose.

In addition to actively coaching older adults to fixate on a target, it is also important to alter the surface under the feet to distort the information provided to the somatosensory system (see figure 14.4). Have clients perform balance activities while seated with their feet on a compliant or moving surface (rocker board, balance disk) or while standing on the same types of surfaces. Begin to increase the balance challenge by introducing head movements to a particular balance activity. It is still important to verbally cue clients to fixate their gaze, but now they must fixate for a shorter period of time as the head or body turns during an activity. Using vision more effectively helps older adults perform a number of daily activities with greater efficiency. Examples include walking with greater confidence and stability when they are out in the community, maintaining their balance more effectively when the head or body is turned to greet a friend, or watching for approaching cars as they cross a two-way street.

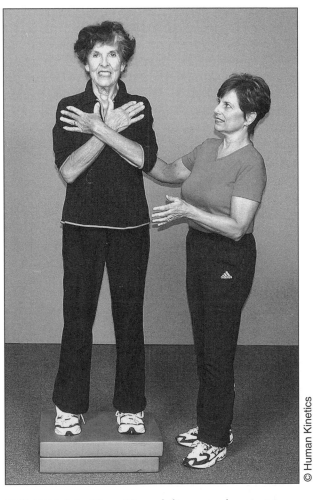

FIGURE 14.4 The older adult must rely on vision to maintain balance when standing on a compliant or moving surface.

Vestibular System Activities

The third sensory system important for balance is the vestibular system. Unfortunately, many older adults experience balance problems that are related to changes in this system. These changes are caused not only by advancing age or the medical conditions described earlier but also by the tendency for older adults to engage less frequently in physical activities that require high-velocity head movements (e.g., spinning, jumping, certain sports) as they grow older. This reduced head movement likely compounds the age-associated changes in the peripheral and central components of the vestibular system.

To tune up the vestibular system, it is necessary to practice activities that make it difficult to get the information needed for balance from either the visual or somatosensory systems. Have your older adult clients perform various balance activities while their feet are in contact with a compliant or moving surface (foam, rocker board) and their eyes are either involved in a second, non-balance-related task (e.g., reading aloud, tossing and catching objects) or closed. Because it is now difficult to use two of the three sensory systems for balance, you will observe higher levels of sway during these activities. It is therefore important both to know your clients' abilities before they try any of these more challenging activities and to provide a safe practice environment in which to perform them. Start with less-challenging seated activities, or position clients close to a wall or behind a chair for additional support when performing standing exercises.

Improved use of the vestibular system positively affects the performance of a number of daily activities, including walking on uneven surfaces at night, maintaining balance when the head is tilted back in the shower, and maintaining balance when turning the head quickly. In some cases, repeating vestibular system activities can result in less susceptibility to dizziness during activities that require fast head or body turns.

Each of the three sensory systems can be improved by manipulating the environmental demands associated with a balance activity. Ways to do this are summarized in table 14.2. Because many of the activities described are challenging for many older adults who have medical conditions that affect one or more sensory systems (e.g., macular degeneration, diabetes, Ménière's disease), extra safety precautions are needed to ensure the safety of your clients. In this section of your balance and mobility component, it is particularly important to apply the principles of challenge and accommodation discussed in chapter 9.

Selecting and Scaling Postural Strategies

At least three clearly defined postural strategies have been described in the research literature (Horak, 1994; Nashner & McCollum, 1985). These are referred to as the ankle, hip, and step strategies and are used either to control sway in a forward and backward direction or to reestablish a new base of support when the limits of stability have been exceeded (see figure 14.5). These postural strategies are used individually and in various combinations to help maintain or control balance while performing a variety of tasks. For example, the ankle strategy controls sway while standing, the hip strategy is used when leaning into a cupboard or dishwasher to retrieve an item, and the step strategy when tripping over a pet or a child's toy.

TABLE 14.2 Environmental Manipulations for Sensory Systems

Sensory system	Environmental manipulation
Vision	Verbally encourage gaze fixation (i.e., keeping eyes on a target at eye level); alter surface under buttocks and feet in seated activites and under feet during standing and moving activities
Somatosensory	Reduce or remove vision (e.g., dimmed room lights, dark glasses, closed eyes) or engage vision in a second task (e.g., reading, reaching for objects); perform all activities on a firm, broad support surface
Vestibular	Reduce or remove vision or engage vision in a second task; perform all activities on a compliant or moving support surface

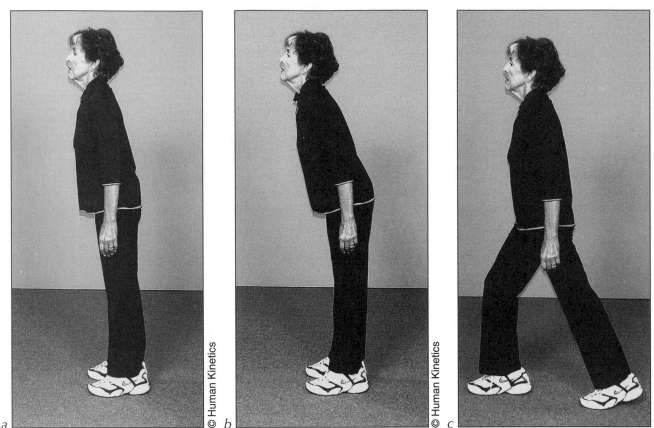

FIGURE 14.5   Three postural strategies have been identified: *(a)* ankle, *(b)* hip, and *(c)* step.

Manipulating either the task or the environment in at least four different ways enables your older adult clients to practice each of these strategies: (a) maintaining balance while standing on different support surfaces (e.g., firm, compliant, moving, narrow), (b) voluntarily swaying farther away from midline in different directions and while standing on different support surfaces, (c) trying to minimize the amount of sway when the body is externally perturbed, and (d) making adjustments in body position in anticipation of a destabilizing limb movement (e.g., stepping over an obstacle).

Ankle Strategy

Voluntarily swaying in a forward and backward direction is one way to practice the ankle strategy. To ensure that the ankle joints are controlling the sway, the speed of the sway must be slow and the distance leaned in either direction small. Check that the upper and lower body are moving in the same direction during this activity and that the heels do not lift off the floor. This is a nice activity to include in a cool-down segment. It is also an excellent means of reinforcing somatosensation or kinesthetic sensibility by verbally cuing clients to focus on the changing pressure under the feet as they sway forward and backward. Chairs can be placed in front of and behind the client so that he or she can focus on touching the chair in front with the hips on the forward lean and the chair behind with the buttocks on the backward lean. This reinforces moving the upper and lower body together during the activity. Place the chairs close enough to ensure this type of movement.

This activity can be combined with another one called the "honey pot." Clients are asked to imagine that their bodies are stirring sticks and their job is to stir the honey forward and backward, side to side, and then in a circular motion, first clockwise and then counterclockwise. The application of small, unexpected perturbations (pushing or pulling action) at the level of the hips is another way to practice using the ankle strategy more subconsciously. A person with good balance can respond to the perturbation with a quick countermovement initiated at the ankles.

Hip Strategy

The hip strategy can be practiced by simply swaying in a forward and backward direction at a faster speed and over a larger distance than for the ankle strategy. Manipulating the task demands in this way necessitates the use of the larger hip muscles to control the sway. Unlike the coupled movement of the upper and lower body that characterizes a movement controlled by the ankles, the upper and lower body become uncoupled during the hip strategy and move in opposite directions: The upper body moves forward as the lower body moves backward. This is an excellent follow-up activity to the ankle strategy activity just described. You can clap your hands or use a metronome to pace the sway.

You can also force a more subconscious use of the hip strategy by having clients stand sideways on a narrow beam or on top of a half foam roller (see figure 14.6). Because the support surface is now narrower than the length of the feet, it becomes more difficult to use the ankle strategy to control sway. You can elicit the use of a hip strategy in your stabler clients by having them reach for an object held at various distances at or above eye level. A progressively larger perturbation at the hips also forces the client to counter the loss of balance using the hip rather than ankle muscles.

Step Strategy

Finally, activities that force your clients to exceed their **limits of stability** (i.e., the maximum distance a person can lean away from a centered position in any direction without moving the feet) require the use of the important step strategy to prevent falls. Simply increasing the challenge of balance activities performed on different surface types is usually sufficient to stimulate the use of this strategy. You can also apply progressively larger external perturbations at the hips to force a step.

No matter which postural strategy your clients practice in a session, carefully observe whether they select the appropriate strategy and scale it appropriately for the task demands. For example, watch to see if a client begins to use a hip strategy even when swaying at a slow speed over a small distance. Watch also to see if the size and type of postural response match the amount of force you applied in

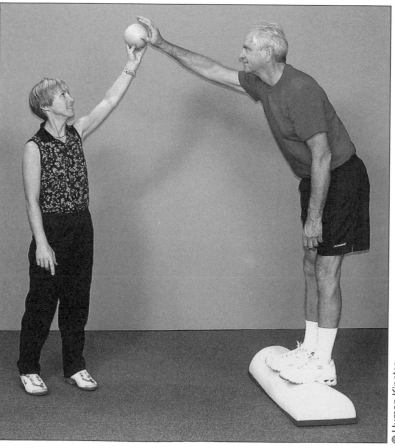

© Human Kinetcs

FIGURE 14.6 Reaching for objects while standing on top of a half foam roller encourages the use of a hip strategy to control balance.

an external perturbation. Many older adults, even healthy ones, often choose to take multiple steps in response to a perturbation, even though the force applied could have been managed using a hip or ankle strategy.

With sufficient practice and increased confidence in their balance abilities, your older adult clients likely will require fewer steps to restore balance or will resort to a step strategy less often. Given that very few older adults voluntarily practice losing their balance on a daily basis, it will likely take some time for them to reacquire an efficient step strategy. The more often you present activities that require them to lose their balance, the more quickly they are likely to learn how to restore it. Just be sure to provide a safe and confidence-building practice environment, and do not increase the difficulty of balance activities too quickly. A summary of how to manipulate the task or environmental demands to elicit each of the movement strategies described is provided in table 14.3.

Gait Pattern Activities

Perhaps the best way to help your older adult clients achieve a flexible and adaptable gait pattern and also improve their overall coordination and agility is through activities that require them to walk at different speeds using a variety of different gait patterns. For example, have them walk around the room on their toes, on their heels, or using a longer and wider than normal stride, side-step, braid, stop quickly or change directions on command, and even walk backward. You can use the tempo of music very effectively here to set different gait speeds and pause it periodically to see how quickly the client stops walking. These are wonderful activities for the warm-up routine, and if they are performed long enough, they can also improve aerobic endurance.

Manipulating the Challenge in a Group Setting

By carefully manipulating the balance challenge for each client during the balance and mobility component of the program, you can have a group of older adult clients perform the same balance activities at the level that best matches their individual abilities. For example, a group can perform the same set of seated weight-shift activities but at different levels of task difficulty; simply manipulate the task or environmental demands appropriately for each individual. For example, to make it easier for some clients to perform seated dynamic weight shifts, they can perform the activity while sitting on a balance disk placed on a chair and holding on to the chair (a stabler support surface). Conversely, more advanced clients can perform the same set of dynamic weight shifts while sitting on a stability ball with arms folded across the chest. This illustrates applying the exercise principle of challenge by matching the task demands to the individual's current capabilities (see figure 14.7). You can also manipulate the challenge of this group activity by manipulating the environmental demands of the activity. Some clients in the group may only be ready to perform the dynamic weight shifts with their eyes open and feet in a wide base of support on a firm surface, while others may be able to do the same activities with their eyes closed and their

TABLE 14.3 Manipulations to Elicit the Ankle, Hip, or Step Strategy

Strategy	Manipulation of task or environment
Ankle	Forward-backward sway over short distance at slow speed (voluntary control) Small external perturbations (involuntary control)
Hip	Forward-backward sway over large distance at fast speed (voluntary control) Standing sideways on narrow beam or half foam roller Forward reaching if standing position is stable (voluntary control) Medium-sized external perturbations (involuntary)
Step	Leaning forward, backward, or to the side until limits of stability are exceeded (voluntary control) Large external perturbations in standing position (involuntary control) Walking against resistance band that is unexpectedly released (involuntary control)

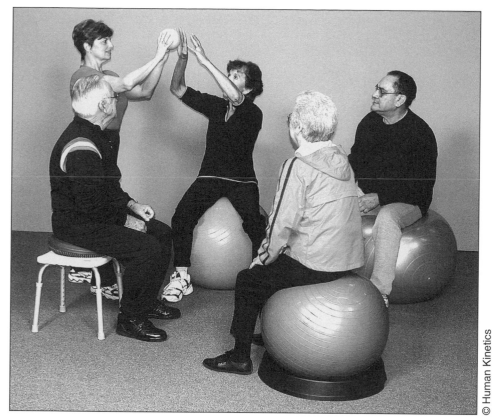

FIGURE 14.7 Different levels of challenge can be achieved in a group setting by having clients sit on different support surfaces.

© Human Kinetics

feet in a narrow base of support or with foam under their feet. Through careful manipulation of the task and environmental demands, you can accommodate many different functional levels of most of the activities in the balance and mobility component of the program.

Summary

Given that balance abilities are critical to safe mobility and the prevention of falls, it is essential that specific activities targeting the multiple dimensions of balance and mobility be an integral component of a well-rounded physical activity program. These activities should address four essential skills needed for good balance and mobility: the voluntary and involuntary control of the center of mass, sensory integration and organization, selection and scaling of postural strategies, and development of a flexible and adaptable gait pattern. Two guiding principles for the effective implementation of activities designed to improve each of these essential skills were presented in this chapter: To tune up the motor system, alter the task demands, and to tune up the sensory sys-

tems, alter environmental demands. Progressively increasing the balance challenge for each essential skill by adding non-balance-related tasks (e.g., counting backward, reading aloud, catching objects), the cognitive contributions to balance (i.e., attention, memory, and executive control) are also enhanced.

Hopefully, this chapter has expanded your knowledge about balance and mobility and has provided you with a good rationale for choosing balance activities for an exercise program for older adults. Of course, to become really proficient in this specific area of exercise programming requires more specialized knowledge and practical training. Reviewing the recommended readings and completing additional training to become a certified balance and mobility specialist can help you obtain this additional expertise.

Key Terms

Recommended Readings

Rose, D.J. (2003). *FallProof! A comprehensive balance and mobility program.* Champaign, IL: Human Kinetics.

Tennstedt, S. (Ed.). (2003). Falls and fall-related injuries. *Generations, 26*(4).

Study Questions

1. In which of the following situations is adaptive postural control most likely to be needed?

   a. during an unexpected loss of balance
   b. when changing from a firm to icy surface
   c. when carrying a load of laundry up a flight of stairs
   d. b and c

2. The combined role of the sensory systems is to

   a. determine the visual layout of the environment
   b. assist in the planning of actions
   c. create sensory conflict that must be resolved by the CNS
   d. determine where our body is in space

3. Sensory conflict occurs when

   a. the sensory information provided by the three sensory systems is not congruent
   b. the sensory systems become overloaded with sensory inputs
   c. the vestibular system provides inaccurate information
   d. vision has been reduced or removed

4. Healthy older adults tend to sway most when

   a. vision is reduced or absent
   b. vestibular information is distorted
   c. somatosensory inputs are distorted
   d. vision is not available and somatosensory inputs are distorted

5. If your goal is to improve the motor system's contribution to balance and mobility, which of the following variables should you manipulate first?

   a. environmental demands
   b. task demands
   c. the individual's capabilities
   d. a and b

6. Which of the following is *not* an example of manipulating a task demand?

   a. altering the position of the arms during an exercise
   b. reducing the base of support
   c. adding a second non-balance-related task
   d. altering the support surface

7. To improve the use of the somatosensory system for balance, you should

   a. remove vision and alter the support surface
   b. alter the support surface only

    c. remove vision and distort vestibular inputs
    d. reduce or remove vision only

8. Which of the following activities will encourage the older adult to use a hip strategy to control balance?

    a. reaching for objects while standing sideways on a narrow balance beam
    b. a perturbation of large intensity
    c. swaying forward and back over a large distance at a fast speed
    d. a and c

Application Activities

1. Describe *one* balance activity you would use to improve the use of the (a) somatosensory system, (b) visual system, and (c) vestibular system. Develop a seated, standing, and moving version of the activity.

2. Design a balance and mobility program component for a class of community-residing older adults who have been enrolled in your class for approximately four weeks. Describe how you would manipulate the challenge of each exercise to accommodate the different functional levels of your clients.

Part IV

Specialty Programs and Training Methods

TRAINING MODULE 1:
Overview of Aging and Physical Activity

TRAINING MODULE 2:
Psychological, Sociocultural, and Physiological Aspects of Physical Activity and Older Adults

TRAINING MODULE 9:
Ethics and Professional Conduct

TRAINING MODULE 3:
Screening, Assessment, and Goal Setting

TRAINING MODULE 8:
Client Safety and First Aid

International Curriculum Guidelines for Preparing Physical Activity Instructors of Older Adults

TRAINING MODULE 4:
Program Design and Management

TRAINING MODULE 7:
Leadership, Communication, and Marketing Skills

TRAINING MODULE 6:
Teaching Skills

TRAINING MODULE 5:
Program Design for Older Adults With Stable Medical Conditions

Now that you know how to apply core programming principles and training methods to design physical activity programs for older adults, it is time to learn the basics of some specialty programs for older adults. Part IV introduces you to mind–body exercise, aquatics program principles, and the more specialized training methods that are used in the training of master athletes. Chapters 15, 16, and 17 provide information recommended in training modules 4 and 5. Module 4 includes information about how to use results from screening, assessment, and client goals to make appropriate decisions regarding individual and group physical activity and exercise program design and management. Chapter 17 also introduces you to a new topic not included in the international curriculum guidelines—how to develop a sport-specific training program for master athletes.

• Chapter 15 describes two popular mindful exercise forms, yoga and tai chi, and discusses their relevance to contemporary exercise programming for older adults. The fundamental components of traditional mindful exercise, its benefits, and important precautions for imple-menting mindful exercise programs for older adults are also discussed. Finally, chapter 15 presents helpful strategies and sample mind-body exercise sequences and relaxation techniques that can easily be incorporated into any well-rounded physical activity program for older adults.

• In chapter 16 the topic of aquatic exercise is discussed, including how it can be used to address the special needs of older adults with dif-ferent functional levels and medical conditions that preclude their participation in land-based exercise programs. Special considerations for teaching aquatic exercise and important safety precautions for working in aquatic settings are also discussed.

• Chapter 17 introduces you to specialized training techniques for older adults who want to participate in competitive sports and athletic events. The chapter begins with a description of age-related changes in competitive sport perfor-mance and their physiological and psychological underpinnings. The chapter then describes how to develop sport-specific training programs for master athletes, including strategies for prevent-ing overtraining and injury.

15

Mind–Body
Exercise Training

Ralph La Forge

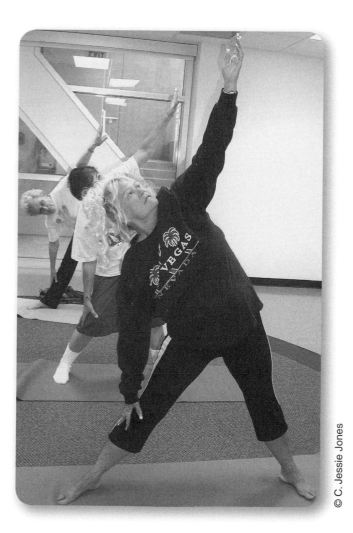

In recent years the popularity of what has come to be called mind–body exercise, or mindful exercise, has burgeoned. Conventional body-centered aerobic and muscular fitness exercise programs clearly enhance cardiorespiratory endurance, musculoskeletal fitness, and psychological well-being, but they most often neglect qualities of mind and spiritual development. In contrast, mind–body exercise integrates a disciplined contemplative or introspective process with moderate-level physical exercise to enhance mental development, self-observation, posture, muscular flexibility, and balance. Mindful exercise is characterized by an intentional and non judgmental mental focus, breath, and the perceptive movement of positive energy. Rather than focus on performance, choreography, or improving fitness, the center of attention with most forms of mindful exercise is kinesthesis (awareness of body movement) itself. Your clients will find these qualities beneficial in addressing specific concerns of aging, such as depression, decreased self-efficacy, a deterioration of musculoskeletal health and balance control, and an increase in fall-related injuries.

The purpose of this chapter is to briefly introduce the essential tenets of mindful exercise, describe several forms of mindful exercise appropriate for older adults, and provide a list of useful education and training resources. It is not the intent of this chapter to disseminate all that is necessary to competently teach yoga, tai chi, or qigong exercise classes per se. Each form of mindful exercise addressed here requires hundreds of hours of personal exploration to attain a sufficient level of teaching skill and knowledge of that system's tradition. Therefore, please consider this chapter to be a brief and hopefully inspiring introduction to these ancient forms of expressive and contemplative exercise.

Mindful Exercise

A mind–body orientation to exercise combines a cognitive or mindful component with low- to moderate-intensity physical effort or movement. Although it has eluded a precise, universal definition, **mind–body exercise,** or **mindful exercise,** is defined in this chapter as physical exercise executed with a profound, inwardly directed, contemplative focus. This inwardly directed attention is nonjudgmental of self. Self-focus includes specific attention to breathing and proprioception, or "muscle sense." Clearly, any exercise modality can integrate this inner attentiveness; however, this is the key process in mindful exercise. Mindful exercise prioritizes this meditative state for self-observation. From the viewpoint of someone who is unfamiliar with yoga, the popular cobra pose may appear to be nothing more than a back extension exercise. Internally, however, the yogi's cognition is entirely and deeply entrained on the simple kinesthesis of the pose and breath centering—noth-

> Mind–body exercise, or mindful exercise, has often been described as a moving meditation or introspection where intentional physical movements are coordinated with the breath.

ing more and nothing less. Many older adults find these attributes beneficial in managing fitness and health concerns.

Over the last century, numerous forms of mindful exercise have grown out of the classic traditions of **qigong,** tai chi, and **yoga. Pilates,** neuromuscular integrative action **(NIA),** the **Alexander technique,** and the **Feldenkrais Method** are among the more mature mindful exercise methods in that they have been reasonably well studied or their techniques have been largely standardized. Figure 15.1 provides a simple taxonomy and description of some of the mindful forms of exercise that have gained considerable popularity in recent years.

Component Criteria for Mindful Exercise

For mindful exercise to be optimally fulfilling, it will require more than merely adding a cognitive component to conventional physical activity. Ideas about what constitutes mindful exercise, at least in a contemporary sense, are likely to metamorphose over the next decade as newer interpretations and programs evolve. A number of authorities have suggested the following criteria for mind–body exercise; that is, mindful exercise should integrate the following features:

- **Meditation** or **contemplation.** Mindful exercise is noncompetitive, focused on the present moment, nonjudgmental, and introspective and is process centered rather than strictly outcome or goal oriented.

- **Proprioceptive awareness.** Mindful exercise is characterized by relatively low-level muscular activity coupled with mental focus on muscle and movement sense. Kinesthetic imagery has also been used to describe this component.

- Breath-centering or breath work. The breath is frequently cited as the primary centering activity in mind–body exercise. Many breath-centering techniques are used in yoga, tai chi, and qigong exercise.

- Anatomic alignment (e.g., spine, pelvis) or proper physical form. Disciplined practice of a particular movement pattern or spinal alignment is a characteristic of many forms of mind–body exercise such as hatha yoga, Alexander technique, Pilates, and tai chi. Note that not all mindful exercise forms use set, sequential choreography or disciplined anatomical alignment. Exceptions include NIA and expressive ethnic dances (e.g., Native American spiritual dance or hula) that exhibit free-form movement.

Classic	Contemporary
Qigong, also known as Chinese health exercise, is a simply choreographed exercise for regulating internal energy (qi) to improve health, calm the mind, and improve fitness.	**Neuromuscular integrative action (NIA)** uses an internally directed approach inspired by yoga, tai chi, aikido, Alexander technique, and jazz dance movements. Unlike most other mindful exercise programs, NIA also includes moderate-level aerobic endurance activities.
Tai chi chuan is a complex martial arts choreography of 108 movements that is practiced for health, meditation, and self-defense. There are many forms and styles of tai chi chuan.	**Pilates** is an orderly system of slow, controlled, distinct movements that demands a profound internal focus. This method can be performed with using special pieces of equipment (e.g., Reformer cadillac) or without equipment (floor and mat work).
Hatha yoga, the physical aspect of yoga, includes a vast repertoire of physical postures, or *asanas,* done seated, standing, or lying prone or supine on the floor. The effort to maintain equilibrium ultimately becomes the stimulus for self-empowerment.	The **Feldenkrais Method** includes both verbal (Awareness Through Movement) and nonverbal (Functional Integration) methods of gentle, nonstrenuous exercise designed to reeducate the nervous system.
	The **Alexander technique** is a method that transforms neuromuscular habits by helping an individual focus on sensory experiences to correct unconscious habits of posture and movement that may be precursors to injuries.

FIGURE 15.1 Simple taxonomy of mindful exercise.

- Focus on **energy.** The perceptive movement and flow of one's intrinsic energy, vital life force, **chi,** or other positive energy are described in many classic mindful exercise programs.

Benefits of Mind–Body Exercise

Over the last decade, a growing body of scientific evidence has supported various mindful exercise modalities as a means of significantly improving various aspects of health, particularly cardiovascular risk factors, psychological well-being, and disease-related symptoms. For example, some yoga and tai chi programs have been shown to be particularly beneficial for older adults with chronic conditions such as arthritis, asthma, and chronic fatigue syndrome (Garfinkel, 1994; Manocha, Marks, Kenchington, Peters, & Salome, 2002; Manchanda, 2000). The slow, contemplative nature of these exercise forms has also been shown to reduce stress-related symptoms such as anxiety, high blood pressure, and depression while improving neuromuscular control (Ray, Mukhopadhyaya, Purkayastha, Asnani, Tomer, Prashad, et al., 2001; Murugesan, Govindarajulu, & Bera, 2000; Janakiramaiah, Gangaadhar, Murthy, Harish, Subbakrishna, Vedamurthachar, et al., 2000; Savic, Pfau, Skoric, Pfau, & Spasojevic, 1990). Because of the relatively low heart rate and blood pressure response to many mind–body exercise forms (e.g., tai chi), such exercises offer a relatively safe alternative to higher-energy-cost activities for older adults who are deconditioned or disease prone. The following list summarizes the research-supported benefits of yoga and tai chi practice (Berger & Owen, 1992; Schell, Allolio, & Schonecke, 1994; Province, Halley, Hornbrook, Lipsitz, Miller, Mulrow, et al., 1995; Telles, 2000; Schmidt, 1997; Wang, Lan, & Wong, 2001; Wolf, Barnhart, Kutner, McNeely, Coogler, & Xu, 1996):

Cardiorespiratory Benefits

- Decreased resting blood pressure
- Increased pulmonary function (e.g., increased one-second forced expiratory volume)
- Improved respiratory function in patients with asthma
- Increased parasympathetic tone, increased heart rate variability
- Decreased blood lactate and resting oxygen consumption

- Enhanced arterial endothelial function
- Increased maximal oxygen consumption and physical work capacity
- Slowed progression of coronary artery disease
- Improved cardiovascular disease risk factor profile (e.g., reduced blood lipids)

Musculoskeletal Benefits

- Increased muscular strength and flexibility
- Increased neuromuscular balance
- Improved posture
- Decreased fracture risk and fewer falls for older adults

Psychobiological Benefits

- Increased cognitive performance
- Improved relaxation and psychological well-being
- Decreased stress hormones (e.g., cortisol)
- Decreased anxiety and depression scores
- Reduction in frequency of panic episodes
- Reduced physiological and psychological response to threat or stress
- Decreased symptoms associated with pain, angina, asthma, and chronic fatigue

Other Benefits

- Increased physical functioning in older people
- Improved glucose tolerance
- Decreased glycated hemoglobin and C-peptide levels in type 2 diabetes
- Improvement in baroreflex sensitivity
- Decreased obsessive-compulsive disorder symptoms
- Decreased osteoarthritis symptoms
- Decreased carpal tunnel symptoms

Mind–Body Exercise Programs

This chapter briefly explores three forms of mindful exercise: basic **hatha yoga, taiji qigong,** and **pranayama** (breathing training). Young and old alike have practiced each of these mindful exercise arts for centuries in many countries throughout the world, and each has spawned numerous styles that are well-suited for older adults.

Yoga

Perhaps the origins of all mind–body exercise programs lie in the Eastern disciplines of yoga and qigong. The focus of these disciplines is to open up the body to a vital life force with balance (i.e., a harmonious state of being). In yoga, this energy is called **prana,** the masculine energy, which resides above the diaphragm, and **apana,** the feminine energy, residing below the diaphragm. It has often been said that the highest goal of yoga is recognition of self. Yoga translated means *union* but also *discipline* or *unitive discipline.* The union refers to an integration of mind, body, and spirit. Hatha yoga is the physical aspect of this discipline and includes a vast repertoire of physical postures, or **asanas,** that are performed while seated, standing, or lying prone or supine on the floor. The effort to maintain equilibrium ultimately becomes the stimulus for self-empowerment. Hatha yoga itself is centuries old, and most of the yoga styles that are practiced in the West today are derived from these early forms.

The principal challenge of nearly all styles of hatha yoga is proficiently handling increasing amounts of resistance (i.e., complexity and degree of difficulty) in the various postures and breathing patterns while maintaining a steady and comfortable equilibrium of mind and body, which is quieting of thoughts and relaxing body tension. A beginning 20-minute hatha yoga session for an apparently healthy older adult may blend several yoga styles into one program. The session starts and ends with a **savasana** (corpse pose) to ensure deep mental and physical relaxation. The yoga poses between the two savasanas should sequentially exercise a variety of spinal, postural, and limb muscle groups and are held for 30 seconds to one minute each. It is paramount that yogic breathing, of which there are many different techniques, be synchronized with each pose so that there is no time during the asana that the breath is held. As a general rule, yogic breathing is combined with yoga exercise in a very logical way. Whenever a yoga movement or pose expands your chest or abdomen, you inhale. Conversely, when a movement contracts or compresses your chest or abdomen, you exhale. It is also important that the yoga instruc-

Although there are many forms of yoga, restorative yoga, a derivative of the Iyengar yoga tradition, is most appropriate for older adults because of the elementary nature of the poses. Restorative yoga uses props such as blankets, pillows, and bolsters.

tor manually guide each participant through each pose during the first few sessions to ensure proper musculoskeletal alignment, safe body positioning, and proper breathing. Props (e.g., blankets, neck and lumbar rolls, and bolsters) are very helpful in the early stages of hatha yoga training to help the individual achieve safe and proper alignment while minimizing musculoskeletal stress.

There are many styles of hatha yoga that differ in their historical derivation, poses, difficulty, and depth of integrated breath work and mindfulness. The restorative, vini, Iyengar, and Kripalu forms of hatha yoga are relevant styles for older adults. For example, **restorative yoga,** a derivative of the Iyengar yoga tradition, is appropriate for older adults who are just embarking on a yoga program because of the use of props and the elementary nature of the poses. Judith Lasater (1995) and others have popularized this style of hatha yoga for a variety of populations, including older adults, with much success.

We should differentiate a *yogic lifestyle* from participation in hatha yoga, Iyengar yoga, and power yoga classes such as those taught in yoga studios and fitness centers in the United States. Those who engage in yogic lifestyles, while perhaps not in full compliance with the historical yogic teachings, generally engage in daily dietary practices, meditation, spiritual centering, and regular yoga exercise, whereas the routine practice of hatha yoga poses may or may not include dietary or other lifestyle changes. This is an important point because some reported outcomes in yoga research are based on following yogic lifestyle principles, which clearly transcend the mere practice of yoga exercise.

Yogic Breathing

In the yogic and qigong traditions, breathing is seen as an intermediary between the mind and body. Breath centering itself is an independent method of reducing anxiety and increasing relaxation in the short-term and increasing psychological well-being in the long term. For this reason, breath work is beneficial to older adults as a simple but important means of integrating mind and body. In the beginning stages of breath training, the physical activity instructor should help the participant develop the ability to (a) sustain relaxed attention to the flow of the breath, (b) refine and control respiratory movements, and (c) integrate awareness and respiratory functioning in order to reduce stress. Quiet **diaphragmatic breathing** (deep abdominal breathing) through the nose rather than the mouth is optimal. Each breath is intentionally slow and deep with an even or smooth effort. Sovik (2000) describes optimal breathing as diaphragmatic, nasal (inhalation and exhalation), deep, smooth, even, quiet, and free of pauses. Breathing needs to be coordinated with movements. Inhaling accompanies opening movements (e.g., arms opening away from the body), while exhaling accompanies closing movements (e.g., arms moving back to the body).

Following is a simple introductory diaphragmatic breathing exercise that is therapeutic in and of itself:

1. Lie flat on your back, and place one hand on your chest, the other on your abdomen (i.e., corpse pose, or savasana). Place a small pillow or folded blanket under your head.

2. Take 10 to 15 slow, deep breaths. Expand your abdomen during inhalation, and contract your abdomen during exhalation while keeping your chest as still as possible.

3. Keep inhalations and exhalations smooth without pauses in between.

Hatha Yoga Sequences for Older Adults

There are countless yoga poses and sequences that can be effectively incorporated into a well-rounded fitness program for older adults. Examples of poses that are appropriate for apparently healthy older adults in a beginning hatha yoga program are shown in figure 15.2. It is important that you provide close supervision and clear instructions when first introducing these routines to your clients.

Each pose should be held for three to six breaths. The beginning and ending savasana pose (figure 15.2a) should be held for four to five minutes. More poses can be added as the participant progresses. Each pose requires individual mental, musculoskeletal, and breathing adjustments to be properly executed with minimal stress on the joints, muscles, and spine. Increased relaxation, psychological well-being, muscular strength, flexibility, and balance can be realized after only two to three weeks of yoga practice. Months to years of regular practice may be required to achieve optimal benefits.

Figure 15.2 illustrates hatha yoga poses (asanas) that are appropriate for most older adults. The hatha yoga poses can serve as a component of a warm-up before aerobic or resistance exercise or as a cool-down. However, five to eight minutes of low-level aerobic exercise before the yoga poses increases muscle temperature and improves the initial muscular flexibility that is required by even the most basic pose. It is also important to screen your participants for existing musculoskeletal problems, especially in the neck and low back. Remember, with yoga, slow progression is good!

Tai Chi and Taiji Qigong

Tai chi (short for tai chi chuan or taijiquan) is only one form of the more ancient practice of qigong (Chinese health exercise). **Tai chi chuan** involves learning a progressive series of movements eventually comprising 108 flowing, graceful movements (in the Wu style). It can be practiced for health, meditation, and self-defense. There are numerous styles of tai chi (e.g., Chen, Yang, Wu). Some styles include a short form that may be more appropriate for older adults.

When teaching tai chi movements, it is important to help your clients understand how to integrate and synchronize breathing with their movements, for the breath is a principal pathway for energy **(qi)** to flow throughout the body. As in hatha yoga, the movements and breathing must be coordinated so that your students can achieve an unimpeded flow of energy. **Tai chi chih,** developed by American Justin Stone, is a simpler form of tai chi chuan and consists of a series of 20 movements and one ending pose. Qigong exercise, also known as Chinese health exercise, also involves a simpler set of movements than its martial arts relative tai chi. Many qigong styles are named after animals whose movements they imitate (e.g., dragon, crane, snake, wild goose, and animal frolics styles).

Another mind–body exercise that is especially appropriate for older adults is taiji qigong, a blend of tai chi and qigong exercises (Tse, 1995). One form of taiji qigong consists of only 18 movement forms that can be easily incorporated into your activity program. Figure 15.3 illustrates a series of basic qigong exercise movements that can be

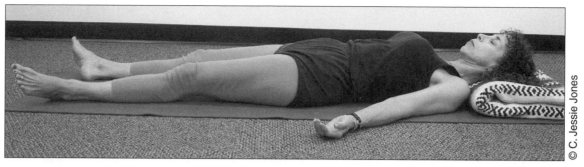

a savasana

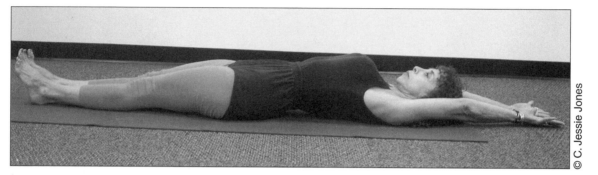

b arm raise

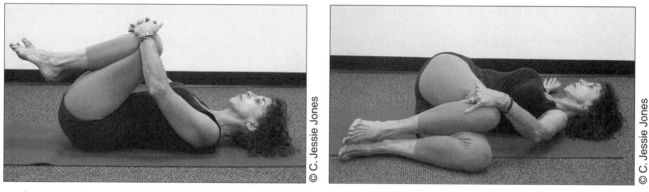

c knees to chest

d lying twist

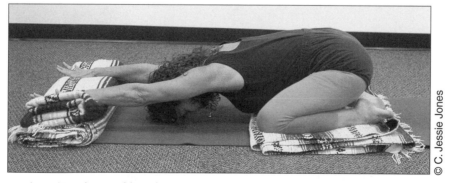

e kneeling forward bend

FIGURE 15.2   Hatha yoga poses (asanas): (a) savasana, (b) arm raise, (c) knees to chest, (d) lying twist, (e) kneeling forward bend (half-tortoise), (f) mountain pose, (g) half-moon pose, (h) one- and two-leg supine leg stretch, (i) standing forward bend with wall support, and (j) downward-facing dog.

(continued)

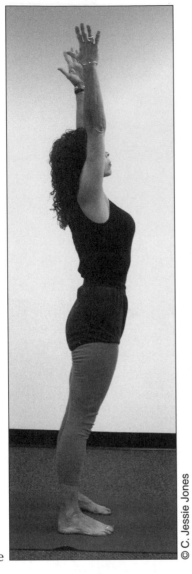

_f_ mountain pose

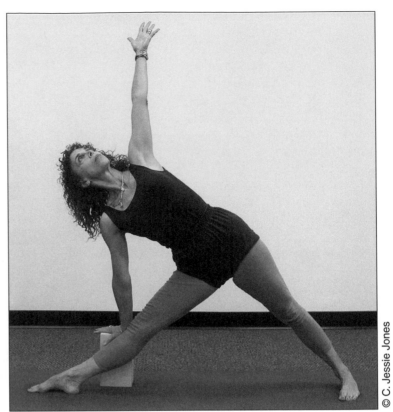

_g_ half-moon pose

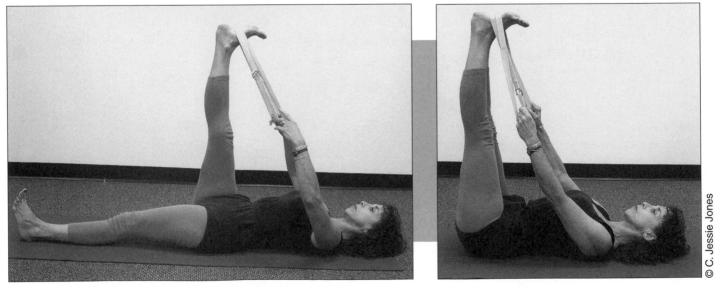

_h_ one- and two-leg supine leg stretch

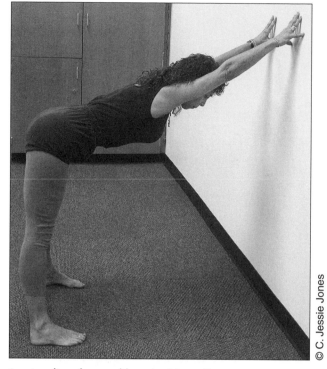

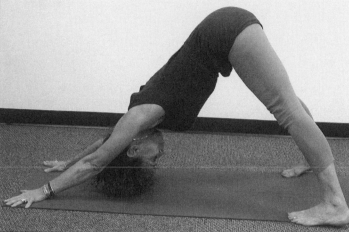

© C. Jessie Jones

© C. Jessie Jones

i standing forward bend with wall support

j downward-facing dog

practiced in the early stages of learning qigong or tai chi. As in almost all mind–body exercise, breathing should be coordinated with the movements. According to qigong tradition, inhaling brings positive qi into the body and usually accompanies an opening movement, while exhaling releases negative qi and accompanies a closing movement. Like the yoga sequence illustrated earlier, taiji qigong is ideal as a preparation for higher-intensity aerobic exercise or as a cool-down.

Implications for Program Design and Management

Select characteristics of mindful exercise can be effectively integrated into conventional exercise routines to further improve relaxation, mental focus, and musculoskeletal health. These are some methods to incorporate mindful exercise characteristics into an existing exercise program for older adults:

• Create the atmosphere for mindful exercise by exercising in a quiet and moderately illuminated space or outdoor area. Such settings are conducive to settling the mind and reducing unnecessary

mental tension. The instructor should use a low but clear voice and display a supportive, caring attitude. Music that is appropriate for the intensity and cadence of the movement can be relaxing and inspiring.

• Meditation and breathing exercises can be added to an existing warm-up and cool-down. For example, begin the warm-up session with three to five minutes of quiet contemplation or meditation, and then progress to low-level aerobic or flexibility exercise. One to two minutes of breathing exercise can also be added here. End the entire exercise session with a similar meditation component.

• Incorporate mindfulness in the aerobic or strength phase of an exercise session. This works best with low- to moderate-intensity aerobic or strength exercise (e.g., 30 to 60 percent of maximal effort or aerobic capacity). Doing flexibility exercise, low-level cycling, slow muscular contractions during strength training, or walking more mindfully can be quite rewarding. For example, during low-level cycling exercise, ask participants to focus nonjudgmentally on present muscle sensations while synchronizing slow abdominal breathing with every two or three pedal revolutions.

• Add any of the yoga poses illustrated earlier in this chapter to the flexibility or strength-training components of the program. Alternative reclining or sitting postures illustrated in *Lasater's Relax and Renew* reference effectively inserted between resistance-training exercises can increase flexibility and offer a welcome period of relative rest and energy restoration (Lasater, 1995).

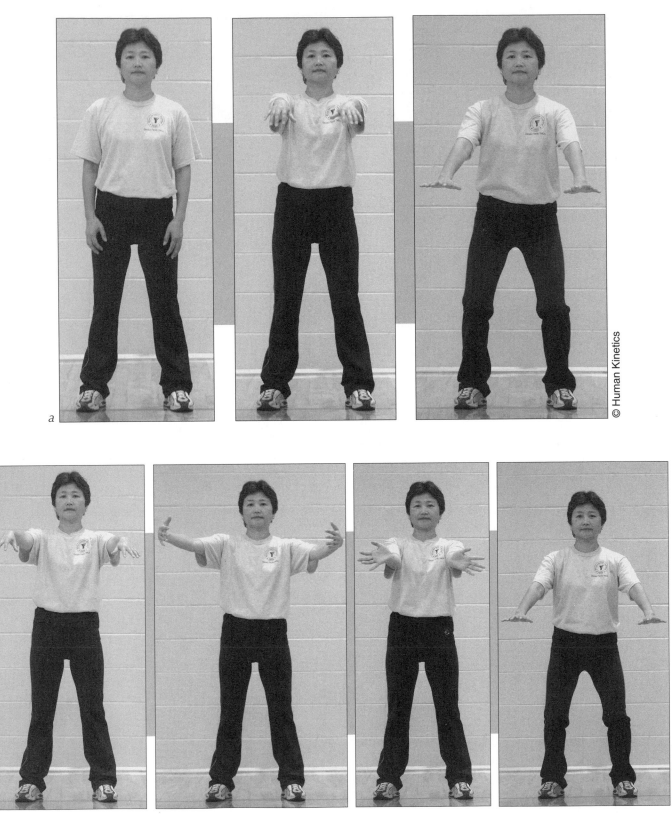

FIGURE 15.3   Basic qigong exercise movements: (a) taiji start, (b) opening the chest, (c) shou gong (balancing qi).

From Michael Tse's book *Qigong for Health and Vitality* (1995).

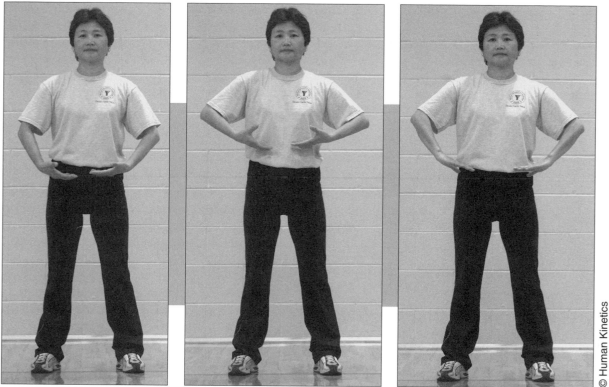

© Human Kinetics

C

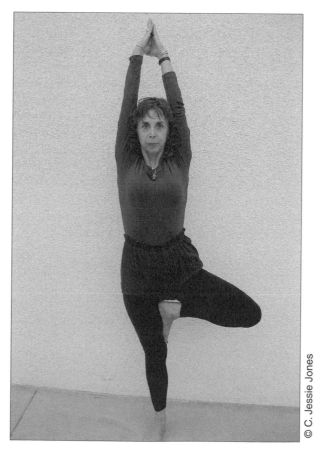

© C. Jessie Jones

FIGURE 15.4   Tree pose.

• Incorporate the popular tree pose as part of a circuit of exercises for your clients. This pose helps stimulate balance control. The tree pose, shown in figure 15.4, starts with a slow exhalation while assuming a one-leg stance on the right foot. Bend your left knee and place the sole of your left foot, toes pointing down, on the inside of your right leg between your knee and your groin. As you inhale, bring your arms over your head and join your palms together. Hold this pose for three to five breaths in the beginning sessions, and six to eight breaths in later sessions. Repeat on the opposite leg. Using a nearby table or wall for support is helpful in early stages of training for this pose.

Mindful Exercise Precautions

Many older adults have suboptimal balance control. Therefore, complex tai chi or yoga choreography that increases the probability of a fall should be avoided, or the choreography should be significantly modified during the early stages of participation. For example, too many consecutive complex yoga poses can exceed older adults' capacity to adequately adjust their foot placement, trunk, and spine alignment in a timely fashion.

Because many styles of hatha yoga involve acute, dynamic changes in body position, it is important to understand the hemodynamic and cardiac ventricular responses to such exercise and how these can alter cardiac function in people with diagnosed cardiovascular disease, hypertension, metabolic syndrome, or diabetes. Inverted poses where the head is below the heart (e.g., downward-facing dog or headstands) and inverted poses that alternate with a head-up pose should be avoided, at least during the early stages of a yoga program. In most cases, individuals who are initially deconditioned or who have chronic disease should (a) minimize acute changes in body position that require the head to be below the heart in early stages of hatha yoga training or (b) use slower transitions from one yoga pose to the next.

Because Ashtanga and Iyengar yoga sequences generally require considerable strength, flexibility, and mental concentration, they should be reserved for the high-functioning older adults in your program (e.g., clients with over 12-MET exercise capacity). Some yoga poses and sequences, such as the rapid sun salutation sequence, that quickly move the body and head down and up can significantly increase blood pressure and may also be inappropriate for older adults with stage II or higher hypertension (i.e., blood pressure equal to or greater than 160/105 mmHg). DiCarlo and coauthors (1995) discovered significantly greater systolic and diastolic blood pressures in Iyengar yoga practitioners than in people who did moderate treadmill walking (less than 3 miles, or 4.8 kilometers, per hour). These findings, however, do not preclude the practice of Iyengar yoga by well-conditioned participants.

Yoga and Tai Chi Teacher Training Resources

There are no less than 1,200 teacher training and certification programs for prospective yoga, tai chi, and qigong teachers. Unlike conventional exercise instructor certification programs (e.g., American College of Sports Medicine, American Council on Exercise, Senior Fitness Association), the vast majority of these programs do not follow consensus standards for exercise and health assessment, program implementation, and exercise safety. This does not mean that no mindful exercise teacher certification programs are competently taught. One promising new professional body governing the training and certification of yoga teachers is the Yoga Alliance. A number of excellent annual conferences and workshops can introduce you to the cultural foundations of, teaching considerations for, and personal experience with hatha yoga, tai chi, and qigong. Several noteworthy examples include *Yoga Journal*'s Annual Yoga Conference, the annual New York City Yoga Conference, the annual IDEA Yoga Conference, and the Annual National Qigong Gathering of the National Qigong Association.

Physical activity instructors of older adults are encouraged to become familiar with the basic tenets of at least the classic forms of mindful exercise for two reasons. First, this knowledge can reduce the unfortunate misconceptions many people still have of yoga, tai chi chuan, and qigong. For example, there is the false assumption that one must be Hindu or an Asian Indian to gain the full benefits from hatha yoga practice or that difficult contorted poses are the basis of all yoga practice. Another incorrect assumption is that slow intentional movements, such as those demonstrated in qigong exercise, are at too low of an intensity level to induce meaningful, health-related benefits. Many contemporary mindful exercise methods, such as NIA and contemporary martial arts, were developed on a platform of qigong or yoga culture and exercise specifically to retain some of the early culture but also to extend the mindful benefits. Second, through a better grasp of the culture and health and fitness benefits of these forms of exercise, physical activity instructors of older adults can more confidently refer clients to qualified mindful exercise teachers, perhaps even inspiring personal interest and participation. Following is a list of selected yoga and tai chi teacher training resources:

- Yoga Alliance, www.yogaalliance.org, 877-964-2255
- Kripalu Center for Yoga and Health, 800-741-7353
- YogaFit International, info@yogafit.com, 310-376-1036
- Yoga for the West Teacher Training Course by Mara Carrico, 760-942-4244
- Wild Mountain Yoga Center, www.wildmountainyogacenter.com, 530-265-4072

- Integrative Yoga Therapy, www.cruzio.com, 800-750-9642
- East West Academy of Healing Arts (qigong), www.eastwestqi.com 415-285-9400
- Qigong Institute, www.qigonginstitute.org
- Qigong Association of America, www.qi.org
- National Qigong Association USA, www.nqa.org, 888-815-1893
- Justin Stone's Tai Chi Chih, www.taichichih.org

Summary

Mindful exercise continues to emerge as an effective exercise modality and nonpharmacologic approach to treating a variety of disorders common in older adults. There is scientific evidence that hypertension, insulin resistance, anxiety, pain, cardiovascular disease, and depression all favorably respond to regular participation in mindful exercise such as tai chi, qigong, and hatha yoga. The core benefits of these programs include increased balance, strength, and flexibility as well as immediate relaxation and mental quiescence. Regular, self-regulated mind–body exercise can be ideal for older adults because of its portability and relatively low intensity. The physical activity instructor can play a role by integrating one or more characteristics of mindful exercises into existing physical activity classes and by encouraging facility management to offer dedicated mind–body classes.

It is not beyond reason that in the near future mindful exercise guidelines and professional resources will be included in respected exercise consensus publications that recommend the appropriate quality and quantity of exercise for primary and secondary prevention. The alliance of conventional health promotion programming with mind–body interventions should further reduce health care utilization and the unnecessary burden of degenerative disease. Given the present mandate to reduce health care costs and inspire self-care through integrated disease prevention and management programs, appropriate mindful exercise programs can reach a much greater percentage of the inactive older adult population than is currently reached without placing this group at undue risk for exercise-related complications or injury.

Key Terms

Recommended Readings

Cohen, K.S. (1997). *The way of qigong.* New York: Ballantine Books.

Lasater, J. (1995). *Relax and renew: Restful yoga for stressful times.* Berkeley, CA: Rodmell Press.

Wilson, S.D. (1997). *Qigong for beginners: Eight easy movements for vibrant health.* Portland, OR: Rudra Press.

Study Questions

1. Which of the following definitions best describes mindful exercise?
    a. exercise integrated with visual imagery
    b. physical exercise executed with a profound, inwardly directed. contemplative focus
    c. physical exercise with disciplined choreography
    d. exercise with a prioritized goal orientation

2. Which of the following is not one of the component criteria for mindful exercise?
    a. contemplation
    b. religious experience
    c. breath work
    d. focus on energy

3. Which style of hatha yoga listed below is *most* appropriate for older adults just beginning a yoga program?
    a. Ashtanga
    b. Kripalu
    c. Iyengar
    d. restorative

4. Which of the following forms of mindful exercise is most appropriate for inclusion in a warm-up or cool-down?
    a. taiji qigong
    b. Iyengar yoga sequences
    c. sun salutation
    d. headstand

5. Which of the following has *not* been scientifically shown to be a benefit of hatha yoga or tai chi training?
    a. decreased resting blood pressure
    b. decreased low-back pain in those with chronic low-back pain
    c. decreased depression and anxiety scores
    d. increased longevity

6. According to the yogic and qigong traditions, what is the function of breathing?
    a. an intermediary between the mind and body
    b. a means to enhance lucid thinking
    c. a problem-solving tool
    d. none of the above

Application Activities

1. Breath centering is the most fundamental component of all mindful exercise programs and should precede the development of choreography. Set aside several 45-minute sessions with other physical activity instructors to practice the simple introductory breathing exercise described in this chapter. Appoint a session leader to lead the participants through each phase of the breathing exercise. Another useful practice session is described in *The Way of Qigong* (Cohen, 1997, chap. 9).

2. Choose an existing physical activity class that you now teach (or wish to teach as a pilot mind–body exercise program), and add a three- or four-minute meditative component to the cool-down. Participants can focus their minds on relaxed breathing sounds and sensations to ensure simplicity of technique. After the cool-down meditation, spend four or five minutes discussing with your participants how they felt during this meditative segment. Let them disclose their own feelings and state of mind.

3. If mindful exercise is an entirely new modality for you, attend a yoga conference or beginner class at a yoga center near you to obtain first-hand kinesthetic and classroom experience with the various hatha yoga styles and forms. Yoga conferences are not to be confused with yoga teacher certification programs, which generally assume that the student has prior hatha yoga experience. Many yoga centers and studios regularly hold hatha yoga classes. Beginner classes in restorative, Iyengar, and Kripalu yoga are recommended.

16

Aquatic Training

Ruth Sova

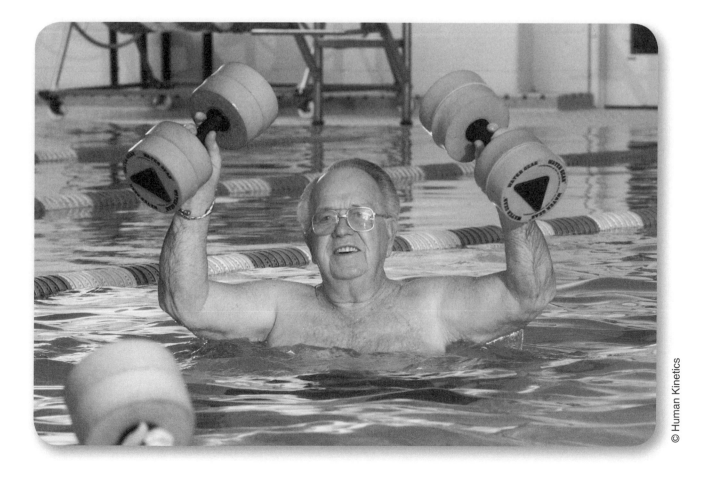

After completing this chapter, you will be able to

1. describe the physical properties of water and the related exercise benefits;
2. develop aquatic exercises that are appropriate for older adults of different functional abilities;
3. describe the exercise techniques that are appropriate for the aquatic environment and how they can be manipulated to alter the exercise intensity; and
4. identify aquatic safety precautions for older adults with common aging disorders.

Aquatic training is an idea whose time has come. The jogging craze of the late '60s and '70s, the aerobic dance frenzy of the '70s and early '80s, and the pursuit of total fitness through cross-training that characterized the '90s have matured into an intelligent pursuit of health and fitness in the new millennium. Like almost everything in life, jogging, aerobic dance, and cross-training have proven to be less than perfect methods of achieving fitness. As more people joined in the bouncing, jumping, jogging, and pumping, reports of minor injuries became more frequent. These activities' adverse impact on the joints also resulted in countless dropouts. As baby boomers move beyond middle age, there is an increasing need for physical activity programs to enable them to continue exercising for the rest of their lives, despite the joint problems and reduced flexibility they will eventually experience. Thus, aquatic exercise has become a major exercise option in our fitness-conscious society.

In this chapter you will first be introduced to the benefits of aquatic exercise and how the unique properties of water contribute to those benefits. Important safety considerations and special guidelines unique to aquatic training environments are reviewed in the next section of this chapter. The final section of the chapter addresses the important components of an aquatic training program and how they can be manipulated to increase or decrease the exercise intensity. Sample activities are also provided for each section of a typical aquatic exercise class.

Benefits of Aquatic Exercise

Over the course of the past decade, several studies have demonstrated numerous health, fitness, and rehabilitative benefits of aquatic exercise for older adults (D'Acquisto, D'Acquisto, & Renne, 2001; Norton, 1997; Takeshima et al., 2002). The physiological benefits documented include increased maximal oxygen uptake, lowered blood lipid levels, increased muscle strength and endurance, and improved flexibility. In addition to providing healthy older adults with health benefits, the unique properties of water also make it a safe and effective exercise environment for clients who have chronic medical conditions such as obesity, multiple sclerosis, arthritis, and osteoporosis (Bravo, Gauthier, Roy, Payette, & Gaulin, 1997; Hall, Skevington, Maddison, & Chapman, 1996; Suomi & Lindaur, 1997; Templeton, Booth, & O'Kelly, 1996). Although the changing of clothes, the wearing of a swimsuit, and the possibility of dry skin may be deterrents to aquatic exercise, the benefits of exercising in the water may outweigh any inconvenience. Exercising in water also causes less impact on the joints and therefore allows clients to exercise without the biomechanical stress experienced on land. Balance challenges are also more easily and safely achieved in an aquatic environment.

The benefits of aquatic exercise go well beyond the physical. Older adults need to feel capable, independent, and successful and to have connections with other people. Research has shown that exercising in the water, a playful environment, provides many psychological and social benefits for older adults (Hall, Skevington, Maddison, & Chapman, 1996; Norton, 1997; Krist, 2000). The improved self-confidence that comes from being able to successfully move through a more complete range of motion and to move in ways not thought possible is also beneficial to the older adult (La Forge, 1995; Maybeck, 2002; Nakanishi, Kimura, & Yokoo, 1999). Because of the playfulness most people associate with aquatic environments, people are also more likely to break down barriers, socialize more freely, have fun, and create connections with other people. The socializing aspect of aquatic exercise creates a feeling of community.

Understanding how the physical properties of water affect the exercise response in older adult populations is fundamental to the successful planning and implementation of aquatic training programs. This knowledge can be used to manipulate the intensity of the exercise, ensure that the client exercises in the correct water depth, establish safe entry and exit procedures, and generally create a more effective program. This section of the chapter first describes each of the important properties of water: hydrostatic pressure, buoyancy, and resistance. It then discusses both the advantages and disadvantages of each of these properties and how each of these properties influences program planning.

Hydrostatic Pressure

Perhaps the best way to visualize the water property known as **hydrostatic pressure** is to imagine wearing a garment against your body that acts like a support stocking. This is how it feels to stand in waist- to chest-deep water. The water exerts pressure uniformly over the entire surface of the body. This water property aids **venous return** (i.e., the amount of blood returning to the atria of the heart) and also increases the range of motion possible by reducing **edema,** or swelling, particularly in the feet.

Advantages

Hydrostatic pressure decreases swelling (thus improving range of motion), increases blood circulation (just like support stockings), increases the strength of the respiratory muscles (because the intercostal muscles must work harder against the pressure of the water), and improves the breathing of older adults (Herfert, 2000). In fact, no movement is necessary to gain the benefits of hydrostatic pressure. Simply being submersed in the water is sufficient (Schoedinger, 2002).

Disadvantages

Clients with high blood pressure or breathing disorders may experience discomfort as a result of hydrostatic pressure. Hydrostatic pressure initially

> No movement is necessary to obtain the benefits of hydrostatic pressure.

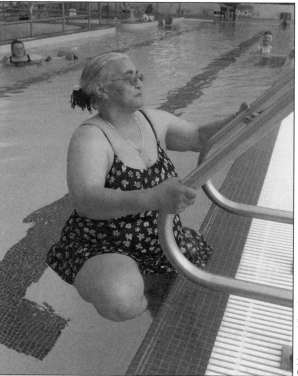

Clients with high blood pressure should be instructed to enter the water slowly.

© Human Kinetics

increases blood pressure. To minimize this problem, clients who have high blood pressure should be instructed to enter the water slowly. This allows the body to adapt without overloading the vascular system. The good news is that as the body adapts to being in the water, blood pressure normalizes. Clients with breathing disorders may also experience difficulty inhaling (getting enough air) because of the pressure of the water. Exercising in shallow water minimizes these breathing difficulties and reduces the likelihood that the client will panic.

Implications for Program Design

All older adults can benefit from entering and exiting the water slowly to allow all body systems to adapt to the hydrostatic pressure. Circulation increases *before* movement occurs, so the warm-up should be gradual to allow clients to adapt to both the water and the activity. Be sure to position clients toward the shallow end of the pool if they have breathing difficulties or high blood pressure.

Buoyancy

Buoyancy is a property of water that can be described as an upward thrust, opposite the force of gravity. Archimedes' principle states that when a body is wholly or partially immersed in a fluid at rest, it experiences an upward thrust equal to the weight of the fluid displaced.

Advantages

The buoyancy of water decreases the weight-bearing impact of exercise. When submersed to shoulder level, a person experiences an apparent weight loss of 90 percent, while in waist-level water, the apparent weight loss is approximately 41 percent (Davis & Harrison, 1988). Because of decreased weight bearing, joint **compressive forces** (i.e., gravitational and biomechanical forces that press components of a joint capsule together) decrease, enabling older adults to move more freely in the water than on land. Moreover, the **biomechanical stress,** the pressure on the body created by the interaction of internal and external forces, also decreases, so there is less impact on the joints during movement and less likelihood of injury (Becker, 2001). Fear of falling also decreases, and clients are more willing to move through a more complete range of motion. As was the case with hydrostatic pressure, no movement is necessary for these reactions to occur. Simply being submersed in the water allows clients to realize these benefits.

Disadvantages

Buoyancy reduces stability. Clients who are standing in water that is too deep may lose control of their movements or their footing. This is particularly true for clients who have excessive amounts of adipose tissue and are therefore more buoyant. Older adults with limbs that more flaccid or less toned, for instance, as the result of a stroke, may also experience stability problems because of the limbs' tendency to float. These problems can often be remedied by moving the client to the shallow end of the pool.

Implications for Program Design

Clients who have pain should keep the affected area submerged to reduce the effect of weight bearing and biomechanical stress, while clients with balance deficits should begin in shallow water where stability is easier to maintain. As your clients become more familiar with exercising in the water, they can eventually move to deeper water to challenge

> One disadvantage of increased buoyancy is that it reduces stability.

their balance more. Conversely, clients who have experienced strokes and have trouble standing independently should begin exercising at a deeper level and exploit the property of buoyancy to gain added support. As they gain the ability to stand in deep water, they should move to shallower depths that require them to bear more weight. Ankle weights can also be used to assist a client whose stroke has resulted in the limbs' tendency to float.

Viscosity and Resistance

The **viscosity** of water, which is defined as the friction between the molecules of a liquid that causes them to tend to adhere to each other and the surface of the body moving through it, creates **resistance** (i.e., load, force, or weight against which muscle must work) against the body as it moves through the water. The resistant forces created by water increase the amount of work required of the muscles and can be particularly helpful in reducing muscle imbalance.

Advantages

There is resistance to all movements performed in the water. The increased resistance to movement increases muscular tone, oxygen consumption, and number of calories burned because more muscle fibers have to be recruited for each movement. Moreover, working against the liquid resistance of water as opposed to weight machines or free weights allows more equalized resistance in both the concentric and eccentric directions of the movement, providing better muscle balance as a result (Arient, 2002; Hurley & Turner, 1991). This means that the biceps muscle works when the elbow is flexed, and the triceps muscle works when the elbow is extended, whereas on land the biceps works during both flexion and extension. Note that the benefits of resistance accrue only when the body is moving.

Disadvantages

Some frailer clients can have difficulty moving the body or even the limbs through the water because of the increased resistance. The speed and sometimes the range of motion of a given exercise need to be decreased to minimize this problem.

Implications for Program Design

Clients who are frail or weak benefit from the resistance created by moving through the water just as they do from resistance training on land. Encourage

> The benefits of water resistance accrue only when the body is moving.

a full range of motion if possible, but instruct your clients to perform movements more slowly to adjust for the increased resistance. Remember also that clients cannot move as quickly in water as an instructor demonstrating an exercise on the pool deck. You should therefore consciously slow down your movements on land so that clients can perform the exercise safely in the water. Movements done as quickly in water as on land can cause joint pain and muscle injury. Also, clients who have muscle balance problems in the back, hips, or shoulders benefit more from water resistance if movements are performed slowly and with control.

Considerations Unique to Aquatic Exercise

There are a few extra safety considerations for working with clients in the water. Some are related to the facility, others are specific to your clients, and others involve teaching methods and the use of equipment. Physical activity instructors must be aware of the properties of water and how they affect exercise conditions to ensure that aquatic exercises are safe and as effective as possible.

Safety of the Facility

The building and pool should be appropriate for your clientele. The ambient air temperature and humidity within the pool facility must be carefully regulated for maximal comfort, and the water temperature of the pool should be monitored to ensure that it meets the needs of groups with different health concerns. A trained lifeguard should be on duty at all times when the classes are in session. Because aquatic exercise is usually performed in waist- to chest-deep water, it is also important that the pool bottom be graded.

Accommodating Clients' Abilities and Health Conditions

Special care must be taken to avoid accidents in aquatic exercise settings. Because most injuries in

aquatic facilities occur on the deck from slips and falls, clients should wear slip-resistant shoes at all times: in the locker room, on the pool deck, and in the water. When using stairs, ramps, or ladders to enter and exit the pool, your clients should also be reminded to move slowly. A slow entrance into the water allows time for body systems to adjust to the change in hydrostatic pressure. This is especially important for clients who have medical conditions such as fibromyalgia, heart disease, and high blood pressure. A lift is essential for clients with chronic medical conditions that limit ambulation (e.g., multiple sclerosis, Parkinson's disease, severe arthritis, osteoporosis).

Many older adults prefer to exercise in warm water (84 to 88 degrees Fahrenheit, 29 to 31 degrees Celsius). Older adults who are easily chilled can wear neoprene gloves, vests, or shorts to conserve body heat. Conversely, it is preferable for clients who are overweight or obese and clients with multiple sclerosis to exercise in cooler water (78 to 84 degrees Fahrenheit, 26 to 29 degrees Celsius). Clients who are obese have difficulty dissipating body heat, and the cool water assists their thermoregulation. Clients with multiple sclerosis may overheat and experience a temporary loss of function in water that is too warm because of their inability to regulate their core body temperature adequately.

Although exercising in deeper water reduces the weight bearing required, it is more important that obese clients be able to control their movements. They are more buoyant because they have more adipose tissue, so they should exercise in shallow water for better control of their movements. In contrast, clients with arthritis should submerge the affected joints. If the shoulders are affected, the client should move to deeper water, and the exercises should be performed more slowly. People who have arthritis in their hands cannot easily grip equipment for a long time. They can use gripping equipment for very short periods (about a minute), but then they should be given the opportunity to rest the hands before using the equipment again.

Clients with balance problems, particularly those who have experienced a stroke, find it particularly difficult to exercise in deeper water due to increased buoyancy. They are better served by exercise in shallower water early in the program. Water exercises can be especially challenging and thus beneficial for clients' balance. One-footed exercises, long-stride exercises, and exercises performed with

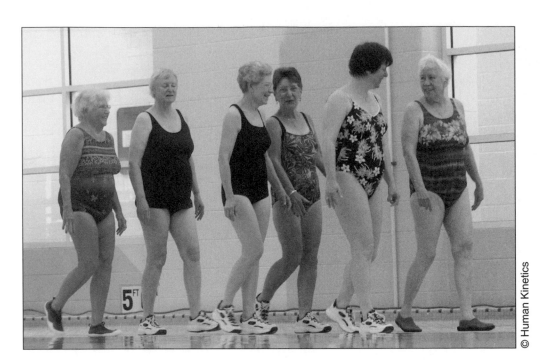

© Human Kinetics

A number of slips and trips can be eliminated by wearing slip-resistant shoes.

feet together rather than hip-width apart effectively challenge your clients' balance. Performing isolated arm movements while maintaining a stable lower body further challenges balance.

Instruction in Aquatic Settings

Teaching in an aquatic setting offers special challenges for the physical activity instructor. For safety, clients should be taught how to recover to a standing position during the first few sessions. If clients slip and end up face down or face up in the water, they should know how to get their feet back under them to regain upright positioning. Whether face down or face up, clients should practice tucking the knees to the chest, rolling until the head is up, and then pushing the feet to the pool bottom.

The water's buoyancy and hydrostatic pressure support the body, so rather than standing upright, clients may lean forward to let the water do the work for the trunk muscles. Encourage an upright posture stabilized by the core trunk muscles, which transfers to stronger standing and sitting skills on land. It is also important that clients use their muscles rather than the water to produce movements. Encourage them to control their bodies while performing each exercise. Although it is important to increase range of motion by having your clients exercise with the arms above the head, most arm movements should be performed underwater so that your clients expend more calories and increase their muscle tone as they move against the water's resistance. If equipment is used, the movements should always be toward and away from the core of the body. Circling the arms to the sides (circumduction), for example, may injure the shoulder joint.

Not all older adults prefer music during their exercise sessions. Hearing loss does not diminish all sounds equally. Background sounds, such as music, interfere with primary sounds, such as the instructor's directions. If clients complain that the music is too loud, turn it down or turn it off. Clients often are unable to stay with the beat of the music; if so, it is fine to simply use music in the background. If music is played, select something from clients' youth or earlier adulthood that they are familiar with, whether swing, big band, or music from the '40s or '50s.

Equipment for Aquatic Exercise

Equipment can be used to increase the intensity of an exercise or simply to add variety and fun to a workout. Resistive devices can range from simple webbed gloves for increasing resistance to a Hydro-Tone system, which includes handheld resistance devices with fins in three dimensions and multi-finned boots. While most aquatic equipment provides buoyancy (hand bars, belts, "noodles," ankle cuffs), some pieces offer resistance (gloves, paddles, finned boots, winged ankle and wrist devices). Weights (e.g., wrist and ankle) are the least often used equipment in aquatic settings.

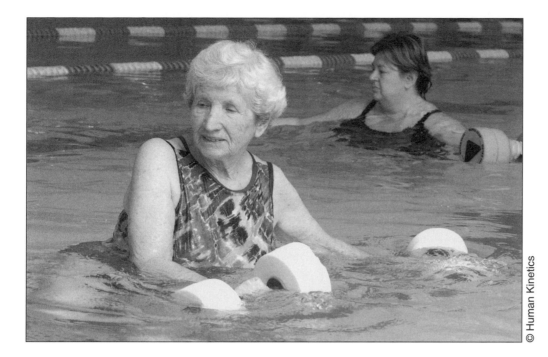

Apply the principle of progressive overload by adding equipment for resistance training gradually.

© Human Kinetics

It is important to follow some additional safety precautions when using equipment. First, avoid activities where clients hang or are suspended (i.e., feet not touching the pool bottom) from equipment. Whether the equipment is placed under the armpits or in the hands, hanging from equipment places unnecessary stress on the shoulder joint capsule. If introduced at all, hanging exercises should be performed briefly, and then the equipment should be removed. This precaution also applies to hanging from the edge of the pool. Second, equipment should not be allowed to "wag" the body. For example, if body parts other than the limb being exercised also move, the exercise is no longer safe or functional. Only the limb being exercised should change position; the rest of the body should remain in good alignment. Finally, be sure to apply the principle of progressive overload by adding resistance gradually. For example, light-resistance equipment (such as gloves) should always be added before heavy-resistance equipment (such as Hydro-Tone handheld devices). In addition, the equipment should be used only for five to ten minutes during the first session, and the duration gradually increased in subsequent sessions. The exercises should also be performed through a small range of motion early in the program and then gradually increased to a full range of motion as the program continues. Clients who have high blood pressure or coronary artery disease may not be good candidates for equipment use. Gripping equipment and high-intensity, forceful movements increase blood pressure and therefore the load on the heart.

Aquatic Training Components

In general, the aquatic workout should follow the format of a traditional land-based program. It should consist of the following components: warm-up, aerobic conditioning, resistance training, specific balance activities, flexibility, and cool-down. The following sections discuss some water-specific issues regarding the warm-up, intensity levels during the aerobic and resistance-training components, and the cool-down.

Warm-Up

Older adults should complete a longer warm-up (approximately 10-20 minutes) when exercising in water than on land. This is because the older adult's **thermoregulatory system** (i.e., system responsible for regulating body heat) does not adapt as quickly while in water. Your clients therefore need to spend more time warming up thermally and also getting blood and oxygen moving through the body. Lengthening the warm-up also allows more time for synovial fluid to be released into the joints. An example of an appropriate warm-up is provided in figure 16.1.

Water Walking

Objective: Increase internal body temperature in preparation for more vigorous exercise. Become familiar with the aquatic environment.

Duration: 15 minutes

Music suggestions: "String of Pearls," "Tuxedo Junction"
Tempo: 130 beats per minute (used at half tempo)

Activities: Perform all activities using an 8- to 12-count sequence in multiple directions (e.g., forward, backward, side to side).

- Walk forward and backward at a tempo that is half that of the music.
- Repeat walking sequence (a) while lifting knees high on each step, (b) with knees crossing midline (internal hip rotation), and (c) with knees turned out (external hip rotation).
- Repeat walking forward and backward without the additional activities but in time with the music.
- Walk forward and then backward, performing side leg lift before each step.
- Repeat walking forward and backward with a lunge each time the foot contacts the pool floor.
- Walk sideways, emphasizing hip abduction by lifting lead leg off pool floor.
- Walk forward and backward using normal arm swing and stride length, then alternating fast and slow steps, and then alternating long and short steps.

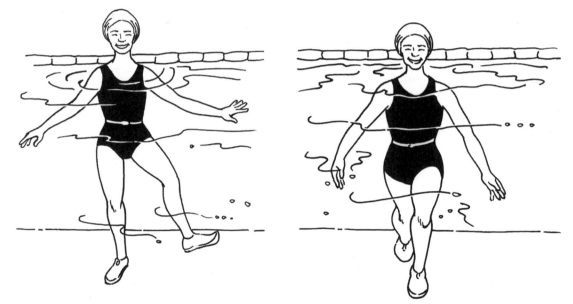

Intensity

- High: Swing arms in extended position while walking; try to propel the body forward or backward using the arms. Increase stride length. Perform walking activities at deeper water level (i.e., chest to shoulder height). Add a momentary pause at end of each side lift movement. Increase the force exerted with each side lift or lunging movement.
- Low: Swing arms in flexed position. Reduce stride length. Perform activities in waist-deep or shallower water. Move at a tempo half that of the music.

Verbal cues

- Emphasize upright body alignment. Balance should be challenged by these activities.
- Emphasize keeping toes and hips pointed forward during side step and side lift activities.

Equipment: None.

Program note: The duration of the aquatic warm-up should be longer than that in a land-based exercise program.

FIGURE 16.1 Aquatic warm-up exercises.

Aerobic Exercise

During this portion of the exercise class, your primary objective is to elevate the heart rate through a series of continuous activities performed at different intensities. Alternate the muscle groups that are working during this segment of the class so that clients do not become overly fatigued. Also intersperse 15- to 30-second intervals of high-tempo work with similar periods of lower-tempo activities so that clients can recover. Examples of aerobic conditioning exercises are presented in figure 16.2, along with ideas for manipulating the intensity to accommodate different fitness levels.

Intensity

If you are using heart rate to monitor intensity during the aerobic conditioning portion of the class, be aware that heart rates in the water do not correlate with heart rates on land. The heart rates of clients exercising in a cool pool (78 to 83 degrees Fahrenheit, 26 to 28 degrees Celsius) are approximately 15 percent lower than heart rates when performing at the same level of oxygen consumption on land, and 10 percent lower than when exercising in warm water (84 to 88 degrees Fahrenheit, 29 to 31 degrees Celsius). The heart rate is also 8 to 11 beats per minute

---

Objective: Improve cardiovascular efficiency and increase caloric expenditure using water jogging, dance, and calisthenic movements.

Duration: 10 to 15 minutes

Music suggestions: "Yankee Doodle Dandy," "Stars and Stripes Forever," "William Tell Overture"
Tempo: 130 to 140 beats per minute (used at half tempo)

Activities: Perform movements 8 to 12 times in one direction and then 8 to 12 times in the opposite direction.

- Jog forward, backward, and side to side with (a) high knee lift, (b) knees crossing midline, and (c) knees turned out.
- Rock side to side, first in place and then moving side to side. (Right foot lifts off pool floor as the right hip abducts.)
- Jog forward, backward, and side to side with (a) toes pointed down (when knee lifts), (b) toes pointed out, (c) toes pointed in. Arms swing forward and back during jogging movements.
- Jumping jacks. Variations include (a) bringing feet together at end of each jump, (b) crossing ankles at end of each jump, and (c) tilting trunk to right (lateral trunk flexion) and then to left on each jumping jack. Perform in place, then moving forward, backward, and side to side.
- "Cross-country skiing" (a) without and (b) with center bounce between forward and backward movements. Perform in place, then moving forward, backward, and side to side.
- Slow heel kickbacks (knee flexion with knee pointed down). Alternate fast and slow movements. Perform in place, then moving forward, backward, and side to side.
- Slow leg kickbacks. Alternate fast and slow movements. Perform in place, then moving forward, backward, and side to side.

Intensity

- High: Lift knees higher on knee lifts. Move arms and legs more forcefully. Change directions (e.g., forward, backward) more frequently. Travel farther to each side on side-to-side rocks. Use arms to propel the body by pushing to the left as the body moves right, and vice versa. Perform exercises in deeper water. Create more water turbulence by forcefully swinging arms forward, backward, and side to side.
- Low: Shorten stride length, reduce height of knee lift. Decrease force applied against pool floor during jumping or jogging movements. Reduce range of motion on jumping jacks and side-to-side rocking movements. Change directions less frequently. Perform movements in place rather than moving. Move at a slower tempo (half-time to music).

Equipment: None.

FIGURE 16.2 Aquatic aerobic conditioning exercises.

lower when exercising in chest-deep water than in waist-deep water. Heart rate during water immersion is influenced by many factors (e.g., air temperature and humidity, ventilation, direct sunlight) and can be highly variable, especially for clients who take certain types of medications. Heart rate is therefore not a good indicator of the level of exertion or how well the client is adapting metabolically to training. Borg's rating of perceived exertion scale (see chapters 7 and 13) is more useful for making day-to-day comparisons of intensity. The intensity of a water exercise program should certainly not be based on the target heart rate or oxygen consumption recommended for land-based exercise.

Resistance Training

The viscous properties of water (i.e., resistance) make it an ideal environment for improving muscle strength and endurance. Resistance occurs as soon as the client begins moving through the water. Increasing or decreasing the range through which the limbs move in any exercise, the speed of limb movements, and the amount of force that is applied during each movement are easy ways of manipulating the exercise intensity. To further increase the resistance, special aquatic resistance devices can also be used during this segment (e.g., aquatic dumbbells, resistance gloves). An example of a resistance-training component is presented in figure 16.3.

Objective: Improve muscle endurance and strength.

Duration: 10 to 15 minutes

Music suggestions: "All that Jazz," "Phantom of the Opera," "Someone Like You"
Tempo: 120 beats per minute (used at half tempo)

Activities: Perform movements at half the music's tempo. To improve muscle endurance, repeat movements 12 to 16 times with no equipment. To improve muscle strength, reduce number of repetitions to 8 to 12 per set and use resistance equipment. Perform exercises at the edge of the pool.

- Knee lifts with right leg (8 to 16 repetitions) then left leg (8 to 16 repetitions)
- Heel kickbacks (knee flexion with knee pointed down) with right then left leg
- Side lifts (hip abduction and adduction) with right then left leg
- Biceps curls below water level (unilateral or bilateral)
- Side arm raises below water level (unilateral or bilateral)

Intensity

- High: Press knee down to floor with greater force during knee lifts; increase height of knee lifts. Add more force as heel kicks back during heel kickbacks. Add a momentary pause after each side lift. Perform movements with no external support so as to challenge balance.
- Low: Lift and lower knee gently on knee lifts. Use a swinging rather than stop–start movement during heel kickbacks. Alternate legs during side lifts and reduce the height of the lift. Do fewer repetitions of each exercise.

Verbal cues

- Maintain upright position during each exercise.
- Isolate movement to limb being exercised.
- Perform movements slowly and with control.
- Point hips and toes forward during side lifts.

Equipment: Buoyancy devices such as ankle cuffs, water wings, knotted noodles; resistance devices such as finned boots, webbed gloves, finned dumbbells.

FIGURE 16.3   Aquatic resistance-training exercises.

Cool-Down

The cool-down phase of an aquatic exercise class is especially important because of the hydrostatic pressure of water. If a participant exits the pool with higher heart rate and blood pressure from an inadequate cool-down, dizziness can occur. This is because exercising at a challenging intensity makes the blood vessels dilate to increase blood flow during the workout. In water exercise classes, it is thought that the blood vessels are compressed by the water and do not dilate to the same extent as during land-based exercise (Becker, 2001). On exiting the pool, air pressure that is lower than water pressure results in the blood vessels' dilating further and causing the blood pressure to drop. This can cause the participant to feel light-headed or dizzy or to pass out in extreme circumstances. It is therefore important to include gentle activities designed to lower the heart rate and blood pressure before the client exits the pool.

The cool-down component of a class is the ideal time to introduce flexibility as well as relaxation exercises. One particular advantage of performing flexibility exercises in the water is that buoyancy makes them much easier to perform than on land. For example, it is much easier to perform leg straddles or side stretches in the water than on land. Simple yoga and tai chi exercises are excellent relaxation exercises that can easily be performed in a pool (see chapter 15 for exercise ideas). In addition, a set of mind–body exercises called Ai Chi has been designed specifically for an aquatic environment. A sample set of Ai Chi exercises is described and illustrated in figure 16.4.

Summary

Aquatic training provides a perfect mix of water and workout. Since the movements are performed in waist- to chest-deep water, these programs can be done by swimmers and nonswimmers alike. The buoyant support of the water effectively cancels out approximately 90 percent of the weight of a person submerged up to the shoulders. This dramatically decreases compression stress on the weight-bearing joints, bones, and muscles. Moreover, since most movements performed in the water are believed to involve only concentric muscular contractions, muscle soreness is minimal. As long as movements are not done too quickly, the possibility of muscle, bone, and joint injuries is almost completely eliminated. Individuals concerned with excess pressure on their ankles, knees, hips, and back can increase their muscle strength and endurance, flexibility, and cardiovascular efficiency with no discomfort and increased safety in an aquatic environment.

Aquatic exercise programs are ideal for many older adults who have painful joints due to arthritis, muscle weakness, poor balance, and other medical conditions (e.g., obesity, chronic back pain) that make traditional land-based exercise programs less well suited for them. With the body submerged in water, blood circulation automatically increases to some extent. The pressure that water exerts against the body also promotes deeper breathing and improves respiratory efficiency. Flexibility exercises can be performed more easily in water because the effects of gravity are countered by buoyancy. The resistance of water also makes it a perfect exercise medium for the well-conditioned individual who is looking to accomplish a challenging workout in less time. Water resistance elevates a simple walk to a challenging workout, developing muscular endurance and strength and cardiorespiratory efficiency simultaneously.

Aquatic training techniques can broaden your teaching opportunities by allowing you to teach clients who may not function well in land-based programs. Aquatic exercise provides older adults with the opportunity to move more freely, with less pain, and with less likelihood of injury than a land-based exercise program. In fact, aquatic exercise can be an ideal mode of exercise for many of your older adult clients. Before you begin teaching in aquatic environments, however, you should know some basic facts. First, you need to be familiar with the unique properties of water and how they can be exploited to improve the exercise experience. Second, you must understand how the body responds at different water depths and with different movement intensities. Finally, you must learn how to manipulate the intensity of the various types of exercise to accommodate the different fitness levels of your clients. The good news is that aquatic exercise is a simple and safe way for older adults to gain the benefits of exercise. Use it and enjoy it!

Objective: Combine dynamic stretching (to increase flexibility) with relaxation.

Music suggestions: Instrumental music that creates a relaxing atmosphere
Tempo: If there's a beat, you'll move to it naturally. Slow, relaxing music with no definite beat is best for allowing the body to let go.

Activities: In Ai Chi, the emphasis is on flowing movements and equal force application during all phases of the movement.

Preparatory position
Begin with feet in a long stride stance with back straight. Both arms are extended forward at shoulder height, palms down with thumbs touching each other. Bend knees until the water is at shoulder level and the arms are resting easily at the water surface. Chin is relaxed and slightly down.

Use diaphragmatic breathing for these exercises.

Accepting
1. Inhale through your nose, turn your palms up, and pull both arms to the sides and back (arms straight and still at shoulder height) so that your rib cage feels fully open. At the same time, shift your weight to the back leg so that you lean back slightly.
2. Exhale through your mouth, turn your palms down, and bring both arms together so that the thumbs touch. At the same time, shift your weight onto the forward leg so that you lean forward slightly.
3. Repeat steps 1 and 2, flowing smoothly, four to eight times.
4. Step back with the front foot on the next inhalation, and repeat steps 1 and 2 four to eight more times with feet in this position.

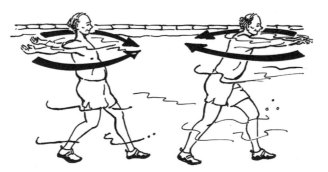

Rounding
1. Inhale through your nose, turn your palms up, and pull both arms to the sides and back (arms straight and still at shoulder height) so that your rib cage feels fully open. At the same time, shift your weight onto the back leg and lean back slightly.
2. Exhale through your mouth, turn your palms down, and bring both arms together so that the thumbs touch. At the same time, shift your weight to the forward leg and do a leg lift to the front with your back leg, toes toward the fingertips.
3. Repeat steps 1 and 2, flowing smoothly, four to eight times.
4. Put the lifted foot down in front on the next inhalation, and repeat steps 1 and 2 four to eight more times with feet in this position.

(continued)

FIGURE 16.4   Sample Ai Chi flexibility and relaxation exercises.

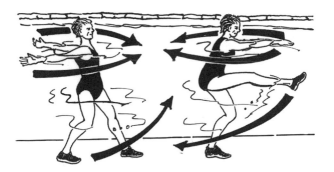

Balancing

1. Inhale through your nose, turn your palms up, and press both arms down and back (next to the body). At the same time, lift your back leg to the front and lean forward slightly.

2. Exhale through your mouth, turn your palms down, and lift both arms forward and up. At the same time, press the lifted leg behind you, leaning forward slightly.

3. Repeat steps 1 and 2, flowing smoothly, four to eight times.

4. Put the lifted leg down in front on the next inhalation and repeat steps 1 and 2 four to eight more times with feet in this position.

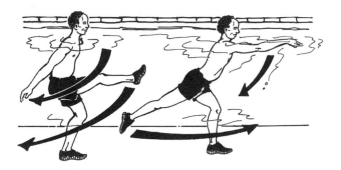

Folding

1. Step out to the side with the lifted leg into a wide stance, inhale, turn palms up, and lift arms to the sides.

2. Exhale easily through your mouth, and turn your palms down while letting your arms lower and cross in front of your body.

3. Inhale through your nose, keep your elbows in at your waist, turn your palms up and open your forearms to the sides.

4. Repeat steps 2 and 3 four to eight times.

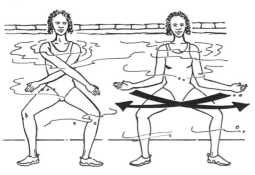

FIGURE 16.4   *(continued)*

Key Terms

Recommended Readings

Lepore, M. (1998). *Adapted aquatics programming.* Champaign, IL: Human Kinetics.

Sova, R. (2001). *Aquatics—The complete reference guide for aquatics fitness professionals* (2nd ed.). Port Washington, WI: DSL.

Study Questions

1. Aquatic exercise offers all the benefits of land-based fitness programs plus

    a. more toning capabilities

    b. less impact

    c. improved breathing skills

    d. all of the above

2. In which of the following ways does circulatory system function change in the water?

    a. Breathing is easier when a person is submerged to neck level.

    b. Circulation decreases when a person gets into the water.

    c. Circulation increases when a person gets into the water.

    d. All of the above

3. Hydrostatic pressure is best described as

    a. an upward thrust opposite gravity

    b. like wearing a support stocking

    c. equalized resistance training

    d. a muscular endurance benefit

4. The benefits of hydrostatic pressure are achieved

    a. as a result of being submersed in water

    b. when movement occurs

    c. after being submersed in water for at least 15 minutes

    d. in reverse proportion to amount of body fat

5. Buoyancy is best described as

    a. like wearing a support stocking

    b. an upward thrust opposite gravity

    c. equalized resistance training

    d. a muscular endurance benefit

6. The benefits of buoyancy are achieved

    a. as a result of being submersed in water

    b. when movement occurs

    c. after being submersed in water for at least 15 minutes

    d. in reverse proportion to amount of body fat

(continued)

7. Participants in an aquatic exercise class experience less biomechanical stress than in a similar land-based exercise class because
    a. the surface friction minimizes exercise-related pain
    b. participants have more density in the water
    c. participants are cushioned by the water's buoyancy
    d. water dissipates heat faster than air

8. The aquatic warm-up should be longer for older adults because
    a. they move more slowly than younger adults
    b. their thermoregulatory systems take longer to adapt to the aquatic environment than in land-based programs
    c. they usually have balance deficits
    d. their increased density makes them heavier

Application Activities

1. To experience the additional training stimulus for muscular endurance that the water provides, walk 15 to 20 steps on the pool deck, and then walk 15 to 20 steps in the water. Which activity is more difficult?

2. On land, jump, tucking both knees toward your chest. Now repeat the same activity in the water. Which activity results in less impact on landing?

3. Perform kicks on land at any tempo. Identify the muscles that are activated most during this activity. Perform kicks at the same tempo in the water. Identify the muscles that are activated most in this environment. Are the same muscles activated in water and on land?

Training Master Athletes

Steven A. Hawkins

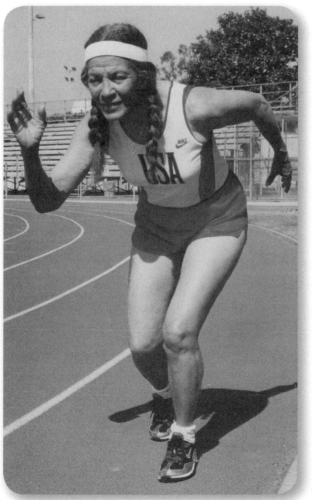

Objectives

After completing this chapter, you will be able to

1. define *master athlete,*
2. describe age-related changes in sport performance and the physiological and psychological factors that might explain those changes,
3. develop a sport-specific training program for a master athlete, and
4. describe the risk and prevention of overtraining and injury in master athletes.

Sport competition has traditionally been seen as the realm of youth. Increasingly, however, that perception is changing as we become aware of the marvelous athletic achievements of adults in their 60s, 70s, 80s, and even 90s. These individuals, representing the upper end of the functional spectrum of older adults, are master athletes. Knowledge about master athletes and master athletics is important for physical activity instructors who may be involved in coaching or training master athletes or may be asked to refer clients interested in competing to relevant organizations and opportunities for competition.

This chapter begins with a definition of *master athlete* and then describes sport performance of older adults, factors that influence performance, and sociocultural aspects of sport participation. A detailed explanation of how to develop a training program for master athletes is also provided. The chapter concludes with a discussion of important training precautions.

Master Athletes

Master athletes have been defined as "competitors who exceed a minimum age specific to each sport and who participate in competitive events designed for masters athletes" (Spirduso, 1995, p. 390). The minimum age varies by sport: Swimmers can compete as masters at age 25, rowers at age 27, female track and field athletes at age 35, weightlifters and male track and field athletes at age 40, and softball players and golfers at age 50. Competition in athletic events provides a clear delineation between master athletes and healthy, active older adults. Competitions, which generally take place in highly motivated situations, provide a perfect setting in which to compare the physical perfor-

mance of younger and older adults (Spirduso, 1995). These comparisons help gerokinesiologists better understand the effects of and limits imposed by aging on physical performance.

Masters athletics is a relatively new phenomenon. The Senior Olympics began in 1969, followed the next year by the inaugural masters swimming meet. Masters track and field began in 1975 with the World Championships and the World Veterans Games. Despite the relative infancy of masters athletics, participation in masters competitions is significant and growing. Currently, over 160,000 adults are registered as master athletes with various organizations, and most organizations report rapid growth in the number of competitors. Moreover, large numbers of older adults train and compete but do not join masters organizations, and sports such as golf, bowling, tennis, and softball involve significant numbers of older competitors. The Senior Games, offering a wide range of games and sports, boast the participation of over 250,000 individuals annually at various levels of competition.

Sport Performance of Master Athletes

It is clear that sport performance declines with age. However, the rate of decline varies as a function of the demands of the event or sport (see figure 17.1). Running, swimming, cycling, and rowing performances gradually decline with age at a rate of approximately 0.5 to 1 percent per year until the age of 70, after which declines in performance accelerate (Tanaka & Seals, 1997; Bortz & Bortz, 1996). The rate of decline is greater for distance than for sprint events (Stones & Kozma, 1981). Events that require power or complex movements, such as throwing and jumping in track and field, Olympic lifting, and power lifting, show performance declines with age of 1 to 2 percent per year

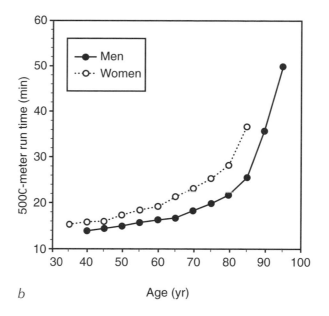

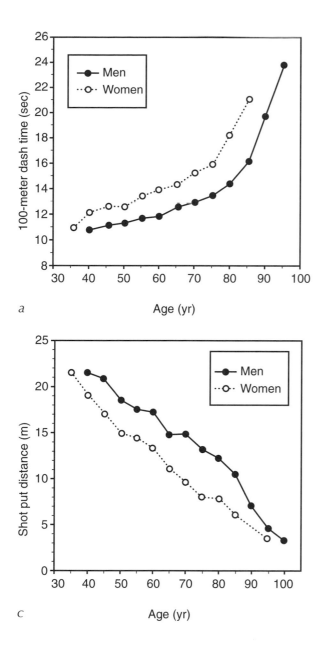

FIGURE 17.1   Masters world records for men and women in *(a)* the 100-meter dash, *(b)* the 5K run, and *(c)* shot put.

Data from National Masters News for 2000, 2001.

sections. Some of the age-related changes in physiological function that can be expected to reduce sport performance and that account for the wide range of physical capacities evident in aging athletes are illustrated in figure 17.2.

Maximal Aerobic Capacity

Maximal aerobic capacity (**$\dot{V}O_2$max**) is considered a key indicator of cardiorespiratory endurance, and it declines approximately 10 percent per decade after the age of 25 years in sedentary adults. Maximal aerobic capacity has been extensively studied in master athletes (Rogers, Hagberg, Martin, Ehsani, & Holloszy, 1990; Trappe, Costill, Vukovich, Jones, & Melham, 1996; Pollock et al., 1997), and its decline is clearly associated with reduced endurance performance (Bortz & Bortz, 1996). Cross-sectional research (different age groups studied at the same point in time) has generally demonstrated rates of decline that are 50 percent lower in master athletes than in sedentary adults, findings that were confirmed by early longitudinal studies (the same athletes tested over time).

In contrast, more current longitudinal studies have demonstrated rates of decline in master athletes' $\dot{V}O_2$max that are similar to or even greater

(Meltzer, 1996; Spirduso, 1995). However, as elite performers continue to compete as master athletes and as the number of competitors increases, particularly at the older ages, it is likely that decreases in sport performance with age will be less than currently reported (Spirduso, 1995).

Sport performance is influenced by similar physiological and psychological factors regardless of age (Maharam, Bauman, Kalman, Skolnik, & Pearle, 1999). However, physical activity specialists must understand age-related changes in these factors to effectively assist master athletes with their training. Important age-related changes and other factors most likely to affect the sport performance of master athletes are described in the following

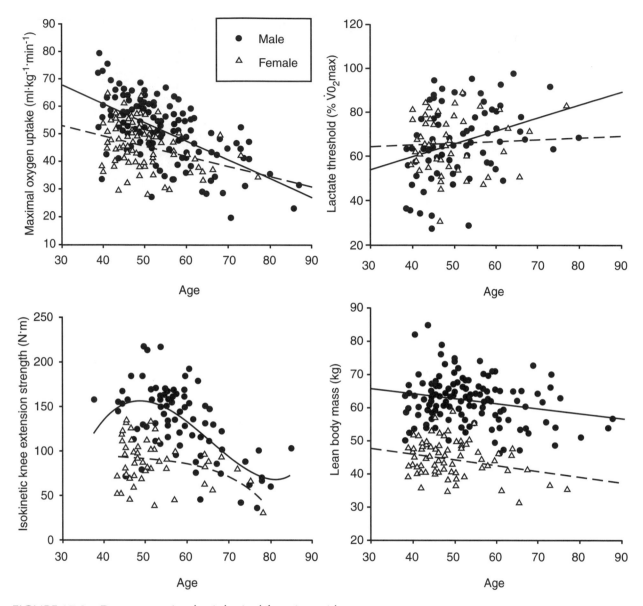

FIGURE 17.2   Decrements in physiological function with age.

Adapted, by permission, from R.A. Wiswell et al., 2001, "Relationship between physiological loss, performance decrements, and age in master athletes," *Journal of Gerontology: Medical Sciences* 56A(10): M618-M626.

than sedentary adults' (Hawkins, Marcell, Jaque, & Wiswell, 2001; Eskurza, Donato, Moreau, Seals, & Tanaka, 2002). It is likely that these more current findings reflect alterations in training patterns. Several researchers have shown that $\dot{V}O_2$max can be maintained for 7 to 10 years in master athletes who maintain the same level of training volume and intensity. However, these same athletes experienced rapid declines in $\dot{V}O_2$max when they eventually decreased or ceased training (see figure 17.3). This suggests the need to avoid dramatic or lengthy interruptions in training if at all possible.

Lactate Threshold

The **lactate threshold (LT)** is associated with endurance performance in older athletes (Allen, Seals, Hurley, Ehsani, & Hagberg, 1985); trained athletes have greater functional use of their maximal aerobic capacity during endurance exercise. In sedentary individuals, LT generally occurs at 50 to 60 percent of $\dot{V}O_2$max, whereas endurance athletes can have LTs of 80 to 90 percent of $\dot{V}O_2$max. Aging is also associated with raised LT, independent of endurance training, which is most likely due to a loss of fast-twitch muscle fibers. LT increases with

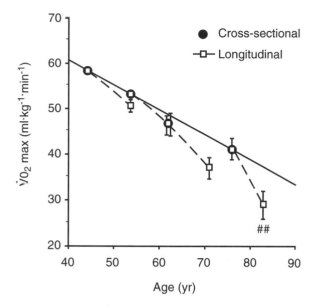

FIGURE 17.3   Change in maximal aerobic capacity with age in male master athletes. ## = Significantly different rate of loss compared to cross-sectional.

Reprinted, by permission, from S.A. Hawkins et al., 2001, "A longitudinal assessment of change in VO_2max and a maximal heart rate in master athletes," *Medicine and Science in Sports and Exercise* 33(10): 1744-1750.

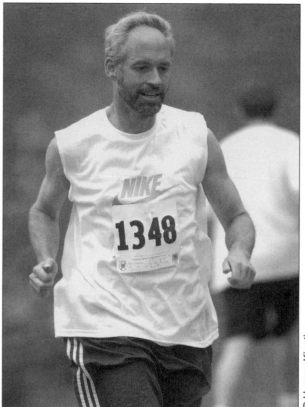

A number of age-related changes in physiological function influence the level of performance that this older male runner can achieve, even with training.

age in master athletes also, but this may represent an adaptation to long-term endurance training (Wiswell et al., 2000). The higher LT of master athletes than of younger athletes has been shown to compensate for lower $\dot{V}O_2$max, accounting for equivalent performances of older and younger athletes.

Muscle Mass and Function

Aging is associated with dramatic changes in skeletal muscle. Studies suggest that chronic exercise delays loss of muscle mass, strength, and power. Resistance and speed training have been shown to be particularly effective. Strength- and sprint-trained older athletes have greater muscle mass, strength, and power and more and larger fast-twitch muscle fibers than untrained peers have (Sipila, Viitasalo, Era, & Suominen, 1991; Klitgaard et al., 1990). In contrast, older endurance-trained athletes are generally weaker or at best no stronger than untrained peers. However, endurance athletes usually have lower body mass, and they are generally stronger than untrained older adults when these differences are accounted for. Additionally, it has been shown that older endurance athletes maintain thigh muscle strength over time and thus retain strength in relation to body mass, which may be more important in terms of physical function

than absolute strength. However, master endurance athletes also lose whole-body muscle mass at rates that are similar to untrained older adults, most likely because the musculature of the upper body is not used in their training.

Body Composition

Endurance-trained master athletes have lower body fat percentages than sedentary individuals of similar ages; however, they tend to have higher levels of fat mass than young athletes and levels similar to those of young, untrained adults (Pollock et al., 1997; Wiswell et al., 2001). This could be explained by aging as well as nutrition, training changes, and lean body mass changes in master athletes.

Training

Training volume and intensity decrease in master athletes, with the greatest decreases occurring in intensity. Master swimmers and runners reduce

> Changes in physiological and psychological function with aging combine to reduce the exercise performance of master athletes. In general, these declines in function are reduced by chronic exercise, although rapid declines occur during periods of diminished exercise. Both the trainer and the athlete should use this knowledge to develop safe and effective training programs and to set realistic performance goals.

practice time by up to 50 percent and focus more on endurance training than younger athletes (Starkes, Weir, Singh, Hodges, & Kerr, 1999; Weir, Kerr, Hodges, McKay, & Starkes, 2002). These reductions occur not only because of functional losses but also because of greater obligations to family and work that consume both time and energy (Menard & Stanish, 1989). Moreover, master athletes are more likely to experience injury and take longer to rehabilitate than younger athletes (Spirduso, 1995). In fact, a majority of significant alterations in the master athletes' training might be due to chronic injury.

Motivation

Motivation decreases in master athletes for various reasons (Carron & Leith, 1986). Striving to win becomes less important for many, partly because victories become relative (winning within an age group) rather than absolute (winning overall; Spirduso, 1995). Demands on time and energy diminish the enjoyment and relaxation of exercise, making it more difficult for the master athlete to train or compete hard (Menard & Stanish, 1989). Injury, fear of injury, and change in health status also affect the motivation of the master athlete.

Sociocultural Aspects of Masters Competition

In addition to reducing or delaying losses of physical fitness and function, participation in masters sport is also associated with other aspects of positive aging. Surveys have shown that master athletes are very interested in maintaining good health and consider their quality of life to be much better than their sedentary peers, in spite of a similar incidence of chronic disease (Shephard, Kavanagh, Mertens, Qureshi, & Clark, 1995; Magee & D'Antonio,

2001). Master athletes also tend to visit a physician regularly and are compliant in taking medications. They focus on family, friends, and relationships and are avid readers and Internet users, helping them stay socially connected (Magee & D'Antonio, 2001).

Principles of Training

There is currently no evidence to suggest that training principles for master athletes differ significantly from those for younger athletes. Hard training is required for sport success, no matter the age of the athlete. However, the correct application of exercise principles and guidelines can minimize many of the declines previously described, reduce the risk of acute and chronic injury, and maximize sport performance. These principles and guidelines are discussed in the following sections.

Individualization

Because of the large variation in physical function among older adults, **individualization** of the exercise prescription is essential for this population. This remains true for the master athlete for several reasons. Master athletes have generally not participated in sports continuously from youth into older age, and many participate in sports with which they have little previous experience. Master athletes also vary widely in their approach to competition. While some master athletes exercise for physical fitness and compete simply to provide incentives, goals, and inspiration for hard training, others consider the competition to be of primary importance. Also, not all master athletes are elite competitors, and many may not demonstrate higher levels of physical function than noncompetitive clients. Training programs should be based on the health, functional capacity, experience, and expectations of the individual master athlete.

Specificity

In athletics, the principle of **specificity** applies primarily to the chosen sport and targeted energy system. To improve in a particular sport (e.g., running, swimming, track and field), that activity should be a primary focus in training. Likewise, the energy system that is the major determinant of success in a particular sport or event should be a focus in training. The three energy pathways to be considered are determined by the duration of the competitive event (see table 17.1). The anaerobic alactic pathway is utilized primarily for activities lasting only a few seconds. These include sprints, throws and jumps in track and field, weightlifting, and many team and racket sports. The anaerobic lactic pathway is the primary energy source for activities lasting between 10 and 90 seconds, which include the long sprints in track and field,

swimming, and cycling and some team and racket sports (depending on the skill level of the players). Beyond 90 seconds, the aerobic pathway becomes the major contributor of energy for exercise. All endurance activities in any sport rely on the aerobic pathway.

Additional characteristics of the event and the energy pathway further specify the type of training that is appropriate (see table 17.1). Power represents the maximal capacity of an energy pathway and determines the success of shorter-duration performances in an energy pathway (lactic, 10-60 seconds; aerobic, 2-30 minutes). Training the power of an energy pathway expands its maximal capacity and allows the athlete to exercise longer at or very near that maximal capacity. Efficiency is a characteristic of the lactic and aerobic energy pathways and determines success in longer-duration events in those energy pathways. Training for efficiency allows the athlete to exercise at a greater percentage of the maximal capacity of the pathway for longer periods of time. Capacity is primarily a quality of the aerobic system and reflects training

> Individualization of training is important for the master athlete. The trainer should avoid a cookbook approach to prescribing exercise and instead develop training programs that reflect each athlete's current level of physical fitness, experience in the chosen sport activity, and motivation for competing. In general, less well-trained athletes should focus on training volume over intensity, whereas better-trained athletes should place greater emphasis on training intensity.

TABLE 17.1 Training Strategies

Event duration	0-10 sec	10-90 sec	40 sec-4 min	2-30 min	20 min-5 h	3+ h
Training goal	Alactic power	Lactic power	Lactic efficiency	Aerobic power	Aerobic efficiency	Aerobic capacity
Training strategy	Speed work and weightlifting	Speed endurance	Special endurance	Intensive tempo	Extensive tempo	Continuous tempo
Percentage of effort*	95%-100%	95%-100%	90%-95%	90%-100%	80%-90%	60%-75%
Training duration	3-10 sec	10-60 sec	40-90 sec	15 sec-10 min	90 sec-1 h	10 min-2 h
Repetitions	3-4	1-5	1-4	4-20	1-5	1-6
Sets	3-4	1-3	1	1	1	1
Recovery between repetitions	1.5-3 min	2-20 min	20-30 min	2:1	1:1	1:1
Recovery between sets	8-10 min	8-10 min				

* Percentage of effort is based on 100% for each energy system: 100% of the alactic system represents maximal short-duration (< 10 sec) speed or strength; 100% of the lactic system represents maximal longer-duration (10-90 sec) speed or strength; 100% of the aerobic system represents $\dot{V}O_2$max.

Data from T. Bompa, 1985, Theory and methodology of training - the key to athletic performance (Dubuque, IA: Kendall Hunt).

performed at the minimal training stimulus. This is often referred to as the aerobic threshold and reflects the minimum intensity required to influence fitness of the cardiovascular system. For the athlete, aerobic capacity training is useful primarily for general conditioning and recovery.

Overcompensation and Recovery

Positive adaptation to training involves a process of correctly timed work and recovery; adaptation occurs during recovery. The overcompensation curve, illustrated in figure 17.4, defines that process. Intense or long-duration exercise leads to fatigue; during the following period of recovery, physical fitness improves beyond the previous level. The process is characterized by both adequate recovery and the proper application of the next intense training stimulus. Adequate **recovery** is very important to the older athlete, as it ensures proper adaptation to training and helps avoid overtraining and injury. Recovery from vigorous exercise takes longer for people who are older, less fit, or overstressed. Moreover, women generally recover more slowly than men. Recovery periods should be built into the weekly, monthly, and yearly training plans (discussed in greater detail later in this chapter) in the form of both low-volume and low-intensity training and complete rest. The exercise performance of many older athletes very likely suffers because they do not allow adequate recovery from training. The next intense training stimulus following fatigue should be timed to coincide with

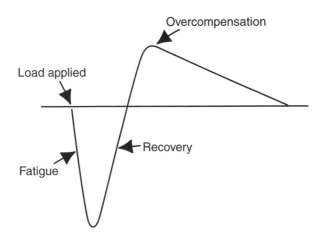

FIGURE 17.4 Overcompensation curve. The next training stimulus should be applied at the peak of overcompensation.

Reprinted, by permission, from F. Dick, 1984, *Training theory* (London: British Amateur Athletic Board).

the peak of overcompensation for maximal adaptation to occur. Determining this point is part of both the art and science of coaching, as general guidelines of two to three days rest between hard efforts must be confirmed by trial and error for individual athletes.

Gradual Adaptation to Physiological Stress

The principles referred to as overload and progression are applied by manipulating training intensity and volume. The gradual application of overload and progression is a cornerstone of proper exercise prescription for any client. Several basic guidelines for training intensity and volume can assist the athlete in adapting gradually to stress. **Training volume** is a product of frequency and duration and can be quantified as distance, time, repetitions, or weight per day, week, month, or year. Volume should be low for beginning athletes and early in the training cycle, and it should increase gradually by not more than 10 percent per week.

Multiple training sessions in a day to achieve high volume is rarely a good practice for master athletes, particularly in weight-bearing activities. While there are currently no guidelines for optimal volumes, younger elite master athletes can attain training volumes similar to those of young elite athletes, and older athletes generally need to use lower training volume. For example, among younger elite master athletes who trained daily, self-selected training volumes reported by runners were 90 to 120 miles (145-193 kilometers) per week, cyclists 150 to 200 miles (241-322 kilometers) per week, and swimmers 14 to 17 miles (25,000-30,000 yards, or 23-27 kilometers) per week (Wiswell et al., 2001). However, most older athletes in the same study trained only three to five days per week, and self-selected training volumes for runners were 25 to 45 miles (40-72 kilometers) per week, cyclists 40 to 80 miles (64-129 kilometers) per week, and swimmers four to six miles (8,000-10,000 yards, or six-ten kilometers) per week.

Training intensity refers to the strength of the stimulus or quality of the effort. For alactic exercise, intensity can be quantified as speed, percentage of one-repetition maximum (1RM), or rating of perceived exertion (RPE). For lactic and aerobic exercise, intensity can be quantified as speed, percentage of $\dot{V}O_2max$, percentage of maximum heart rate (HRmax), percentage of heart rate reserve (HR reserve), lactate threshold (LT), or RPE. In older sedentary adults, percentages of $\dot{V}O_2$max and HRmax accurately estimate training intensity, whereas HR reserve and RPE have been shown to underestimate intensity (Kohrt, Spina, Holloszy, & Ehsani, 1998). In contrast, percentages of $\dot{V}O_2$max, HRmax, and HR reserve effectively predict exercise intensity in master athletes. Although no data currently exist concerning the accuracy of RPE for monitoring training intensity in older athletes, it is likely that RPE is accurate, as athletes are more accustomed to hard exercise than sedentary adults. Recall that LT represents a greater percentage of $\dot{V}O_2$max in older adults independent of training status, so you should exercise caution when using LT to prescribe exercise intensity for inexperienced older athletes.

Training intensity should start low early in the training cycle and gradually increase. Peak training intensity is generally determined by the intensity or pace of the competitive event. That is, peak training intensity for 5K runners should be 5K racing speed. Master athletes are able to train at the same relative intensities as younger athletes but not as often within a training cycle. In addition, volume and intensity should have an inverse relationship: As intensity increases, volume should decrease. Many master athletes reduce training intensity because they are unwilling to reduce training volume. Some successful older athletes maintain high-intensity training by reducing training frequency and duration to allow adequate recovery.

Components of Master Athlete Training Programs

There is currently very little research on effective training practices for master athletes. However, this is true of training practices for younger athletes as well. Most of the information published concerning training methods for athletes is derived from professional practice. Thus, information presented in this section is derived from sources such as the *USA Track and Field Coaching Manual* (Gambetta, 1981) and coaching certification program materials (USA Track & Field, 1991), as well as the author's and others' personal experience coaching, training, and testing master athletes (P. Daland, personal communication, May 2002; D. McLoughlin, personal communication, March 2002).

Perhaps the best way to demonstrate how to develop a training program for a master athlete

is by looking at a case study. The client is a 60-year-old male runner with 10 years of running experience whose primary events are 5K and 10K road races. His previous season's bests for the two events were 23:20 and 49:35, respectively, and he hopes to run under 23 minutes for the 5K and 49 minutes for the 10K. He has averaged 30 miles (48 kilometers) and five sessions per week for the past several years, with little variation in intensity or volume throughout the year. He has not experienced any major injuries or breaks in training. Figure 17.5 gives a sample training program for this client. The following sections explain many of the concepts introduced in this sample program.

Assessment

Several methods for assessing older adults are described in part II of this text. The accurate assessment of the physical fitness parameters of master athletes is important to optimize their training. It is also important to be aware that predictions of master athletes' physiological variables, particularly $\dot{V}O_2$max and HRmax, generally underestimate the actual values. Therefore, direct measures are always preferable when possible (see chapter 7 for a discussion of appropriate methods).

Planning

Planning is a key element in developing a training program for the master athlete. Athletes cannot be in peak condition all throughout the year, and planning prepares the athlete to reach top form for the most important competitions of the season. **Periodization**—or dividing the year into specific periods, each with a different focus, volume, and intensity—is commonly used in the training plan for athletes. The year is divided into four training periods: active rest, general fitness, specific fitness, and competition. Each period has a different focus, progressively building on the training performed in previous periods and ensuring the appropriate timing of training throughout the year. The focus of each training period is described later in this chapter. The sample training program in figure 17.5 uses periodization.

Unfortunately, few master athletes periodize their training, even though most would benefit if they did. Many master athletes spend the entire year in specific training and competition phases, thereby neglecting the active rest and general fitness

A series of 5K and 10K races next May and June are the target competitions. It is now early August, and the client has been training throughout the summer.

Step 1. Outline the periods and determine peak volume and intensity.

Macrocycle 1 (August)—Active rest

Macrocycles 2-3 (September-October)—General conditioning

Macrocycles 4-9 (November-April)—Specific conditioning

Macrocycles 10-11 (May-June)—Competition

Peak volume—40 miles (64 km) per week, in five days' training each week; peak intensity—race pace for 5K in under 23 minutes (7:25 per mile, 4:36 per kilometer). If assessments are possible, aerobic efficiency training is performed at the lactate threshold running pace, and aerobic power training is performed at $\dot{V}O_2$max running pace. If assessments are not possible, training paces are based on $\dot{V}O_2$max pace, which can be approximated from 5K race pace.

Step 2. Outline specific volume, intensity, and training strategies for each period.

Active rest

(1) Volume and intensity should be low, no more than 15 miles (24 km) of running per week.

(2) Training strategies

(a) Aerobic capacity 60%-70% (10:30-12:30 per mile, 6:34-7:49 per kilometer)

(b) Complementary training

(c) Cross-training

(d) Recovery one to two days per week

General conditioning

(1) Volume builds gradually from 20 to 35 miles (32-56 km) per week.

Macrocycle 2—Microcycle volume 20, 22, 25, 20 miles (32, 35, 40, 32 km) per week

Macrocycle 3—Microcycle volume 25, 28, 30, 20 miles (40, 45, 48, 32 km) per week

(2) Intensity builds gradually from current 5K race pace.

(3) Training strategies

(a) Aerobic capacity one to three days per week, 60%-75% (10:00-12:30 per mile, 6:15-7:49 per kilometer)

(b) Aerobic efficiency one to two days per week, 80%-90% (8:20-9:15 per mile, 5:12-5:46 per kilometer)

(c) Aerobic power introduced in microcycle 4, one day every two weeks, 90%-100% (7:30-8:20 per mile, 4:41-5:12 per kilometer)

(d) Complementary training two to three days per week, focusing on strength and flexibility weaknesses

(e) Cross-training one to two days per week in place of aerobic capacity training

(f) Alactic (speed) training one day every two to three weeks

(g) Recovery one to two days per week

Specific conditioning

(1) Volume builds to 40 miles (64 km) per week, then declines as intensity increases.

Macrocycle 4—Microcycle volumes 30, 32, 35, 25 miles (48, 51, 56, 40 km) per week

Macrocycle 5—Microcycle volumes 32, 35, 37, 30 miles (51, 56, 60, 48 km) per week

Macrocycle 6—Microcycle volumes 35, 37, 40, 30 miles (56, 60, 64, 48 km) per week

Macrocycle 7—Microcycle volumes 40, 37, 35, 30 miles (64, 60, 56, 48 km) per week

Macrocycle 8—Microcycle volumes 35, 32, 30, 25 miles (56, 51, 48, 40 km) per week

Macrocycle 9—Microcycle volumes 32, 30, 30, 25 miles (51, 48, 48, 40 km) per week

(2) Intensity builds toward goal race pace.

(continued)

FIGURE 17.5   Training program development: A case study.

(3) Training strategies

(a) Aerobic capacity one to three days per week, 60%-75% (9:00-12:00 per mile, 5:38-7:30 per kilometer)

(b) Aerobic efficiency one to two days per week, 80%-90% (8:10-9:10 per mile, 5:06-5:44 per kilometer)

(c) Aerobic power one day every one to two weeks, 90%-100% (7:20-8:10 per mile, 4:35-5:06 per kilometer)

(d) Complementary training two to three days per week for weaknesses

(e) Cross-training one or two times per week in place of aerobic capacity

(f) Alactic (speed) training one day every one to two weeks

(g) Recovery one to two days per week

Competition

(1) Training volume is reduced to 15 to 25 miles (24-40 km) per week.

(2) Intensity is limited to one hard training session the week of a competition and two during weeks without races. Intense workouts should focus on goal race pace for the 5K and 10K races (7:25 and 7:54 per mile, or 4:38 and 4:56 per kilometer, respectively), followed by one to two recovery days.

(3) Training strategies

(a) Aerobic capacity one to three days per week, 5 to 10 miles (8-16 km) total running, 60%-75% (9:00-12:00 per mile, 5:38-7:30 per kilometer)

(b) Aerobic efficiency one day per week if no competition

(c) Aerobic power one day per week

(d) Cross-training one to two times per week in place of aerobic capacity

(e) Alactic (speed) training one day every one to two weeks

(f) Recovery one to two days per week

Step 3. Develop the daily workouts within each microcycle as the plan proceeds.

Step 4. Be flexible.

FIGURE 17.5   *(continued)*

periods. For example, an older athlete who focuses on one race each year, plans his or her training to peak for that particular race in an organized fashion, and then takes several months off from structured training to recover can achieve and maintain a high level of performance over many years.

Period durations described in the literature are for younger athletes and may not accurately meet the needs of master athletes. In general, more-experienced athletes can spend shorter periods of time in general training (1-4 months) with longer periods of time devoted to specific training and competition (6-10 months). Inexperienced athletes require a longer general training period (4-12 months), however, so that they can build the base of fitness necessary for hard training. Competition periods are generally two to four months in duration. All master athletes, regardless of experience, should incorporate a planned active rest period of at least one month in duration. Note that the period durations described in figure 17.5 (i.e., one month

of active rest, two months of general training, six months of specific training, and two months of competition) are for an experienced athlete.

Active Rest

Active rest is not a time without any physical activity but rather a time for training at a low intensity and volume to allow recovery. Cross-training is particularly useful during active rest, as long as volume and intensity remain low. For example, rowers may alternate long walks, bicycle rides, and light running with several days of rest per week, with maybe an occasional bout on a rowing ergometer. However, it is often advisable to minimize exercise involving the athlete's mode of competitive activity to allow psychological as well as physiological recovery.

General Conditioning

General conditioning develops a base of endurance, strength, and flexibility that enables the athlete to achieve the high-intensity training required in later periods. Training during this phase need not be event or sport specific, as the basic goal is building fitness. Volume is more important than intensity during this phase. Circuit training and complementary training (described later) are useful, as is aerobic capacity training (see table 17.1). For beginning athletes, this phase is a good time to introduce technique work.

Specific Conditioning

Specific conditioning develops the technique and conditioning required for success in a particular event, and training should focus on the specific activity and its primary energy systems. Table 17.1 outlines specific training strategies and guidelines based on event duration and training goal. The training strategy should encompass both goals for events whose duration falls under two overlapping columns (e.g., the training goal for an event of 60 seconds' duration should be to improve both lactic power and lactic efficiency). Non-weight-bearing sports such as swimming, cycling, and rowing have longer durations at higher intensities than running and other weight-bearing activities.

To train for power, the athlete should perform exercise at or near 100 percent of the target energy system's capacity. For example, to improve the power of the alactic pathway, use near maximal strength or speed exercise. Developing the power of an energy system is very intense and requires longer recovery periods, especially for the lactic and aerobic pathways. This type of training should be scheduled no more than once a week and should not represent more than 5 to 8 percent of the weekly volume. Training the efficiency of an energy system is also intense, but less so than power, so it can be done once or twice per week. Efficiency training should be no more than 10 percent of the weekly volume. Capacity training can be done either continuously or with long intervals and is considered intense when a single workout is very long.

In the specific conditioning phase, volume peaks early, after which intensity starts to build as volume declines. In addition, while specific conditioning is of primary concern, all training strategies that contribute to the athlete's success should receive attention. For example, endurance athletes should do training that targets the alactic system because most competitions, regardless of distance, require sprinting at some point during the race. However, training at greater than competition intensity should

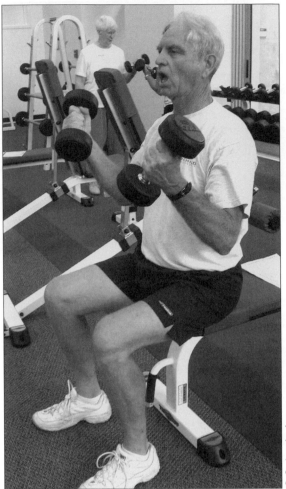

Maximal strength training is important for improving the power of the alactic pathway.

be minimal (one to three times per macrocycle), as it reduces functional capacity and lowers performance. In contrast, training at lower than competition intensity allows recovery but provides a minimal training stimulus.

Using various levels of training intensity in each period has been shown to be the most effective means of maximizing fitness and recovery. For example, during the specific conditioning period, 5K runners focus on aerobic power training, but they should also incorporate a few sessions aimed at developing aerobic capacity, aerobic and lactic efficiency, and alactic power. When entering competitions during this period, the master athlete should focus on developing a particular aspect of fitness or on a particular strategy rather than on outcomes such as speed or ranking. Training takes precedence over competing.

Competition

The focus of the **competition period** is to bring the athlete to peak condition for sport performance. Volume during this period is low to moderate, while intensity reaches its peak. Almost all training during this phase is event specific, followed by long recovery periods. The competitions are more important than training during this period.

Microcycles and Macrocycles

Within each period, training is organized into smaller units known as cycles. A **microcycle** is one to two weeks in length, and a **macrocycle** is a group of two to four microcycles (one month). The cycle method of planning allows effective management of hard and easy training sessions to optimize physical adaptation and recovery (Bompa, 1985; Gambetta, 1981). A microcycle should include one to two hard training sessions, each followed by easy to moderate sessions. Master athletes may need two or more easy days to recover from hard workouts. Figure 17.6a represents a microcycle plan with one high-intensity training session in the week and two rest days.

Macrocycle plans allow the trainer to progress volume and intensity in an organized fashion and also to enhance recovery by reducing volume and intensity every third or fourth microcycle. Figure 17.6b demonstrates this technique: Training volume and intensity build during microcycles 1 to 3 and are then reduced in microcycle 4. Periodization is particularly appropriate for the master athlete. Training that does not vary in intensity or volume throughout the year and does not include adequate time for recovery leads to fatigue, overtraining, and injury, all significant concerns for the master athlete.

Putting the Plan Into Practice

Start by developing a yearly training plan. After identifying the most important competitions of the year, establish time frames for each period. In the sample training schedule in figure 17.5, the important competition period is May and June. Period durations are determined from the active rest month of the previous August. Next, establish the peak volume and intensity to be achieved during the training year, then establish the beginning volume and intensity. Remember that volume and intensity should increase gradually, no more

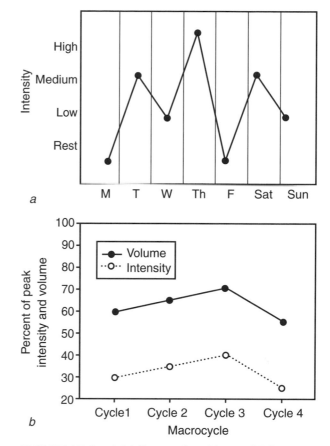

FIGURE 17.6 *(a)* Microcycle with one high-intensity workout. Points represent training intensity for each day of the week. *(b)* Macrocycle with progressive increase in volume and intensity followed by one rest microcycle (reduced volume and intensity). Volume and intensity are indicated as a percentage of the yearly maximum.

Reprinted, by permission, from T. Bompa, 1985, *Theory and methodology of training- The key to athletic performance* (Dubuque, IA: Kendal Hunt).

than 10 percent in one microcycle, and as intensity increases, volume should decrease.

In the example in figure 17.5, 40 miles (64 kilometers) per week and the target 5K race pace are selected as the peak volume and intensity. Peak volume is not achieved until the 11th week of general conditioning (macrocycle 4) and beginning volume is set at 20 miles (32 kilometers) per week. Beginning intensity is based on the client's current 5K race pace. Finally, the training goals and strategies to use in each period are identified (refer to table 17.1). Specific microcycles are developed throughout the training year, based on the yearly plan. Trainers and athletes should remember that plans can and should be adapted as required.

Peaking

The goal of planned training is to ensure the athlete is in peak condition for the most important competitions of the year. **Peaking** is a product of proper training, an adequate number of competitions, and unloading or recovery. In track and field, it has been estimated that 10 to 20 competitions are required for younger athletes to peak. One competition every other week throughout the specific conditioning and competition periods is ideal. Peaking also requires adequate recovery, usually called *unloading*. This is accomplished by reducing volume by 50 percent or more while maintaining the same intensity, with a long recovery period between hard sessions and competitions. Two weeks is generally required for adequate unloading for younger athletes, but this may need to be longer for master athletes. In the example presented in figure 17.5, unloading occurs throughout the entire competition period, with the greatest reductions in the week before a target competition.

There is currently no research that documents the benefits of peaking for master athletes. However, a recent study demonstrated that the endurance performance of master athletes was much stabler over time than that of younger athletes (Hopkins & Hewson, 2001). Whether this reflects a fault in training or older athletes' inability to peak is unclear.

Cross-Training

Cross-training involves exercise to enhance the energy system critical to success in the athlete's sport or event but that is not specific to the activity of the event. Endurance runners, for example,

> Periodized training involves dividing the year into segments with specific training goals that build on training performed in earlier segments. In a periodized training program, plans based on weekly microcycles and monthly macrocycles allow proper progression of volume and intensity and alternation between hard and easy training for optimal training adaptation and recovery. Periodization ensures that the athlete is in peak condition for the most important competitions of the year and reduces the risk of injury and overtraining.

can train the aerobic energy system by cycling. Activity specificity remains essential, as athletes lose event-specific fitness despite retaining general fitness through cross-training. However, several advantages of cross-training make it not only advisable but in many cases essential for the master athlete. Cross-training minimizes the risk of overuse injuries, allows complete upper- and lower-body fitness, and enhances recovery while still providing a training stimulus. Therefore, cross-training should be included in the training plan.

Complementary Training

Complementary training is not specific to the athlete's event but is aimed at improving general fitness and preventing injury. Complementary training, particularly flexibility and resistance training, is extremely important for the master athlete and should be part of the training plan. As described in chapter 11, aging is associated with alterations in connective tissue that lead to greater stiffness, reduced flexibility, and diminished joint range of motion. Although physical activity minimizes the changes, loss of flexibility still occurs in master athletes. The increased risk of injury posed by diminished range of motion clearly demonstrates the need for flexibility training. The training program should include regular, static flexibility exercises for the major muscle groups of the body. These exercises should be done as a stand-alone flexibility training component, not simply as a component of the warm-up or cool-down.

Resistance training should also be included in a well-rounded training program. Loss of muscle mass and strength contributes to many of the functional changes and the increased risk of injury experienced by master athletes. Resistance training is essential for older athletes to maintain muscle mass and strength, yet many master athletes, particularly endurance athletes, do not include resistance exercise in their training program. Athletes whose performance depends on maximizing muscle strength and power (e.g., for weightlifting, jumping, and throwing) require high-intensity strength training. But resistance exercise of moderate intensity (50-70 percent of 1RM) as complementary training is likely to improve the overall performance of any master athlete. Refer to chapter 12 for specific resistance-training protocols. Circuit training, also described in chapter 13, is another form of complementary training that has the unique advantage of addressing aerobic endurance, flexibility, and strength in the same workout.

Training Precautions

Training for sport performance requires hard exercise, regardless of the athlete's age. However, hard exercise by older adults requires several precautions that affect not only sport performance but also athletes' safety and enjoyment of their chosen activity.

Medical Screening

The American College of Sports Medicine (ACSM, 2000) recommends that older adults considering participation in vigorous exercise should be medically screened and cleared. More recently, however, it has been suggested this advice may be inappropriate for older adults considering physical activity for several reasons. It could act as a deterrent to participation, it is expensive, and it seems of little benefit for identifying individuals at risk of significant health problems from exercise (Gill, DiPietro, & Krumholz, 2000). However, this argument seems aimed at screening for moderate physical activity. Athletic participation involves high-intensity exercise in both training and competition, which is justification to advise all your athletes to undergo a medical screening before training for sport participation. You should also obtain a medical release signed by the examining physician for each master athlete.

Overtraining

Overtraining occurs when excessive volume or intensity, coupled with inadequate recovery, leads to chronic fatigue, staleness, and injury. Overtraining leads to decreased exercise capacity and exercise performance (Moore, 1999). Improper training, life events, social environments, inadequate nutrition, and health problems can contribute to overtraining. Training faults include excessive workload, inadequate recovery, too rapid an increase in workload, and scheduling too many competitions. However, training alone is rarely the cause of overtraining. Demands of daily life, insufficient sleep, poor nutrition, and poor health also contribute to overtraining.

Older adults are more likely to face these additional stressors that, when combined with exercise,

lead to overtraining. In addition, older adults take longer to recover from stress. Therefore, overtraining is a common and significant issue for master athletes, and it is crucial for the physical activity instructor or personal trainer to recognize the signs and symptoms of overtraining (see figure 17.7) and know how to prevent it. One of the early signs is decreased exercise performance, which may occur before physical symptoms of overtraining appear (Moore, 1999). Exercise may seem harder than usual and cause rapid exhaustion. Heart rate can be dramatically affected: Resting and recovery heart rates can increase, while maximal heart rate decreases. For this reason, a master athlete's heart rate should be closely monitored, both at rest and during training. Other symptoms of overtraining include extreme tiredness, mood and personality disturbances, weight loss, loss of appetite, sleep disturbances, chronic muscle soreness, and increased injuries and illness.

Overtraining is best avoided by following a planned training schedule with controlled increases in volume and intensity and periodized recovery. Good nutrition and adequate hydration are also important. Cross-training is an effective way of avoiding overtraining. Finally, master athletes should be encouraged to take it easy when they are feeling run down or when they are experiencing significant stress from sources other than training.

Injury Prevention

Acute and overuse injuries occur with much greater frequency among master athletes than younger

---

- Chronic muscle soreness
- Decreased appetite
- Decreased exercise performance
- Decreased maximal heart rate
- Depression
- Increased irritability
- Increased recovery heart rate
- Increased resting heart rate
- Injuries and illness
- Loss of motivation
- Sleep disturbances
- Weight loss

FIGURE 17.7 Signs and symptoms of overtraining.

athletes (Maharam et al., 1999). The type of injury usually depends on the activity or sport. Swimmers commonly injure their shoulders, whereas rowers tend to suffer back and knee injuries. Cyclists suffer more upper-extremity injuries, whereas runners tend to injure the lower extremities, particularly the knees. Older athletes are more susceptible to injury as a result of age-related changes in connective tissue, bone, and muscle. Tendons are more likely to rupture, cartilage is more likely to tear, and stress fractures are more likely to occur.

Additionally, the healing process is prolonged in older athletes, and they often never achieve complete recovery. Athletes over the age of 60 years take twice as long to heal as younger adults, while athletes over the age of 75 years take three times as long (Brown, 1989). For this reason, injury prevention is essential for the master athlete. The most effective means of preventing injury is through gradual progression of volume and intensity, adequate recovery time, and effective use of complementary and cross-training. Proper equipment, technique, and nutrition also play an important role in reducing the likelihood of injury.

Physical activity instructors should recognize that many master athletes are reluctant to discontinue training and competing despite being injured. This trait is common to athletes of any age. Master athletes must be made to recognize that relatively short periods away from activity to allow an injury to heal or supplementing their sport-specific training with cross-training increases the likelihood of their lifelong participation in sport. On the other hand, continuing to train with an injury creates the potential for damage that might permanently end sport participation (Menard & Stanish, 1989).

Summary

Master athletes embody the potential for truly successful aging. Although athletic performance declines with age as a result of changes in physiological and psychological function, sport-specific exercise training can significantly reduce the loss of physical function normally associated with aging. Participation in masters sport is growing, and physical activity specialists should understand the needs and characteristics of older competitive athletes. Key steps for the effective training of master athletes include individualizing the program, developing a training program specific to the sport and energy demands of the event, and gradually increasing volume and intensity to allow optimal adaptation.

An individualized exercise program must consider the athlete's current level of physical fitness, his or her experience in the chosen sport, and his or her motivation for competing. Adequate planning, a process known as periodization, involves yearly phases during which the focus of training varies in weekly and monthly cycles. Active rest allows the athlete to recover and rebuild from a previous training cycle, after which training builds in volume and intensity in general and specific conditioning phases. The competition period coincides with the most important events of the training cycle and allows the athlete to peak at those events. Perhaps the most important component of the master athlete's training is adequate recovery, without which the athlete is highly susceptible to overtraining, overuse, and injury. Recovery involves both days without exercise training and planned cross-training and complementary training.

Key Terms

active rest 273
competition period 275
complementary training 276
general conditioning 273
individualization 268
lactate threshold (LT) 266
macrocycle 275
master athletes 264
microcycle 275
overtraining 277
peaking 276
periodization 271
recovery 270
specific conditioning 274
specificity 268
training intensity 270
training volume 270
$\dot{V}O_2max$ 265

Recommended Readings

Fee, E.W. (2001). *How to be a champion from 9 to 90: Body, mind, and spirit training.* Mississagua, ON: Feetness.

Sloan, J. (1999). *Staying fit over fifty: Conditioning for outdoor activities.* Seattle, WA: Mountaineers.

Study Questions

1. The master athlete is
   a. an older adult who is very physically active
   b. an adult who exceeds a minimum age and participates in masters competitive events
   c. an older athlete who was an elite performer at an early age
   d. an older athlete who is elite in his or her sport

2. Sport performance with age
   a. declines in a linear fashion throughout the life span
   b. declines to a greater extent in power events than in endurance events
   c. declines at the same rate in men and women
   d. declines to a greater extent in sprint events than in endurance events

3. Which of the following statements is true concerning injury in the master athlete?
   a. Master athletes are more likely to get injured than younger athletes.
   b. Master athletes heal more quickly than younger athletes.
   c. Master athletes tend to injure the knees regardless of mode of activity.
   d. Injuries are best prevented by avoiding cross-training.

4. Adequate recovery for the master athlete
   a. is less important than for the younger athlete
   b. is unimportant for improvements in fitness to occur
   c. can be achieved by following a training program similar to one for young athletes
   d. helps prevent injury and illness

5. At which point in the overcompensation curve should the next training stimulus be applied?
   a. fatigue
   b. recovery
   c. overcompensation peak
   d. return to baseline following overcompensation

6. Planned training involves
   a. organizing the training year into periods, each with a specific training focus
   b. building on the training achieved in the previous period
   c. weekly and monthly plans to optimize the alternation between hard and easy workouts
   d. all of the above

Application Activities

1. Overtraining is a significant concern for master athletes. Describe the common signs and symptoms of overtraining, and discuss strategies to avoid overtraining in older athletes.

2. Outline a training program for an inexperienced master long-distance swimmer and an experienced master track and field sprinter. Explain why these training programs may need to be different.

Part V

Program Design, Leadership, and Risk Management

International Curriculum Guidelines for Preparing Physical Activity Instructors of Older Adults

TRAINING MODULE 1:
Overview of Aging and Physical Activity

TRAINING MODULE 2:
Psychological, Sociocultural, and Physiological Aspects of Physical Activity and Older Adults

TRAINING MODULE 9:
Ethics and Professional Conduct

TRAINING MODULE 3:
Screening, Assessment, and Goal Setting

TRAINING MODULE 8:
Client Safety and First Aid

TRAINING MODULE 4:
Program Design and Management

TRAINING MODULE 7:
Leadership, Communication, and Marketing Skills

TRAINING MODULE 6:
Teaching Skills

TRAINING MODULE 5:
Program Design for Older Adults With Stable Medical Conditions

The final section of the book provides you with additional knowledge and skills needed to become an effective instructor of physical activity programs for older adults. The focus of the five remaining chapters include teaching and leadership skills, understanding motor learning principles, knowing how to develop a risk management plan, and understanding the legal standards and professional ethics of this field. Chapter 18 addresses specific topics included in training modules 4 and 6—applying movement analysis and motor learning principles to the selection and implementation of specific activities designed to enhance the skill-related components of functional fitness. Chapters 19 and 20 address recommended areas of study from training module 7—developing effective motivational, communication, and leadership skills for teaching individual and group classes. Chapter 20 also addresses specific topics in training modules 6 and 7, namely, how to develop safe, friendly, and fun exercise and physical activity environments, the development of lesson plans and elements of instruction, and how to market your physical activity program. Chapter 21 addresses both training modules 5 and 8 of the international guidelines, including how to prevent injury by adapting exercises to suit the fitness levels and medical conditions of your older adult clients, and information on the physiological and psychological effects of common medications. Another recommended area of study from training module 8, knowing how to give first aid and to respond appropriately to emergencies, is covered in chapter 22. The knowledge recommended in training module 9—legal, ethical, and professional conduct—is also addressed in chapter 22.

• Chapter 18 provides an overview of the important tasks associated with a qualitative analysis of movement skills and how to prioritize the methods used to correct errors in performance. Several important motor learning principles on which you can base your decisions about how best to create an optimal learning environment for your older adult clients are presented. You will learn how to use demonstrations and verbal cues effectively to introduce new movement skills, how to structure the practice environment to maximize learning, and how to provide augmented feedback to older adults as they learn skills.

• Building on the skills presented in chapter 18, chapter 19 presents ways to develop your leadership skills and thereby enhance your teaching effectiveness. A variety of techniques and strategies are presented, including how to motivate and effectively communicate with clients in both individual and group settings, how to create a positive learning environment, and how to analyze your effectiveness as an instructor.

• Designing and managing group conditioning classes is the focus of chapter 20. The discussion highlights strategies for becoming an effective instructor, including many ideas for creating a fun environment that will keep your older adult clients motivated. In addition, you will learn how to market your group exercise program, how to create a safe and comfortable exercise environment for older adults, and how to manage group dynamics to promote your class members' success.

• Chapter 21 discusses disabling conditions that can affect older adults and ways to modify exercises that will prevent injury and ensure the safety of your older adult clients with specific medical conditions. Also discussed are the effects of commonly prescribed medications and how they can influence client safety during exercise. You will learn how to recognize the signs and symptoms of overexertion and other conditions and what to do if they occur while your older adult client is exercising.

• Chapter 22 is devoted to a discussion of legal and ethical standards that will minimize your liability as a physical activity instructor. Legal case studies, legal concepts and definitions, and many issues related to lawsuits are introduced, including negligence, types of applicable insurance coverage, and how to develop a risk management plan. This information is provided to help you better recognize the boundaries of your professional competence and know when it is appropriate to refer older adult clients to physicians or other qualified health professionals. The last section of chapter 22 presents the professional ethics of the field today. This information can help you establish an exemplary reputation as a physical activity instructor of older adults and also help you elevate the reputation of the profession in general.

18

Applying Motor Learning Principles to Program Design

Richard A. Magill
Janene M. Grodesky

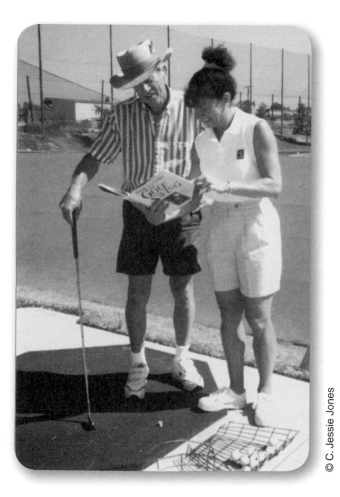

Although physical activity instructors of older adults are taught how to lead group exercise classes, the skill of effectively *teaching* movement skills to older adults is often overlooked in instructor training programs. An essential goal of instruction is to enable class participants to successfully learn skills. Although any instructional environment presents challenges, instructing older adults is particularly challenging. With this in mind, the primary goal of this chapter is to familiarize you with some fundamental motor learning concepts and to describe how to apply them effectively in group exercise programs for older adults. These concepts include movement analysis, the definition of learning as it applies to motor skills, the transfer of skill learning, the assessment of skill learning, and the stages of skill learning. Introducing new skills, providing augmented feedback to class participants, and structuring the class environment in which skills are practiced are also described.

Nervous System Changes and Motor Skill Learning

Changes within the nervous system influence how well the aging population is able to learn and perform movement skills. For example, changes in cognition, memory, and attention deserve special consideration by the physical activity instructor because of their possible effects on motor skill learning. Because many of the age-associated changes in neurological function are discussed in some detail in chapter 4, we briefly highlight only those changes that are likely to influence how the exercise setting should be structured for optimal learning.

Declines in cognitive functioning may have the greatest impact on motor skill learning for older adults. In fact, Salthouse (1991) asserts that these observable declines are sufficient for the instructor to give them special consideration. For instance, the pace of learning becomes slower in the elderly (Shephard, 1997). Also, the capacity to acquire new concepts or to apply existing concepts quickly and accurately to complex movement situations declines. The older adult's capacity to quickly adapt movement patterns in response to environmental conditions also declines (Spirduso, 1995). In addition, older adults typically demonstrate slower **simple reaction times** (i.e., to a single event) and **choice reaction times** (i.e., to multiple events), measures of how quickly they react to environmental stimuli or events. What is especially noteworthy for the physical activity instructor is that physically active elderly people do not exhibit a reduction in reaction times to the same extent as their inactive peers (Spirduso, 1995).

Aging effects on memory and attention are also relevant for motor skill learning. Deficits in memory functioning, especially short-term memory, can reveal themselves in difficulty remembering instructions and feedback and can lead to difficulty learning new movement patterns. Attention means attending to environmental events at a given time. Older adults can experience increased problems with tasks that require them to maintain their attentional focus for a period of time (e.g., reading a book), selectively attend to certain events in the environment while tuning out all others (e.g., the movements of the instructor and not other participants in the class), or divide attention between two different tasks (e.g., exercising or walking while conversing).

Movement Analysis of Skills

On what basis does an instructor decide what to try to accomplish in a teaching session? A comprehensive model of the qualitative analysis of skills proposed by Knudson and Morrison (2002) suggests that these decisions should depend on the results of four tasks for the instructor. As can be seen in figure 18.1, these tasks are sequential and cyclic.

The first task in the model is *preparation*, when the physical activity instructor acquires the prerequisite knowledge about the activities to be taught and the population (i.e., older adults) who will be

taught this information. This knowledge is essential for the physical activity instructor to become an effective analyzer of movement skills performed by older adults. The instructor's second task is the *observation* of the class participants' performance of the skill or activity. This should be done from several different viewpoints and should include several observations of each class participant. From these multiple observations comes the instructor's third task: the *evaluation* or *diagnosis* of the participant's performance. This task requires the instructor first to assess how correctly the critical features of the skill or activity are being performed (i.e., identifying and prioritizing the critical errors involved in the performance of the skill) and then to determine the strengths and weaknesses of the participant's task performance.

Finally, on the basis of the information accumulated from multiple observations and evaluation of the participants, the instructor then determines

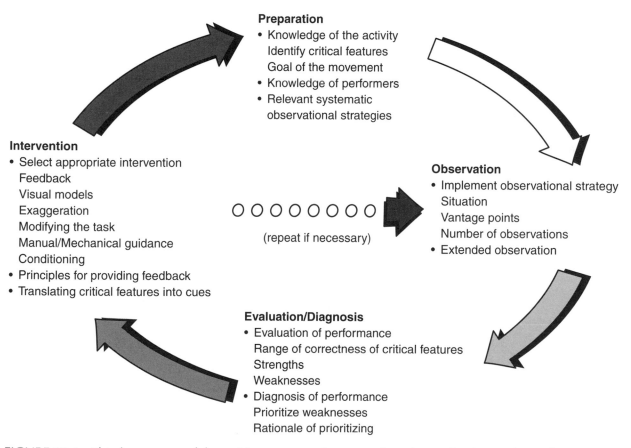

FIGURE 18.1   This four-step model provides a systematic approach to the qualitative analysis of movement skills.

Reprinted, by permission, from D.V. Knudson, and C.S. Morrison, 2002, *Qualitative analysis of human movement*, 2nd ed. (Champaign, IL: Human Kinetics), 9.

the appropriate *intervention* strategies to improve performance of the skill or activity. Because of the cyclic nature of the model, the instructor further observes and evaluates the results of the intervention strategies on the participants' performance and then continues with the same intervention strategies or alters them accordingly.

It is important to note that the evaluation, or assessment, of movement skills immediately precedes the selection of appropriate instruction techniques and practice condition characteristics. How does an instructor analyze movement skills? In the Knudson and Morrison model, this analysis is primarily **qualitative,** which means the "non-numerical analysis of movement . . . or a judgment on the quality of an aspect of movement" (Knudson & Morrison, 2002). To engage in this type of movement analysis, the instructor must have an adequate knowledge of the skill being evaluated. This knowledge is an important part of your preparation as a physical activity instructor. Your knowledge of a skill should include its critical features (i.e., characteristics that a person must perform correctly to achieve the goal of the skill).

Identification of the performance characteristics that are most important for successful performance of the skill results from an analysis of the skill. For example, an analysis of a vertical chest press on a weight machine results in the identification of the five critical features described in table 18.1.

The instructor also should establish an acceptable range of correctness when evaluating a person's performance of a skill or activity. Although the critical features of a skill need to be performed correctly, a certain amount of performance error is acceptable for any given critical feature. Some flexibility is necessary to accommodate for medical conditions your clients may have, such as structural deviations that affect postural alignment (e.g., scoliosis, kyphosis), back pain, joint surgery, or osteoporosis. But performance error that is greater than this acceptable range needs to be corrected. The breadth of the acceptable range of correctness for any critical feature depends on the performance context. For example, a broader range of error is acceptable for an activity that involves sitting than for one that involves standing, especially if loss of balance is of concern. Because the safety of the participants is the number one priority for all activities, the acceptable range of correctness for any activity should be determined according to the risk of injury that could result from a performance error.

The intervention task that follows performance evaluation and diagnosis should be based on the prioritizing of weaknesses identified during the diagnosis. Knudson and Morrison (2002) describe six approaches to determining priorities for correcting errors: (1) relating errors to previous actions, (2) maximizing improvement, (3) correcting errors in order of difficulty, (4) sequential error correction, (5) correcting errors starting from the base of support, and (6) correcting the most critical error first. Each of these six approaches is briefly summarized in table 18.2. No single approach should

TABLE 18.1   Critical Features of the Vertical Chest Press and Associated Verbal Cues

Critical features	Verbal cues
SKILL: VERTICAL CHEST PRESS (ON MACHINE)	
1. Five-point body contact position (left and right feet on floor, upper back and shoulders, lower back and buttocks, and back of head against seat and backrest)	Five points of body contact
2. Grasp handles with closed grip; wrists pronated	Firm hold, palms down, wrists extended not flexed
3. Push handles away from chest (at nipple height) to fully extended position	Push using a 1-2 count, fully extended arms
4. Exhale on concentric phase and inhale during the eccentric phase of movement	Blow out as you push away, inhale as you pull back, four-second count
5. Maintain five-point body contact position during both movement phases	Press down and back with body

TABLE 18.2   Approaches to Determining Priorities for Performance Correction

Approaches determining error correction priorities	Description of approaches
Relationship to previous actions	Errors are symptoms of other movement problems, e.g., not stepping on a step because of not looking at the step rather than because of a leg movement error.
Maximizing improvement	Prioritize error correction that can lead to the most improvement in the practice time available.
In order of difficulty	Correct errors that are the easiest to correct first, and then progress through errors that are more difficult to correct, an effective approach for older adults who exhibit low self-confidence in their ability to perform skills.
In temporal sequence	Correct errors in the sequence of affected skill components; an error in the performance of the first component of a skill (e.g., backswing of forehand tennis stroke) should be corrected first.
Base of support	Correct errors from the base of support up; e.g., for golf swing errors, begin error correction with stance errors.
Most critical first	Correct first errors in the component that is the most important for successful performance of the skill.

be considered the best. The approach you select depends on the goal and type of the skill and the learning stage of your client. (For a more detailed discussion of this movement analysis model, see Knudson and Morrison, 2002.)

Definition of Motor Skill Learning

How do you know when the client you are teaching has learned the skill or activity? To answer this question, it is important to have a working definition of the term **motor skill learning.** Most textbook authors (e.g., Magill, 2004; Rose & Christina, 2005; Schmidt & Wrisberg, 2004) agree that motor skill learning involves several distinct characteristics. (1) Learning results from practice or experience that takes place over a period of time. (2) During this period of time there is an observable improvement in the performance of the skill. (3) As performance improves, it becomes increasingly more consistent from one attempt to the next. (4) The performance improvement remains relatively permanent over time. (5) The learner can perform the skill in a variety of contexts in which the skill needs to be performed. Most of these characteristics are addressed by this working definition of motor skill learning: "a change in the capability of a person to perform a skill that must be inferred from a rela-

tively permanent improvement in performance as a result of practice or experience" (Magill, 2004, p. 193). Although the ability to perform the skill in a variety of situations is not explicitly stated in this definition, it is implied in the phrase "a relatively permanent improvement in performance." This transfer capability is discussed next.

Transfer of Motor Skill Learning

People perform many skills in contexts and situations that differ from those in which they learned them. An important reason that many of the older adults in your class participate is to acquire skills that will enhance their performance of activities of daily living as well as sport or recreational activities. For example, older adults may engage in aerobic and resistance exercises to help them better perform the activities they need or want to do every day, such as go up and down stairs or have better stamina when they play sports such as tennis or golf. In motor learning terms, this application of skills from one performance context to another is known as the **transfer of learning.**

Transfer of learning is typically judged by the degree to which the performance of a skill in one context influences the performance of the same skill in a different context or the performance of a dif-

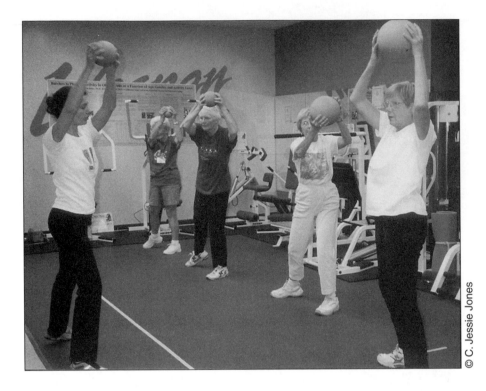

Activities that require older adults in your class to lift and lower balls of different weights will transfer to the performance of daily activities that involve lifting and lowering heavy objects such as wet laundry or packed suitcases.

© C. Jessie Jones

ferent skill. For example, physical activity instructors are often interested in knowing how well the skill they taught in class influences clients' ability to perform the same skill in their everyday lives. The transfer of learning can be *positive,* when the previous skill experience is beneficial, or it can be *negative,* when the previous skill experience hinders performance of either the practiced skill in a different context or a new but similar skill. In general, the greater the similarity between the practiced skill or context and the new skill or context, the greater the amount of positive transfer. This principle of transfer provides a good rationale for the inclusion of aerobic, resistance, and balance activities that mimic real-life skills in any class designed for older adults.

Applying the four steps of movement analysis described earlier is especially important to ensure positive transfer of skills. For example, suppose that a client wants to participate in an exercise class to help his or her tennis game. The instructor needs to determine the characteristics of playing tennis that could be enhanced through exercises and activities presented in the class. Positive transfer to playing tennis can be expected if the class activities help the client increase relevant aspects of physical fitness such as aerobic endurance and strength of the specific muscles involved in playing tennis and relevant motor skills, or performance-related components, such as balance and agility. Or consider a client who

> The physical activity instructor needs to provide class experiences that are as specific as possible to activities outside the class that clients need to improve.

wants to participate in an exercise class to improve his or her ability to go up and down stairs safely and without feeling undue fatigue. Again, the instructor needs to evaluate the movement requirements of stair climbing and then develop exercises and class activities to enhance the client's performance of this activity. The bottom line is that the instructor needs to provide class experiences that are as specific as possible to activities outside the class that clients need or want to improve.

Assessment of Motor Skill Learning

Three important characteristics of motor skill learning should be taken into account when assessing how well a person has learned a skill. One is that learning involves a change in a person's capability to perform a skill at a certain level. Of course, factors in the performance may still influence the person in such a way that his or her performance is worse than he or she is capable of. For example, an older adult may be able to perform an aerobic dance sequence without music but find it more difficult to remember the steps or perform them to the beat once music is added. Second, because learning involves internal processes within the central and peripheral nervous systems that we cannot directly observe, the assessment of learning requires an *inference*. This means that we must depend on repeated observations of a person's behavior to evaluate learning. It is from these observations that we infer the extent to which learning has occurred. Third, it is essential to assess *adaptability* because people typically must use a movement skill in contexts and situations that differ from those in which the skill was practiced.

The most relevant means for the physical activity instructor to assess movement skill learning is a transfer test. A **transfer test** primarily assesses how well the learner adapts to contexts and situations that differ from those in which the skill was practiced. Because transfer of learning is commonly the underlying reason to participate in an exercise class, the physical activity instructor should use some form of transfer test to assess the participants' abilities to perform learned activities outside the exercise class.

One practical and easy way to administer a transfer test is to ask participants in your class to write short anecdotes about changes they have experienced in their daily activities over the course of the exercise program. For example, a client's writing that she can walk more regularly again because she feels more steady when moving about the neighborhood or another's writing that he is now able to walk down a flight of stairs without fear of falling can serve as evidence of the positive impact of the class on motor skills. Clients may write that their tennis or golf performance has improved. Or, you could have your clients complete the Composite Physical Function (CPF) scale introduced in chapter 5 when you conduct your regular screening and assessments.

Why is it worth the instructor's time and effort to develop or use learning assessments? An important reason is *instructor accountability.* If people spend time and money with you to acquire capabilities they did not have previously or to improve their present capabilities, you are accountable to provide evidence to them that their time and money have been well spent. Keeping daily records of class performance and asking clients to write short anecdotes about changes they have experienced in their daily activities over the course of the physical activity class are ways to collect this type of evidence. If these records show improvement, you and your clients can have confidence that the exercise

program you have designed is effective and that their time and money have been well spent.

Stages of Motor Skill Learning

The improvement in performance a person makes when learning a motor skill typically progresses through distinct stages. Although motor learning scholars have proposed several models to identify and describe these stages, one presented by Ann Gentile (1972, 2000) nicely captures the essence of these stages for the practitioner. Gentile described two stages that characterize the learner's progression from being a beginner to being a highly skilled performer. During the initial stage of learning, the primary goal is to acquire a movement coordination pattern that enables the person to experience some degree of success at performing the skill. Some common characteristics of the beginner's performance are presented in figure 18.2.

In the second stage, the learner's goal depends on the type of skill being learned. If the skill is a **closed**

- The movement coordination pattern is not well developed and requires much refinement. This movement pattern is sometimes referred to as "in the ballpark."
- Performance of the skill is inconsistent from one attempt to another, which means the person may be reasonably successful on some but not all attempts.
- The errors the learner makes tend to be obvious errors that are easy for the instructor to observe.
- The learner is aware of making errors but typically does not know what the errors are or how to correct them.
- The learner's attention is devoted almost exclusively to what to do and how to perform the skill. As a result, the learner has difficulty engaging in another activity at the same time, such as listening to instructions or carrying on a conversation.
- Performance of the skill involves an excessive amount of movement because more muscles are activated than necessary, which results in the person using more than an optimal amount of energy to perform the skill.

FIGURE 18.2 Common characteristics of the beginner and the beginner's performance during the initial stage of learning.
Adapted from A.M. Gentile 1972, 2000.

TABLE 18.3   Implications of Gentile's Learning Stages Model for Instructional Settings

| DURING THE INITIAL STAGE OF LEARNING | DURING THE SECOND STAGE OF LEARNING | |
	Closed skills	Open skills
• Emphasize the development of the basic movement coordination pattern for both open and closed skills. This can be accomplished by promoting the achievement of the goal of the skill rather than the correct performance of the critical movement features of the skill. • Expect inconsistent performance of both open and closed skills. • Focus correction on flaws that cause the greatest performance errors.	• Emphasize successful and consistent achievement of the goal of the skill. • Establish practice situations that are as similar as possible to situations in which a test will occur.	• Vary the situations in which the skill must be performed so that the client must adapt to conditions not previously experienced. This improves the ability to adapt movements to the demands of unique situations.

skill, which means that nothing in the environment is changing and the person can initiate the skill at a time of his or her own choosing (e.g., weightlifting or walking in an empty hallway), then the goal is to refine the movement pattern acquired during the first stage so that the skill can consistently be performed successfully. Gentile refers to this process as *fixating the skill.* But, if the skill is an **open skill,** which means that the person must perform the skill in a changing environment (e.g., playing a competitive game of tennis or walking in a crowded mall), then the goal is to be able to modify the movement pattern acquired in the first stage so that it successfully meets the changing demands of a performance situation. Gentile refers to this process as *diversifying the skill.* In this second stage of learning, the person makes fewer and smaller errors, which might be difficult for you to detect, depending on your knowledge of the skill. Some implications of Gentile's two learning stages for instruction are presented in table 18.3.

Motor Learning Principles for the Physical Activity Instructor

The following sections describe specific ways to present a new skill, provide augmented feedback, determine whether a skill should be practiced as a whole or in parts, schedule the activities presented during class sessions, and determine how long participants will be engaged in performing those skills or activities during class sessions. Of course, the best way to learn these skills is to practice teaching motor learning skills and solicit evaluative feedback from your clients and peer instructors.

Demonstration

The most commonly used strategy for communicating how to perform a new skill is to demonstrate the skill. Research indicates that in certain situations a demonstration is likely to be more effective than other forms of conveying a skill. One of these situations is when the skill requires the production of a new movement coordination pattern, which involves a combination of limb and body movements that is unique to each individual. For example, if a physical activity is new and different from any activity the client has previously performed, the client needs to produce a new coordination pattern, and a demonstration can effectively communicate how the skill should be performed.

Demonstration is effective in part because of the relationship between vision and the motor system. When we watch a person perform a skill, our visual system detects the relative motions of the body and limbs. This visually detected information is used by the motor system to enable the observer to move in a way similar to the observed movement. Because of this sensorimotor relationship, the most effective type of demonstration usually is of the correct performance of the skill.

An interesting alternative to a correct demonstration is to have beginners observe other beginners as they practice. Research has shown that beginners can benefit from observing other beginners practice a skill, especially when they can hear the instructor's correct evaluation of the observed person's performance (McCullagh & Weiss, 2001). This strategy can be especially useful in a large class where it is difficult for the instructor to provide evaluative comments on each participant's performance. Whatever type of demonstration you decide to use, these guidelines should be helpful to you:

- Be certain that the class participants observe the demonstration from a location that allows them to see the most critical parts of the skill performed. Everyone should be able to see the skill performed from the same vantage point.

- Demonstrate the correct way to perform a skill several times.

- Demonstrate the skill at a speed that is similar to its actual performance speed.

- Do not provide a lot of verbal commentary during the demonstration.

- If verbal comments are necessary, use verbal cues before the demonstration to direct attention to key features of the skill.

- Allow beginners to observe other beginners practicing a skill; make sure the observers can hear the instructor's corrective feedback.

Verbal Instruction

Verbal instructions are often used to communicate how to perform a movement skill. One important function of verbal instructions is to focus the learner's attention on the critical features of the movement skill or the environmental context that will enhance their performance of the skill. It is particularly important when teaching older adults, however, that the quantity of the instructions does not exceed older adults' limited capacity to attend to or retain the information provided.

Several important factors influence the effectiveness of verbal instructions. These factors include characteristics of the instructions and of the learners:

- Compared with younger adults, older adults typically can pay attention to less information at one time and can remember that information for a shorter amount of time.

- People to whom instructions are directed must be able to interpret the meaning of the instructions. The meaning of a term to the instructor may not match its meaning to the client.

- Instructions influence how and where participants focus their attention as they learn and perform a skill or activity. This is important because a person's focus of attention while performing a skill influences how well he or she learns the skill.

- Instructions can help simplify what may appear to the learner to be a complex sequence of movements. When verbal instructions provide a strong visual image that the learner can associate with performing a skill, learning the complex coordination required by the skill becomes much easier. For example, the coordination between the arms during the sidestroke in swimming can be better visualized with the instruction, "Reach above your head with your bottom arm and pick an apple off the tree, put the apple in your other hand at the level of your waist, and then put the apple in a basket by your hip."

Verbal Cues

A useful technique to help people remember how to perform a skill or activity is to have them repeat **verbal cues** while they perform the skill. Verbal cues are single words or short, concise phrases. When teaching new motor skills, these cues can serve two functions. First, verbal cues can direct people's attention to specific features of their own movements, an object they must do something with to perform the skill, or the environment in which the skill is performed. For example, when you introduce step aerobics exercises, it is important that the class participants look directly at the step as they step on it. The verbal cue "look at the step" tells them where to direct their visual attention.

Second, verbal cues can serve as reminders about critical features or parts of the skill. For example, if the activity involves several parts that must be performed in a specific sequence (e.g., an aerobic dance sequence), one or two words can be assigned to each part as a verbal reminder of what to do in that part of the sequence (e.g., step-kicks, knee lifts). You can use verbal cues to reinforce the critical features of an exercise while the client performs the exercise. A set of appropriate verbal cues associated with the critical features of the vertical chest press are listed in table 18.1. For example, you might present the first two verbal cues as the client prepares to perform the first repetition and each of the subsequent cues with the first few repetitions.

The verbal instructions you provide are the first method by which you introduce a new movement skill to learners. It is therefore important that you choose your words carefully and avoid saying too much before demonstrating the skill or before the learner has had an opportunity to practice the skill. These guidelines can help you effectively use verbal instructions:

- Include no more than one or two points about how to perform a skill or activity.

- Use terminology that all the participants understand; avoid jargon that is commonly used among physical activity professionals but will probably not be understood by the people in your exercise class.

- Give instructions that conjure up well-known visual images that help the learner think about moving in such a way as to produce the image rather than about the many parts of a complicated skill.

- Use verbal cues to direct the participants' attention to the aspects that are critical to performing the skill successfully, such as the height that the foot is lifted when stepping onto exercise equipment, the position of a limb at a key part of the backswing in golf or tennis, or what to look at or for when catching a ball.

Verbal Cues and Demonstration

In some situations it is helpful to combine a demonstration with verbal cues. This strategy can be especially beneficial for teaching older adults a skill that requires performing a series of movements in a specified sequence. Research shows that older adults' reduced short-term memory makes remembering a verbally presented sequence difficult (Landin, 1994). To help older adults overcome this potential problem, you can supplement a demonstration with verbal cues. These cues can be especially helpful for remembering the sequence if they form a sentence or if their first letters spell out a word or phrase. For example, to help participants remember the transitional sequence for moving from one step to another in a step aerobics class, the verbal cue "MOON" can be a signal to "Move Over Onto the Next step." Additional verbal cues will be discussed in chapter 19.

Augmented Feedback

Learners obtain sensory information from the various sensory systems (e.g., vision, somatosensory, vestibular) while they perform a skill. The instructor can provide additional feedback that supplements, or augments, this internal, sensory feedback. This additional feedback is commonly referred to in the motor learning research literature as **augmented feedback.** For example, if you putt a golf ball that does not go in the hole, your own sensory systems allow you to feel the direction and distance of the putter movement during the backswing and the force used to hit the ball, to hear the club and ball make contact, and to see the direction and distance of the ball and by how much it missed the cup. A golf instructor who watched your putt could provide augmented feedback by telling you that the ball did not go in the hole because of the way you initiated the backswing.

Role of Augmented Feedback in Skill Learning

When working with beginners, an instructor should describe the critical error and what should be done to correct the problem. When used in this way, augmented feedback facilitates the learning of the movement skill by not only identifying the error but also clarifying how to correct it on the next attempt. Another role that augmented feedback serves is to motivate the learner to continue striving toward a goal. For example, when an instructor tells a participant in a physical activity class about the amount of progress he or she has made toward achieving a personal performance goal, this augmented feedback motivates the participant to continue to pursue that goal.

Types of Augmented Feedback

Instructors can provide augmented feedback about the outcome, or result, of a skill performance. This type of information is known as **knowledge of results,** for example, telling a participant the amount of time he or she took to complete an activity. Augmented feedback can also provide information about what the person did that led to a performance outcome. The term used to describe this type of information is **knowledge of performance.** For example, knowledge of performance can be information about what a participant is doing that hinders his or her achievement of a performance goal, such as completing an activity in a specific amount of time.

Frequency of Feedback

How frequently should an instructor provide augmented feedback to a learner? A common misconception is that the more often an instructor gives augmented feedback, especially to a client in the initial stage of learning, the more effective it is in helping the client learn a skill. However, research has shown that augmented feedback presented less frequently than on every practice attempt is more beneficial for beginners than feedback during or after every attempt (Magill, 2001). One reason for this is that beginners in the initial stage of learning who receive augmented feedback every time they perform a skill can become dependent on that feedback. This means that receiving augmented feedback becomes a necessary part of performing the skill. When required to perform the skill without the augmented feedback, the learner's performance is worse than with it. Acquiring the capability to perform skills without augmented feedback is important because most motor skills are performed in situations in which the performer cannot receive augmented feedback from an instructor.

Structuring the Practice Environment

Three issues that are especially relevant for determining the best way to practice skills to facilitate learning are discussed in this section: how to decide when to practice a skill as a whole or in parts, how to organize the practice schedule for optimal learning and transfer, and how to allocate practice time, particularly when working with older adults.

Augmented feedback

- is additional feedback that supplements, or augments, sensory feedback;
- can facilitate skill learning or motivate class participants to continue striving toward a performance goal or participating in the fitness class;
- can provide information about the outcome of performing a skill (knowledge of results) or the characteristics of performing the movement that led to the outcome (knowledge of performance); and
- should be given less frequently than on every practice attempt.

Skill Practice

An important decision that physical activity instructors face when introducing a new skill to clients is whether they should practice the skill in its entirety or in parts. Motor learning research indicates that this decision should be based on two characteristics of the motor skill. One is the **complexity** of the skill, which refers to the number of component parts in a skill. A highly complex skill has more parts than a less complex skill. For example, an aerobics dance routine is a more complex skill than putting a golf ball. The other characteristic is the **organization** of the parts of the skill, which refers to the temporal and spatial relationship among the parts. A highly organized skill is one in which the performance of any one part depends on the performance of the previous and succeeding parts. The golf putt is thus more highly organized than the aerobics dance routine. For skills and activities that are low in complexity and high in organization, practicing the whole skill is recommended. For example, a bench press in weight training has only two component parts (pushing the bar above the chest and returning the bar to the chest), which depend on each other to be performed properly. For skills that are high in complexity, the best decision is to practice it in parts.

A problem inherent in making the decision to practice a skill in parts is determining what constitutes a part for practice purposes. The organization of the skill helps solve this problem. You should first analyze the skill by identifying its component parts and then evaluate the extent to which the performance of any one part depends on the performance of the preceding or succeeding part. One common method used to identify the different components of a skill is the basis of certain spatial or temporal characteristics (e.g., leg kick and arm action used in front crawl swimming stroke). Parts that are dependent on each other should be practiced together (e.g., putting a golf ball). Parts that are independent of other parts can be practiced individually (e.g., aerobic dance routine).

An effective way to engage beginners in practicing skill components is to use a strategy known as **progressive-part practice.** Participants practice the first part, then the second part, then the combination of the first and second parts, then the third part, and then the combination of the first three parts. This progression continues until all the parts have been practiced individually and then in

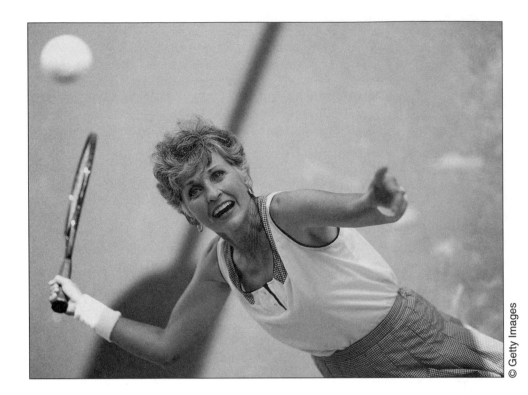

Because the complexity of this tennis forehand skill is low but the organization of its parts is very high, this skill should be practiced as a whole.

© Getty Images

sequence with all the previous parts. Eventually, the whole skill is practiced. This strategy works particularly well when teaching older adults an aerobic dance sequence or certain swimming strokes.

Class Schedule

Physical activity classes typically involve learning and performing several variations of a skill. For example, swimming involves the learning of different strokes; stair climbing includes going up a set of stairs, going down a set of stairs, and going up and down stairs of different heights; step aerobics requires a variety of different movements such as stepping up, stepping down, and side-stepping on and off steps of different heights. You must decide whether class participants practice the variations in the same class session or individually over a series of sessions.

Motor learning research has examined this practice schedule issue from the perspective of a learning phenomenon known as the contextual interference effect (Brady, 1998; Magill, 2004, chap. 15). This effect is relevant in situations when several different skills need to be learned. Research has shown that people learn skill variations better when they practice all the variations in each practice session rather than practicing each variation independently over a series of sessions. For example, if class participants must learn three

different swimming strokes, they will learn them better if they practice all three strokes in every session than if they practice only one stroke for several sessions, then only the second for several sessions, and finally the third for several sessions.

The two types of practice schedules create different amounts of **contextual interference,** which refers to the memory-related interference that results from practicing variations of a skill within the same practice session. The greatest amount of contextual interference occurs when all the skills are practiced in a random order in each practice session, which is referred to as **random practice.** The least amount of contextual interference occurs when each skill is practiced independently in its own block of practice trials, which is referred to as a **blocked practice** schedule. Because the amount of memory-related interference is lower when skill variations are practiced according to a blocked schedule, performance of the skills during the initial practice session often improves more rapidly and to a higher level than when multiple skill variations are practiced according to a random schedule. However, performance on transfer tests, used to assess how well the skill has been learned, are typically better for those who experience random practice. Researchers interested in this motor learning phenomenon believe that when learners practice skills according to random practice schedules the practice is more cognitively effortful and the learning of each skill variation more distinctive and memorable as a result (Lee, Swinnen, & Serrien, 1994).

Blocked and random practice schedules are the extremes of a continuum of possible ways to organize the skill practice within and across class sessions. Figure 18.3 compares some practice organization schedules in terms of the amount of contextual interference they create. Figure 18.4 presents three different schedules for practicing three different bench-stepping skills. The key point to remember is that practice schedules that

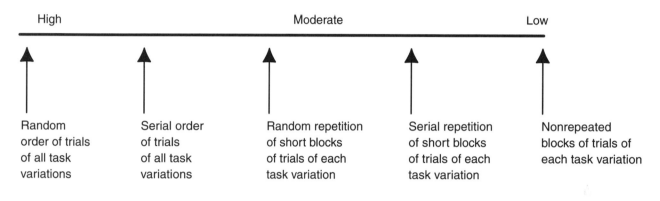

Amount of contextual interference

High	Moderate		Low
Random order of trials of all task variations	Serial order of trials of all task variations	Random repetition of short blocks of trials of each task variation	Serial repetition of short blocks of trials of each task variation	Nonrepeated blocks of trials of each task variation

Practice schedules

FIGURE 18.3 Various practice arrangements along a continuum from high to low for the amount of contextual interference created.

From R. Magill, 2004, "Application of motor learning principles to program design," *Motor learning: Concepts and applications*, 7th ed. (New York, NY: McGraw-Hill Companies), 312. Reproduced with permission of the McGraw-Hill Companies.

Practice schedule	Practice time	DAY					
		1	**2**	**3**	**4**	**5**	**6**
Blocked practice	24 min.	A	A	B	B	C	C
Serial practice	4 min.	A	A	A	A	A	A
	4 min.	B	B	B	B	B	B
	4 min.	C	C	C	C	C	C
	4 min.	A	A	A	A	A	A
	4 min.	B	B	B	B	B	B
	4 min	C	C	C	C	C	C
Random practice	4 min.	B	B	C	B	A	C
	4 min.	A	C	A	C	B	B
	4 min.	C	C	C	C	A	C
	4 min.	C	A	A	A	C	A
	4 min.	A	B	A	B	A	C
	4 min.	B	B	C	B	B	A

Skill A: Step onto and off low benches
Skill B: Step onto and off benches of medium height
Skill C: Step onto and off high benches

FIGURE 18.4   Sample blocked, serial, and random practice schedules for three different skills, A, B, and C. Each schedule consists of six 24-minute sessions.

Adapted from R.A. Magill 2004.

create more contextual interference are better for skill learning than schedules that create lower amounts.

Practice Time

In addition to deciding how best to organize the practice of different skills within a class session, the instructor needs to determine the amount of time to devote to practicing each skill or activity. In the motor learning literature, this decision is called **practice distribution.** Because there is only a certain amount of time available in which to carry out planned activities, the available time must be distributed to allow each of the activities to be carried out and also to provide an optimal learning opportunity for all participants.

The research literature indicates that shorter and more frequent practice periods are better for skill learning than longer and less frequent periods (Magill, 2004, chap. 16). This means that if you determine that participants in your activity class need about two hours to learn to perform an activity properly, the two hours should be distributed across several practice sessions rather than getting it over with quickly in the fewest possible sessions. It is important to keep in mind that the issue of practice distribution relates specifically to the learning of motor skills and not to the physical fitness–related benefits of performing skills. The amount of time that is optimal for learning is specific to the skill or activity. As a rule of thumb, shorter and more frequent practice periods are better for skill learning than longer and less frequent periods. Your experience teaching a particular skill or activity will help you determine the total amount of time participants need to learn it.

How well the practice environment is organized strongly influences how much is learned. You have to decide how best to schedule the practicing of each skill or variation, whether the skill should be practiced in parts or as a whole, and how best to distribute the practice time based on the skill you are teaching and the skill level of your clients. To assist you in making these decisions wisely, this set of guidelines is provided:

- Determine whether class participants should initially practice a skill or activity in its entirety or in parts on the basis of an analysis that identifies its complexity (i.e., number of component parts) and degree of organization (i.e., temporal and spatial relationships among the parts). In general, skills that are high in complexity but low in organization can be practiced in parts, while skills that are low in complexity but high in organization should be practiced in their entirety.

- When class participants must learn several variations of a skill or activity, organize practice sessions so that they create more as opposed to less contextual interference. Practicing each skill variation in each session creates more contextual interference than practicing only one variation in each session.

- Shorter and more frequent practice periods are better for skill learning than longer and less frequent periods.

Applying Motor Learning Principles in Group Settings

Your challenge as a physical activity instructor is to provide effective instruction for older adults with diverse characteristics. Older adults vary in both physical and cognitive abilities as well as stage of learning. The guidelines in the preceding sections provide suggestions for applying each of the four motor learning principles in group settings. However, because of the heterogeneous nature of the groups you will work with, it is important to be prepared to adapt each suggestion to the individual characteristics and needs of the older adults in the group.

Instructional techniques also should be adapted to individual needs. Do not take a "one-size-fits-all" approach to instructing a class; be prepared to individualize your instruction so that learning is optimized for each client. Use the guidelines for each of the four motor learning principles as starting points. Experiment with each suggestion, and then carefully observe the performance of each individual client to determine whether the demonstration or practice method you are using or the feedback you are providing need to be adapted for clients at a different stage of learning or less physically capable of performing the skill being taught. With ongoing conscientious application of the motor learning principles presented in this chapter, you will soon learn how to adapt your teaching methods to meet the individual needs of your clients at different stages of the learning process.

Summary

The motor learning principles described in this chapter are the basis on which physical activity instructors can determine how to use demonstrations or verbal instructions and cues to convey a new skill, how to present augmented feedback, whether clients should practice a new skill or activity as a whole or in parts, how the practice of different skills should be varied, and how to distribute the time available during to the practice of different skills or activities. It is important to design a physical activity program with content that addresses the individual needs of your clients, but it is equally important for optimal learning that you apply each of the motor learning principles described in this chapter. The most successful physical activity instructors are those who combine strong leadership skills with effective teaching strategies.

Key Terms

Recommended Readings

Knudson, D.V., & Morrison, C.S. (2002). *Qualitative analysis of human movement* (2nd ed., chaps. 2, 5, 6, 7, & 8). Champaign, IL: Human Kinetics.

Magill, R.A. (2004). *Motor learning: Concepts and applications* (7th ed., chaps. 10, 11, 14, 15, 16, & 17). New York: McGraw-Hill.

Study Questions

1. According to the Knudson and Morrison model that describes the qualitative analysis of skills, identifying and prioritizing critical errors in the performance of a skill would be a component of which of the four analysis tasks?

   a. preparation
   b. observation
   c. evaluation or diagnosis
   d. intervention

2. Which of the following is an essential part of the definition of motor skill learning?

   a. can be observed during practice
   b. can occur without practice
   c. results in correct performance
   d. results in relatively permanent improvement

3. The greatest amount of positive transfer of learning between two skills can be expected to occur when

   a. the number of component parts of the two skills are equal
   b. a similar amount of practice occurs for each skill
   c. there is a small amount of similarity between the performance contexts of the two skills
   d. there is a high degree of similarity between the component parts of the two skills

(continued)

4. A transfer test assesses primarily which of the following characteristics of motor skill learning?
   a. relatively permanent improvement
   b. adaptability to a variety of situations
   c. increased performance consistency
   d. the degree of correctness of performance of the skill

5. According to Gentile's model of the stages of motor skill learning, which of the following skills is an example of one for which the goal of a learner in the second stage should be to perform the movement pattern consistently each time?
   a. throwing a dart at a target that is mounted on a wall
   b. passing a soccer ball to a teammate who is running down the field
   c. stepping onto a step of a moving escalator
   d. any of these

6. For which of the following skills is a demonstration by a skilled performer most likely to benefit someone in the initial stage of learning?
   a. all motor skills
   b. all motor skills when verbal cues are given also
   c. motor skills that require learning a new coordination pattern
   d. motor skills that can be performed at different speeds

7. Verbal instructions can help simplify the initial stage of learning of a complex skill by
   a. describing how to perform each movement component of the skill in detail
   b. providing a strong visual image that the learner's movement should imitate
   c. describing all the critical features of the skill before the learner practices the skill
   d. directing the learner to think about each movement component as it is performed

8. Which of the following is an example of augmented feedback?
   a. seeing one's golf ball go into a sand trap
   b. being told by the golf instructor what was incorrect about a swing
   c. hearing the sound of the golf club hitting the ball
   d. feeling the position of the golf club at the top of the backswing

9. Practice of a motor skill in its entirety is recommended when the skill is
   a. high in complexity and low in organization
   b. low in complexity and high in organization
   c. high in complexity and high in organization
   d. low in complexity and low in organization

10. Which of the following practice schedules involves the least amount of contextual interference?
    a. random repetition of short blocks of each of three skill variations
    b. random trials of three skill variations
    c. serial trials of three skill variations
    d. serial repetition of short blocks of each of three skill variations

Application Activities

1. Movement analysis. With a partner, select a specific skill or activity to teach to older adults in an exercise class.

   • Analyze the critical features of the selected skill, that is, the parts that must be performed correctly to be successful in the skill or activity.

- For each critical feature, describe the range of correctness that you would permit when an elderly participant first attempts to perform the skill or activity.
- For each critical feature, propose a statement that would provide appropriate knowledge of performance to a class participant whose performance is outside your permitted range of correctness. Explain why this statement would be appropriate.

2. Structuring the practice environment: Variability of practice.

   - Which of the following activities have high complexity and low organization, and which low complexity and high organization? Why?

     A tennis serve

     The sidestroke in swimming

     A six-part tai chi sequence

     An aerobic dance combination

     A chip shot in golf

   - Which of the preceding physical activities can be practiced in parts and which ones should be practiced as a whole? For the activities that you decide can be practiced in parts, how would you organize that practice?

3. Verbal cues. Materials needed: Videotape or voice recorder. With a partner, take turns as instructor and learner in this exercise. Select one physical activity that your partner is not skilled at performing. Determine the critical features of the skill. Record yourself as you provide verbal instructions to your partner for performing those critical features of the skill. Listen to or watch the recording and evaluate the following:

   - Which verbal cues were best to remind your partner of the critical features of the movement?
   - Was the timing of the verbal cues appropriate for the component of the skill being performed?

19

Teaching and Leadership Skills

Ken Alan
C. Jessie Jones

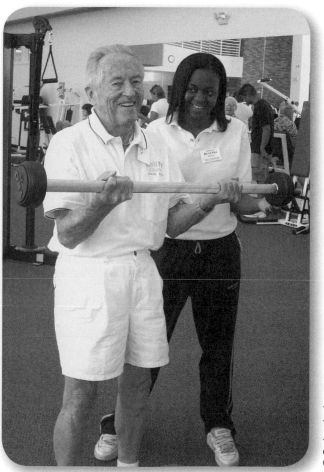

© C. Jessie Jones

The 21st century has ushered in unparalleled expansion of physical activity programs for older adults in both group and individual exercise environments. Although becoming competent in teaching one type of exercise class is an accomplishment, becoming adept in leading a variety of classes (e.g., yoga, Pilates, tai chi, aerobics) is in high demand. Whether your goal is to be a personal trainer or a group instructor of one or a dozen specialized workouts, the art of teaching is central to the successful application of didactic knowledge to practice. This chapter will help you develop and excel in both the art and the science of teaching and leadership, which are essential for skillful and charismatic instruction of physical activity classes. Once you have studied and mastered these teaching and leadership skills, your abilities as a physical activity instructor of older adults will rise from the ordinary to the extraordinary.

Teaching Skills

Think of personal trainers, group instructors, and teachers you admire. What specific skills do you think contribute to their effectiveness? Although at first glance the teaching of exercise may look relatively simple, it actually requires a complex orchestration of many skills used in constantly varying degrees (Poole, 1991). Factors such as skill level, exercise selection, workout environment, and instructional style have an effect on a program. Exercise leaders, especially group instructors, are like orchestra conductors. With numerous movements occurring simultaneously, the instructor needs a sharp eye, a keen ear, and sensitivity to the audience (participants) in order to create a harmonious experience. Excellent physical activity instructors, like orchestra conductors, are not created with just a few days of training. Teaching skills are learned in developmental stages over time through education, observation, planning, preparation, practice, and self-evaluation. The following sections provide an overview of the teaching skills and strategies that can enhance the effectiveness of your physical activity programs.

Lesson Plan Development

After reviewing the information obtained from your preactivity screening and performance assessments (discussed in chapters 5, 6, and 7) and possibly through personal interviews and goal setting (see chapter 8), the next step is to develop a lesson plan for each class. Following are 10 basic steps to help you develop your lesson plans.

Step 1. Begin by setting priorities. Decide what health-related and performance-related components need to be emphasized with these clients, such as balance, strength, power, aerobic endurance, agility, and flexibility.

Step 2. Select specific exercises you want to include for each major component of the class (i.e., warm-up, main conditioning and skill development, and cool-down).

Step 3. Determine the appropriateness of each selected exercise by asking yourself, "Will this exercise efficiently and effectively meet the needs, interests, and goals of my clients?"

Step 4. Group similar exercises together so that your routine begins to develop a logical sequence and progression across each major component of the class.

Step 5. Determine how you will adapt the selected exercises to accommodate the various health conditions, fitness levels, and motor abilities of your clients. You can then establish the safety precautions needed (e.g., monitoring blood pressure, watching for signs of adverse effects of medication, providing special assistance or equipment).

Step 6. Determine what type of music, lighting, space, and participant placement is needed (e.g., lines, semicircle, circuit stations) and what equipment or props are needed for the exercises or to enhance the atmosphere of your class (e.g., ribbons, balls, elastic bands, weights). Following are some sources of music and videos for group exercise classes:

- AeroBeat Music—www.aerobeat.com
- DynamixMusic—www.dynamixmusic.com
- Muscle Mixes—www.musclemixes.com
- Power Music—www.powermusic.com

Step 7. Write down examples of teaching cues to use in each section of the class. Teaching cues are discussed in more detail in the next section of the chapter.

Step 8. Practice your class routine. Nothing takes the place of practicing what you have planned. Practicing will help you develop the best sequencing and transitions for a smooth-flowing workout to music.

Step 9. If possible, for each new class you develop, have a friend, a coworker, or your clients provide you with a critical evaluation of the class structure and your teaching style. In addition, master instructors always conduct a critical self-evaluation. Refer to chapter 13 for a checklist to help you self-evaluate your teaching skills. You may also find it helpful to have someone videotape you leading a class, but be careful to teach as you normally teach. That is, do not do anything differently just because you are being videotaped.

Step 10. Based on self-evaluations and evaluations from others, refine the exercises, class structure, and teaching style as appropriate for each class.

Teaching Cues

To learn an exercise, participants need brief, simple, and clear instructions. Instructions need to include a number of signals to indicate when a movement is going to start, stop, or change. You must give this signal, or cue, *before* starting or changing a movement. **Cuing** is a teaching technique that prepares a participant for what comes next in the sequence of movements in an exercise routine. Cuing, when timed correctly, helps your clients follow you with more confidence and greater ease and facilitates both the learning and the performing of the exercise (Francis & Seibert, 2000; Heitmann, 1989). There are three cuing methods for leading group exercise classes: *physical, visual,* and *verbal* (Kennedy, 2000). Keep in mind that mastering the art of cuing can require a lot of practice.

- A **physical cue** (also called tactile or kinesthetic cue) is very effective for personal trainers. It is a hands-on approach of guiding a limb manually to the proper position or through a desired movement pattern. It is also employed to direct attention to a specific body part. Physical cuing can be the most effective method for learning a challenging movement pattern. Since this method is usually performed one on one, it takes your attention away from the rest of the participants unless you involve the class in a meaningful way. Related to this, appropriate touch and physical contact with clients are discussed later in the chapter.

- A **visual cue,** or visual preview, is a physical demonstration of the upcoming exercise or the next set of movements. Visual cues are effective between exercises and during rest periods. The value of visual cuing is highest among clients with diminished hearing and those who do not easily understand the language you speak.

- A **verbal cue,** or verbal preview, is a vocal description or specific instructions for the upcoming sequence or exercise. Verbal and visual cues (i.e., "show and tell" cues) often are presented together as participants near the end of an exercise movement or between exercises.

Which cuing method is most effective depends on the skill and fitness levels of your clients, their learning styles, and the complexity of the movement pattern you are trying to introduce. A combination of cuing methods and techniques

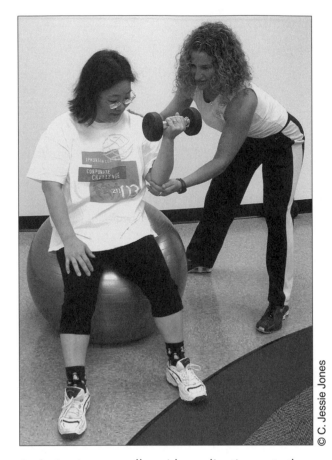

An instructor manually guides a client's arm to the proper position.

best promotes learning because it provides clients with an opportunity to learn using multiple sensory systems (i.e., vision, hearing, and touch). For many fitness professionals verbal cuing is the most daunting cuing method to master. Not only must you put the physical movement into words, but you also need to anticipate and prepare participants for the next exercise.

Following are suggestions to improve your verbal cuing and thus enhance your classroom instruction.

• A common verbal cue to signal that a change in movement is coming up is the **countdown** technique, for example, "Ten more, nine, eight, seven . . ." As you reach the final repetitions or counts, stop counting and instead describe your next movement. It will take time to find just the right way to communicate your message so that your clients can easily understand it. Aim for an economy of words. You should finish your instructions before the final

two repetitions of the current movement so that you can provide a transitional cue.

• **Transitional cues** are used to guide participants specifically through the change from one movement or exercise into another movement or exercise. These cues are succinct, direct, and commonly four or eight syllables in length to correspond with the last four or eight beats in a music phrase or a rhythm pattern. Examples of transitional cues are "OK, now lift," "Rea-dy, let's start," and "Last one and change."

• When you state the quantity of exercise to do, you give a **goal-oriented cue.** This type of cue can help to motivate some individuals by defining the amount of work needed to complete a task. There are two types of goal-oriented cues, *timed* and *numerical.* Here are examples of each type: "I'd like you to be fatigued between the sixth and tenth repetition" (numerical) and "Just 30 seconds more—hang in there" (timed). Make sure the goals you set for participants are obtainable. As a rule, achieving the goal results in feelings of success. When goals are unobtainable and unrealistic, participants may experience a feeling of failure.

• With **process-oriented cues,** numerical goals are downplayed or eliminated altogether. Instead, you direct focus inward on the quality of movement or a purposeful awareness of how the body feels during the exercise. This cuing technique allows you to better accommodate different ability levels in the same class, as it does not push clients to work beyond what is safe for them and makes feelings of failure less likely. Here is how a process-oriented cue works:

1. Determine the maximum number of repetitions for the exercise, but do not tell that number to the participants.

2. Count repetitions silently to yourself during the exercise.

3. Encourage clients to perform the exercise until they no longer can maintain proper technique.

4. Replace the counting of repetitions with a focus on body awareness and the feelings and sensations caused by the movement.

5. As you near the end of your predetermined maximum number, provide an open-ended numerical cue to bring the

Process-oriented cuing allows the instructor to better accommodate different ability levels in the same class, as it does not push clients to work beyond what is safe for them.

exercise to a close, such as "Just a few more repetitions if you can; otherwise, just rest."

• A **mindful cue** can be thought of as "mental fuel" for exercise, a stimulus for movement. A stimulus is a thought, event, or image that temporarily increases the activity of an organism. Mindful cues summon emotions and imagination to help engage appropriate physical action. Visualization and imagery are frequently used as mindful cues to facilitate the desired outcome, as these examples illustrate: "Allow your spine to relax to the floor one vertebra at a time, like the temperature gauge on a thermometer going down one degree at a time," or "Imagine pulling a heavy rope up from the ground."

• Appropriate tone, the last tip for verbal cuing, relates to the effective use of voice inflection. The tone of a verbal cue helps to describe or inspire the appropriate intensity of a movement. For example, a forceful command like a drill sergeant—such as "Lift!" "Push!" or "Keep going!"—emphasizes the need to increase effort, as for a movement requiring power. A soothing tone with a softer voice—saying such words as "Relax," "Nice and easy," "Slow and steady"—encourages people to relax during a cooldown or stretch phase of a class.

Elements of Instruction

Based on several years of teaching group exercise, observing master instructors, and interviewing experts, the following basic tips are recommended for effective teaching in a group exercise setting.

• Arrive early. Whenever possible, be at your facility before participants arrive. If using music, have it prepared, cued, and ready to go. Looking rushed diminishes your professionalism, and without adequate time, preworkout tasks are difficult to do. Promptness grants you time to screen new participants and interact with regular participants.

Welcome each person by name as he or she enters the class.

• Set the mood. Before starting the exercise program, it is important for you to set the mood. Make a couple of statements or announcements (such as identifying today's workout goals and general safety reminders), ask a couple of questions, tell a quick story or joke. This is your opportunity to express the positive elements of your personality and your human relationship skills.

• Introduce the exercise. First, introduce the exercise by *name;* then provide *verbal* and *visual cues* for performing the exercise, for example: "This is called the side bend. Stand with feet shoulder-width apart, toes pointing forward and knees slightly bent. Lean to your right while letting your right hand slide down the outside of your thigh. Lift your left arm up toward the ceiling. Feel a stretch along the left side of your body." The blending of verbal cues with demonstration is extremely helpful for many clients learning a new skill.

• Explain the purpose of exercise. People tend to be more interested in performing an exercise if they understand *why* they are being asked to do it. An explanation educates, which helps increase your clients' motivation. Here is an example: "Performing chair stands will reduce the amount of muscle lost in your thighs and help you remain physically independent longer."

• Help clients develop body awareness. Body awareness improves the kinesthetic ability to execute the exercise properly through (1) positioning or placement, (2) alignment and form, (3) breathing pattern, and (4) movement quality. Helping clients to develop body awareness increases the safety and effectiveness of an exercise. Here is an example to help increase your clients' body awareness during the overhead stretch. "With feet slightly farther apart than your shoulders, toes pointed out [position], slightly bend your knees. Now relax your shoulders, and inhale as you lift your arms up into the air; pause; now while exhaling, lower your arms [breathing pattern]. As we perform this movement again, remember to keep your torso lifted, abdominals in, elbows soft [alignment and form], and move slowly and smoothly [movement quality]."

• Adopt a participant-centered approach. Teaching exercise is more rewarding when you approach it from a people-oriented rather than a task-oriented standpoint. Effective instructors do not teach *exercise;* rather, they teach *people* how to exercise by presenting various types of movements and activities and allowing participants to discover for themselves the physical exercise that is right for them. Exercise itself is important, yet more important is recognizing how a participant relates and responds to the exercise. One important characteristic of participant-centered teaching is to curtail using the word "it," and replace "it" with "you" when appropriate in conversations. Whenever possible, you should also refer to your participants by their names; doing this makes them feel important in your eyes (Hoffman & Jones, 2002).

• Choose words carefully. What you say is often more important than what you do. The importance of the words you choose when teaching is often underestimated, yet what you say makes a big difference in how participants perceive you as a person and as an instructor. It is challenging to become conscious of the words that you habitually use while teaching. Do you use phrases such as "you guys," "good job," and "well done"? Most instructors and trainers get into a verbal rut. If you are serious about improving what you say, here are two suggestions for self-evaluation: (1) Ask your clients to write down any irritating or annoying words or phrases that you use, and put them in a box without signing their names. (2) Video- or audiotape yourself teaching a class. After you or your class participants evaluate your word choices, write down key replacement words on an index card, and place the card on the floor near you when teaching a class or in your pocket when training a client. To help you evaluate and possibly improve your word choices during instruction, consider the examples of overused words and possible substitutions in figure 19.1.

• Create a social connection. Many older adults find it difficult to develop new friendships, especially after retirement. Exercise, particularly in a group setting, helps people to connect with one another. Many participants have reported that the anticipation of seeing the instructor or their exer-

---

"It"

Nothing is more versatile but more nebulous than the word *it.* "Stretch *it* out in front of the hip." "Feel *it* in the shoulder." "Great, you have *it.*" In place of *it,* say what *it* is: "Stretch *your muscles* in the front of your hip." "Feel *the stretch* in your shoulder." "Great, you can *climb the stairs now.*"

"Tiresome Ts"

Also overused are *these, that,* and *those.* "Hold *that* stretch" or "Feel *those* hamstrings starting to work" are examples. The "tiresome Ts" are impersonal and are better relegated to objects than to people. Replace a "tiresome T" with *your,* and see how instructions become more personalized. You talk *to* your participants, not *at* them. Can you hear a difference between "Contract that biceps" and "Contract your biceps"?

"Don't"

When possible, eliminate the word *don't. Don't* is negative in tone and implies a participant may be doing something wrong. It is better to select words that convey your message in a positive manner. It may take months to eliminate *don't* from your instructional cues, but it can make a big difference in how your clients perceive your teaching style. Consider substituting the following words and phrases to use instead of *don't: Avoid, rather than, please, I want you to, are you, focus on, be aware of.*

"Try"

To avoid sounding too rigid or inconsiderate, instructors often cushion their instruction by using the word *try.* But some people interpret *try* as meaning that they do not *really* have to do what's instructed. Rephrase "try" statements for more effectiveness. Instead of "Try to keep your back still," eliminate "try to": "Keep your back still." Change "Try to pull your leg in farther toward your chest" to "Gently pull your leg in toward your chest."

FIGURE 19.1   Overused words and possible alternatives.

cise buddies is the highlight of their week. When you create a supportive environment that brings about socializing, a person's ethnic background and economic status are inconsequential. Your openness and acceptance of every individual create a bond that often becomes an integral part of your client's life. Relationships evolve through personal interactions, similar experiences, empathetic listening, the sharing of life events, and lots of laughter. You can also become the catalyst for social connections among your participants through creative programming. One way to create social connections is to move around often during the class and interact with participants, although you need to be careful walking near some individuals because they may get nervous. Another way to facilitate socializing is to have your clients bring in pictures of themselves as teenagers doing something they enjoyed. At the beginning of one of your classes, collect the pictures and randomly hand them out to half of the participants. Ask those individuals to find the person in the picture. Notice how the atmosphere awakens with energy as people search, interact, inquire, laugh, and learn about each other as they try to find the right match. After the exercise, re-collect the photos and post them somewhere conspicuous, such as on a bulletin board. The interactions continue for weeks afterward as everyone tries to identify one another's pictures.

• Maintain a relaxed, nonthreatening atmosphere. This requires skillful communication, both verbal and nonverbal. A participant may become anxious when you look at her without saying anything, for example. She may worry about your evaluation of her abilities (Price, 2002). Your smile is rarely intimidating, but a blank face can feel unwelcoming. A nod of the head, a wink of the eye, or a positive comment such as, "I'm so glad to have you here today" helps to dissolve any tension instantly.

• Create a friendly exercise environment. Maintaining a friendly exercise environment enhances the overall well-being of your clients, including aspects of their physical, social, mental, emotional, and spiritual health. Following are suggestions for creating a friendly exercise environment:

- Just as you come early to greet clients, plan on staying after class to shoot the breeze.
- Create a designated area that is conducive for gathering and socializing before and after workouts.

> A friendly exercise environment enhances the overall well-being of your clients, including aspects of their physical, social, mental, emotional, and spiritual health.

- Share something about yourself.
- Use humor. Humor is the common denominator that puts everybody at ease. One example of how this can be done is by developing a playful, even childlike zest toward exercise. Childlike does not mean childish, clownish, or becoming a comedian. It means a not-so-serious, light-hearted attitude rather than a regimented, stern approach (Gavin, 1992).
- Build interaction and socialization into exercise. This is easily accomplished by designing moves or steps that do not require participants to continuously watch you, such as walking in a big circle around the room or having them do activity in two lines facing each other. You can pair up participants. Once participants are in pairs, have them walk in various patterns around the room (e.g., corner to corner, snake formations, even the London Bridge formation—this will certainly bring smiles).
- Discourage criticism, gossip, or comparisons with others.

• Use positive affirmations. Offer encouragement throughout the class, during as well as before and after exercise, for example: "You can do it," "Believe in yourself," and "Look at how much you have progressed."

• Provide corrective feedback with sensitivity. Addressing a few people or the class in general helps to draw attention away from any single person, especially if that person is very sensitive.

• The beautiful part of teaching is the opportunity to interact with various personalities. However, communicating effectively with different personality types requires skill and practice. Discretion is needed when approaching certain people such as "loners," "untouchables," and "scaredy-cats." Table 19.1 describes common personalities that you may encounter as a personal trainer or group instructor.

TABLE 19.1 Personality Types

Personality type	Characteristics	Strategy
Untouchable	Does not like to be touched. Nonverbal communication says, "Don't infringe on my space."	Avoid hands-on corrections. Use verbal feedback.
Scaredy-cat	Afraid of getting hurt and of trying anything new. Low self-confidence. "I can't do this" attitude.	Work with the person individually and in private. Provide extra reinforcement to help him or her set and meet goals.
Siren (attention getter)	Loud, boisterous, gregarious. Usually has comment or opinion. Likes to be the center of attention. Enjoys being a "social butterfly."	Acknowledge his or her presence without drawing more attention to him or her. Confine interactions primarily to before or after the workout.
Flirter	Touches, hugs, makes lots of contact. Makes side remarks or insinuations. Wants to help others. Wants to be helped.	Keep a professional boundary. Minimize hands-on feedback.
Ham (hotdog)	Laughs and jokes a lot at him- or herself. Often a risk taker. Shows off, not afraid to stand out.	If others are not bothered by the behavior, no need to take action.
Talker	Always talking to someone.	Suggest that this person move to the side or back of the room so as not to distract others. Incorporate segments that allow clients to interact and talk with each other.
Follower	Wants a tightly organized program. Wants everyone to exercise in unison. Perturbed by those who do not follow instructions.	Acknowledge the consistency he or she is seeking. Encourage the client to focus on him- or herself rather than on others.
Natural leader	Takes the initiative. Offers useful suggestions and feedback. Wants to help you. Frequently boosts or reinforces others.	Allow the participant to contribute in some way. For example, helping with equipment, spotting frailer clients, helping at an exercise station.
Loner	Quiet, stays to him- or herself. Conscientious, often introverted. Blends in; doesn't want to draw attention to him- or herself.	Avoid individual feedback when others are present. Communicate in private and by phone, fax, or e-mail if necessary.
Soloist	Stands out in a crowd. Does his or her own thing. Thinks he or she knows more than you. Comes late or leaves early.	Use creative class organization to keep client from being front and center. Incorporate segments that allow participants a choice of exercise variations.
Hoarder	Selfish, "me first" attitude. Grabs the first seat or saves a spot in class. Takes the best equipment. Distressed when another person is in his or her spot or when the schedule or instructor changes.	Be diplomatic in the ways you distribute equipment to participants. Periodically change the directional orientation of the class. Give plenty of advanced warning of any programming changes.
Complainer	Loud, talks a lot, gossips. Tends to make negative comments. At odds with everything, like the world is against him or her.	Express empathy on a one-to-one basis after the workout. Paraphrase conversations to acknowledge that you heard the client. Avoid giving too much advice. Compliments should be plentiful and sincere.
Pleaser	Will do anything you request of him or her. Wants to help others.	Be judicious and genuine with positive feedback. Self-esteem may need external boosting. Provide leadership opportunities.

Some strategies for interacting with each personality type are also presented.

Leadership Skills

A number of factors are related to and predictive of instructor effectiveness. These include client compliance, client satisfaction, and individual and program outcomes. The single most important variable is the leadership skills of the instructor, especially the ability to cultivate positive relationships with participants. This is accomplished by having a genuine desire to help people, establishing trust, inspiring participants, and helping to improve your clients' well-being—physical, mental, and spiritual. Even the top-selling business leadership books emphasize the importance of developing interpersonal relationship skills (Carnegie, 1981; Carter-Scott, 1998; Goldman, Boyatzis, & McKee, 2002). These books are recommended to help you continue improving your leadership skills.

Responsibility

A trademark of professionalism is responsibility. A physical activity instructor must fulfill a number of responsibilities when working with older adults:

- Follow the physical activity guidelines presented in this textbook for older adults.
- Be on time for classes. Contact participants as far in advance as possible when there are changes to the schedule.
- Update and practice all safety and emergency procedures regularly with staff members and with clients.
- Know each client's personal health, fitness and mobility status, safety precautions, and needed exercise adaptations.
- Conduct periodic reactivity screening and assessments and provide client feedback.
- Be straightforward about what exercise can and cannot do to minimize, stabilize, and improve specific health conditions. This is where realistic goal setting begins.
- Keep confidential, up-to-date client records, documenting participant attendance, notable improvements, unusual reactions, or any atypical behaviors or responses.

- Control emotions by staying calm and clear-headed in times of high stress, crisis, or emergencies in the class.
- Manage your own personal stress, and leave negative moods outside the classroom.

Being Supportive

Many of your clients lack support from family and friends. Here are a few ways you can express support for your participants:

• In every class have at least one verbal exchange with every participant. In a big class, it may only be "hello" or "good-bye," a comment, or a compliment; what matters is that everyone in attendance can say to him- or herself, "The instructor talked to me today."

• Some people have had negative experiences with physical activity. Downplay self-defeating statements, and emphasize the positive aspects with such statements as "It's never too late to improve."

•When participants are absent for more than two classes, contact them by phone or e-mail to find out if everything is OK. You may even want to send a postcard saying, "I missed having you in class this week. I trust you are OK, and if you won't be here next week, please let me know. Your presence is missed." It only takes a few moments to send a message, yet the response from the participant may astound you.

• Supportiveness can also be demonstrated by utilizing the talent and experience of your class participants. As people age, they tend to become more altruistic, wanting to give back to the world in some way. Tap into this wealth of experiences by affording opportunities to contribute to the program. An individual develops greater enthusiasm and takes a more vested interest in the program when you welcome his or her suggestions. Simply considering a participant's suggestion can boost his or her **self-esteem** (the way a person feels about himself or herself) and his or her **self-efficacy** (a person's perception of his or her ability to do, learn, or master something; Sonstroem, 1984). Suggestions will often surprise and enlighten you, from novel music ideas to having grandchildren join in for a special exercise session.

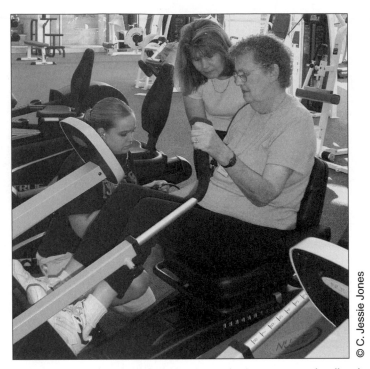

© C. Jessie Jones

A client is able to improve form through constructive feedback.

Care

One of the most basic human needs is knowing that you are cared about by other people. It is therefore important to try to make everybody feel like "somebody." However, be careful of the hoarders, soloists, sirens, and talkers, because they can monopolize your time (see table 19.1). Everyone in the class deserves your attention, not just the gregarious clients. Here are some examples of how to let your clients know you care.

- Bestow generous amounts of attention, acknowledgment, smiles, and even hugs on participants. There is always something to compliment about a person, even if it is just for coming to class.

- Inquire about your participants' activities or family life outside of exercise.

- Use nonverbal communication to express caring and interest in your participants. Many clients say that their favorite part of class is the hug they receive from their instructor at the end of the workout. Of course, you must learn who feels comfortable being hugged and who does not. Although some people do not like being touched and may even read too much into it, for other clients, a caring hug may be the only human contact they experience until the next class.

- Show genuine interest in the goals, interests, strengths, and weaknesses of your clients, and provide constructive feedback. Do not forget the power of referring to your clients by name.

Compassion

Compassion involves being empathetic, or having the ability to appreciate another person's suffering. How do *you* feel about someone who is kind and compassionate toward you? Compassion has the power to touch the heart and soul, to heal wounds, to cultivate inner strength and confidence, and to bring peace to conflict (Dalai Lama & Cutler, 1998). Following are some ways to express compassion.

- Although you do not want to encourage long-term self-pity, you should listen to the worries, pains, concerns, and losses of your clients. Indicate concern through nonverbal gestures and expressions. Hug or pat a person on the back (if appropriate for their values and personality). Learn to be patient with difficult individuals.

- Allow beginners to be beginners. Avoid any insinuation that beginner level is less prestigious than other levels. Trying to make every individual obtain perfect form on each exercise is unrealistic. Sometimes physical activity

> Compassion has the power to touch the heart and soul, to heal wounds, to cultivate inner strength and confidence, and to bring peace to conflict.

instructors forget what the process of learning an exercise is like for a new participant. Beginners must listen, look, follow, attempt the exercise, observe more, listen again, and continue to watch and follow while you instruct and demonstrate. As people learn at different rates and perform at various levels, plan for a liberal and generous learning curve (Heywood, 1989). To help you be empathetic (sensing others' emotions and understanding their perspective) toward beginners, try a new activity yourself at which you are not naturally adept. This will help you to remember or learn what it is like to be a beginner.

- Remind participants to listen to the wisdom of their bodies: "We are all individuals, so it does not matter what anyone else is doing. Do what is right for you." Participants need to be reminded to stay in their comfort zone and to do only what they consider safe. This is an application of the exercise principle of accommodation (described in chapter 9).

Using Positive Reinforcement

Positive reinforcement increases the likelihood that a behavior will be repeated in similar circumstances (Dishman, 1988). Verbal praise for even the smallest improvement in behavior is consistently associated with enhanced intrinsic motivation (Conroy, 2002). Any effort in exercise or physical activity deserves recognition and positive feedback. A pleasant tone of voice conveys that you are not about to reprimand anyone. To diffuse any anxiety students may have from your moving about and observing, you have to communicate verbally or nonverbally to each person with whom you make eye contact. Another strategy for client motivation and reinforcement is providing feedback about changes in health, fitness, or mobility status measured by periodic rescreening and reassessment. Studies show that extrinsic, or external, rewards for adopting healthful behaviors can be reinforcing (Wagman, 1997). Rewards can be anything that is perceived as meaningful, fun, or memorable—T-shirts, key

rings, magnifying glasses, certificates, water bottles, towels, a potluck celebration—you are limited only by your imagination. Ultimately, as people come to find physical activity more fulfilling, material rewards become less important because exercise and being active become intrinsically, or internally, rewarding (Conroy, 2002).

Other Characteristics of Good Leadership

For the most part, leadership style is shaped by one's personality and life experiences, including family environment, education, and training. It is more than likely that some of your leadership characteristics have been shaped by the inspirational teachers or instructors you have learned from yourself. Think about why they were inspirational. What were some of the leadership skills you admired in them?

Adopting the following seven characteristics of good leadership will help you become a master instructor.

- Positive attitude. Many people believe that the single most important factor for health, happiness, success, and quality leadership is having a positive attitude. John Maxwell, the author of the best-selling book *The Winning Attitude* (1993), defined attitude as "inward thoughts and feelings expressed by our behaviors" (p. 20). What qualities do you think of when you hear someone say, "She or he has a great attitude"? Here are examples of what some people consider a sign of a positive attitude: focusing on the positive aspects of life, treating others with respect, not giving up in the face of adversity, being friendly and fun-loving, being mentally tough, being passionate about life, being helpful and caring toward others, being loving and kind. Physical activity instructors with positive attitudes are likely to have more clients, to have higher retention and compliance rates, and to demonstrate more effective outcomes than instructors with negative attitudes. Since attitude is reflected not only in what we say but also by our facial expression and body language, it is helpful to have someone you respect videotape you teaching a class and then help you evaluate how you come across to others. Also, if you want to work at improving your attitude, the recommended readings at the end of the chapter can help get you started.

- Awareness. The skill of client awareness involves recognizing your clients' strengths and weaknesses, fears, likes and dislikes, needs, and values. It is also

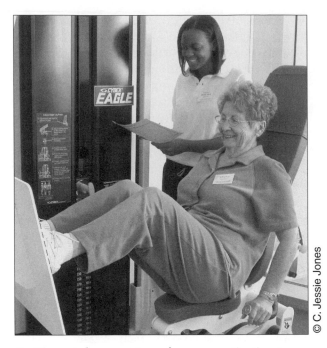

© C. Jessie Jones

Positive reinforcement can be very motivating to your clients because it can help to build their self-confidence.

important to be aware of the changing dynamics of a class environment from day to day. Becoming fully observant requires practice, and being responsive to those observations is even more difficult. For example, if participants start talking to each other immediately after you provide an instructional cue, it may mean that they did not understand or hear you. Remember the teacher you thought had eyes in the back of his or her head or could hear a pin drop? These phrases describe the skill of tuning-in and being fully present in the now. Effective leaders also are emotionally self-aware; that is, they are attuned to their feelings and how those feelings affect them and their clients (Ashforth & Humphry, 1995). They also have an accurate awareness of their limitations and strengths, they are not afraid to say, "I don't know," they welcome constructive evaluations from others, and they are willing to ask for help.

• Enthusiasm. Most people can detect artificial enthusiasm, but genuine enthusiasm can be an instructor's greatest asset. Moving and talking with positive emotion and high energy expresses enthusiasm; it shows a passion for what you are doing. Your passion carries an energy of excitement

that can arouse enthusiasm in those you lead. You can instill the passion of physical activity through your words and behaviors. Being optimistic and helping others to see the positive side of life can be very motivational. When you smile and laugh, others cannot help but smile and laugh with you; it is contagious. Clients connect with your enthusiasm when they look into your twinkling eyes. You can even express enthusiasm while maintaining your professionalism by wearing fun clothing. Pioneering fitness activist Dr. George Sheehan delivered speeches in a suit, a tie, and running shoes, not for novelty, but because it connected him to his fuel for enthusiasm: his passion for running. Remember that enthusiasm is a powerful tool for inspiring others.

• Respect. One of the best ways to show respect for your clients is by sincerely listening to them without passing judgment. Listen with both your ears and eyes. Listen for the message and the feeling behind the message; nonverbal gestures often speak louder than words. A skillful listener picks up on what people are truly concerned about and responds appropriately. Another way of expressing respect is by recognizing the individuality and wisdom of your clients. Contrary to popular belief, people become more unique, not more alike, as they age. Avoid generalizations that keep biases alive. Respect is also expressed through your attention to details such as the selection of workout and background music, the type of magazines available in your center, your interaction with other staff members, accommodating special requests, remembering special occasions, having equipment and supplies available, and so on. A comfortable physical environment coupled with polite, cordial interactions and thoughtful anticipation of preferences sets the stage for positive experiences.

• Creativity. Being prepared for the unexpected is another skill of excellent leadership. Being creative is vital, as you have to juggle many tasks and demands without losing your cool. This takes confidence in your teaching skills. For example, if you notice that a client is having trouble accomplishing a goal, be creative in helping the client modify the goal. This helps remove the stigma that surrounds failing to reach a goal. If a client never stays for on-the-floor exercises, chances are he or she feels vulnerable or unstable getting down to the floor and up again. Work with the client in private to

> Highly competent people are ethical and have a drive to improve their professional skills to meet an inner standard of personal excellence.

teach him or her the steps to safely get down to the floor and up again. Relearning this skill increases capabilities and confidence.

• Flexibility. If you notice clients look bored or down, you may need to vary the activities or the order of exercise on the spot. By being flexible and adding to or slightly altering the program, you can produce unexpected surges in enthusiasm. To spark the atmosphere and mood, use props creatively or incorporate folk, social, or line dancing. Appropriate partner exercise facilitates bonding between participants and increases camaraderie (Hoffman & Jones, 2002). One caveat, however, is that too many changes at once can overwhelm and discourage some individuals.

• Competency. The field of gerokinesiology is a rapidly changing area of study. Competent instructors know that continuing their education is imperative to their long-term success. Ideas for continuing your education include attending workshops and conferences, reading journal articles and books, observing expert instructors, taking classes, completing specialist certifications and college degrees, and regularly conducting participant and self-evaluations. Highly competent people are ethical and have a drive to improve their professional skills to meet an inner standard of personal excellence. Establishing friendly relationships, creating a welcoming atmosphere, and staying competent are the keys to avoid lawsuits. More on this topic is presented in chapter 22. In addition, being competent influences your self-confidence, and your self-confidence affects the confidence of your clients.

Summary

The field of gerokinesiology is a rapidly changing area of study because of the research in the field, the increase in community programs for older adults, and the demand for highly trained physical activity instructors of older adults. Your choice to be a physical activity instructor of older adults carries with it many responsibilities and opportunities to influence the health and well-being of our aging population.

Effective teaching is both science and art. Factors such as skill level, exercise selection, workout environment, and instructional style have an effect on program design and effectiveness. In addition to the steps described in this chapter, information obtained from preexercise screening, assessment, and goal setting helps you to develop effective lesson plans that are targeted and meaningful to your clients.

The teaching and leadership skills described in this chapter are easy to understand, but they must be studied and practiced if you intend to become a master physical activity instructor for older adults. Remember to be participant-focused, learn and practice how to deal with the different personalities you will meet as an instructor, and most important, remember that your enthusiasm and positive attitude are key components of being a successful teacher.

Key Terms

countdown 304
cuing 303
goal-oriented cue 304
mindful cue 305
physical cue 303
process-oriented cues 304
self-efficacy 309
self-esteem 309
transitional cues 304
verbal cue 303
visual cue 303

Recommended Readings

Carnegie, D. (1981). *How to win friends and influence people.* New York: Pocket Books.

Carter-Scott, C. (1998). *If life is a game, these are the rules.* New York: Broadway Books.

Goldman, D., Boyatzis, R., & McKee, A. (2002). *Primal leadership.* Boston: Harvard Business School Press.

Study Questions

1. A cue that guides a person through the change from the end of one movement to the beginning of another movement is referred to as a

   a. verbal cue
   b. transitional cue
   c. physical cue
   d. sequencing cue

2. Which of the following is an example of a goal-oriented cue?

   a. "Imagine pulling a long rope up from the ground."
   b. "Reach up high as if you are trying to get something off the top shelf."
   c. "Keep your feet about 12 inches (30 centimeters) apart in this exercise."
   d. "I'd like you to aim for 6 to 10 repetitions today."

3. You notice that a few participants find it difficult to move to the beat of the music during cardiovascular training. Their facial expressions lead you to believe that they are self-conscious and embarrassed. What is the best action to take?

   a. Give positive reinforcement whether they move on or off of the beat of the music, educating participants that both situations are allowed and beneficial.
   b. Leave the situation as it is, and hope they do not get in anyone's way.
   c. Ask them to move to the side or to the back of the room so that they will not disturb other class participants.
   d. Suggest that they get a personal trainer.

4. The best strategy to respond to a client who talks a lot during exercise classes is to

   a. suggest that the person move to the back of the room
   b. ask the person to leave the class
   c. ask the person to be quiet
   d. don't say anything to him or her

Application Activities

1. You are asked to take over an exercise class for older adults. It is held in a community center multipurpose room. The program has had mixed results since starting two years ago. There have been three interruptions of three to five weeks' duration when one instructor left and another was recruited and trained. You have been informed that the most recent instructor was popular, and participants were disappointed by her departure. The program is scheduled to restart in four weeks. It will be held twice a week at 10:00 a.m. There is a meeting held in the same room that ends at 9:30 a.m. on exercise days. You are informed that 12 participants are returning students, and 11 new participants are registered for the same class. No preactivity screening, testing, or evaluation has been conducted in the past.

   - Describe what additional information about the history of the program would be helpful to you as the next instructor, and explain why.

   - Discuss any obstacles you think you might encounter entering this new position.

   - What elements of instruction do you think would help increase the likelihood of a successful program?

2. Using the description in activity 1, describe how you would develop your exercise lesson plans. What type of activities would you include?

3. A participant in your class is a constant complainer. What strategies would you use to handle this person effectively before, during, and after class?

20

Designing and Managing Group Conditioning Classes

Janie T. Clark

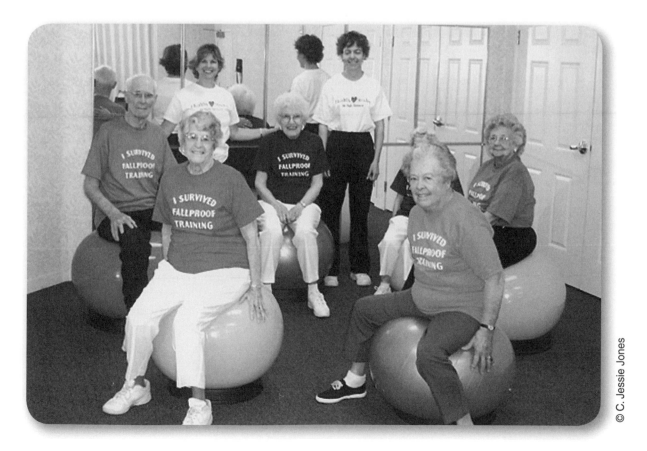

As discussed in chapter 19, instructors who have the ability to teach different types of group classes are in high demand. However, the productive design and management of group conditioning classes require the careful integration of the knowledge and skills discussed in this book, especially part II, "Screening, Assessment, and Goal Setting," and part III, "Core Program Principles and Training Methods." In addition, teaching group exercise classes demands an understanding of group dynamics. This chapter builds on the foundation provided in chapter 19 by providing instructors who teach group physical activity classes with additional principles of group dynamics. Applying these principles can improve your teaching effectiveness and the long-term adherence of your older adult clients. The chapter then provides specific techniques for making the exercise environment fun and for maintaining an efficient record-keeping system. The last part of this chapter discusses strategies to market your physical activity program.

Key Principles of Group Dynamics

Although physical exercise is a serious undertaking that produces important training effects, human nature predisposes us to seek pleasure in what we do. For many older adults, associating exercise routines with social enjoyment can mean the difference between long-term adherence and dropping out (Annesi, 1996; Annesi & Zimmerman, 2001). Instructors who understand the key principles of group dynamics can use the power of team training to help their participants sustain habitual exercise.

Group Versus Individual Motivation

Research indicates that exercise adherence by older people increases when being part of a group promotes feelings of team purpose toward completing a task (Annesi & Zimmerman, 2001). **Team purpose** is the sense of motivation shared by members of a group when working together to accomplish a desired outcome. Applying this finding in practice can be as simple as actively advocating that participants view their exercise class as a group project and bolster one another's persistence. Alternatively, a special group objective can be set, such as improving everyone's endurance enough to hike to a well-known landmark and back (Clark, 1997). Following the group's steady progress toward achieving a common goal (e.g., walking a specified distance) facilitates conversation and camaraderie among the members and reinforces their focus on the desired task. Another means of promoting a sense of team purpose is offering specialized classes to people who share similar challenges and concerns. For example, classes targeting the management of arthritis afford members a strong sense of group identity and an opportunity to provide one another with mutual support (Annesi & Zimmerman, 2001).

Assimilation of New Members

Many older adults perceive exercise classes somewhat differently than do younger adults. Seniors feel more integrated with their group both socially and in terms of task completion. This provides a potential advantage: When group bonding is successfully fostered, aging members can be particularly resistant to dropping out (Annesi & Zimmerman, 2001). For this reason, it is important to provide newcomers with a smooth entry into the group setting and to nurture the beginner's sense of being a part of the group.

The most effective first step is to provide a warm welcome. Introduce the new member to the group, if possible including some information about the person's hobbies and interests. Consider assigning an experienced participant as a temporary "exercise buddy" to help the new member get settled into the group's routine. It may be helpful to have everyone wear name tags when starting a new session or when inducting new members (Clark, 2003).

New group members may have questions such as "What should I wear?" or "What do I need to bring with me to class?" Of course, the instructor should make certain that all such questions are fully answered. However, it is usually the questions a newcomer might not think to ask that can lead to awkward moments if not addressed. Such issues typically involve group customs that have become established over time. For example, do the members have fixed—though perhaps unspoken—positions or seats on the exercise floor? Do they all contribute toward the purchase of weekly refreshments? Not knowing the answers to this type of question can result in embarrassment and may even delay

or obstruct a newcomer's feelings of harmonious assimilation into the group. It is the leader's responsibility to be a troubleshooter, preventing discouraging missteps by anticipating and meeting the needs of new class members. Figure 20.1 provides a new member orientation checklist, including steps to take and points to cover with beginners to help them enter smoothly into their new group.

Instructor-to-Group Feedback

Feedback from the instructor is important to participants. **Instructor-to-group feedback** is your means of providing direction, correction, and validation to participants. Through encouragement and honest praise, you can inspire participants to try their best while reinforcing their motivation to maintain a physically active lifestyle. It is good practice to compliment the group as a whole (e.g., "Keep up the great work, everybody!") and each member by name (e.g., "Good job, Evelyn"; Clark, 2003). On the other hand, a participant may experience acute discomfort if singled out in front of the group for correction. A tactful approach to reforming poor exercise technique is to address the entire class (e.g., "Let's all practice bending from the hips like this"). If that does

---

The following steps will help new members enter their new group setting smoothly.

1. Ask how the person prefers to be addressed: Dr., Mr., Mrs., Ms., Miss, first name? New members may wish to know how others in the group are addressed.
2. Welcome the new member and conduct the introductions.
3. Consider assigning an experienced "exercise buddy" to help the new member settle into the group.
4. Consider the use of name tags until the newcomer learns others' names.
5. Familiarize the newcomer with features of the facility; for example, point out the location of showers, bathrooms, lockers, rest benches, exits, and water fountains.
6. Advise the newcomer about what kind of clothing and shoes to wear.
7. Inform the newcomer about what to bring to class (e.g., a towel, dumbbells, exercise band, water bottle).
8. Advise the newcomer of local retailers where any needed accessories can be purchased.
9. Teach the newcomer any exercises he or she will need to know in order to participate successfully in the next class (e.g., circuit-training routines).
10. Familiarize the newcomer with customs of the group; for example, do members share or rotate certain tasks, such as moving chairs or putting away exercise accessories? When members have out-of-town visitors, are they permitted to bring their guests to class? Do members have fixed positions on the exercise floor? Do they all contribute toward the purchase of weekly refreshments?
11. Assure the new member that you always welcome questions and feedback.

FIGURE 20.1 New member orientation checklist.
Adapted from "Senior fitness instructor training manual," 2002, by the American Senior Fitness Association.

> Instructor-to-group feedback is an instructor's means of providing direction, correction, and validation to participants.

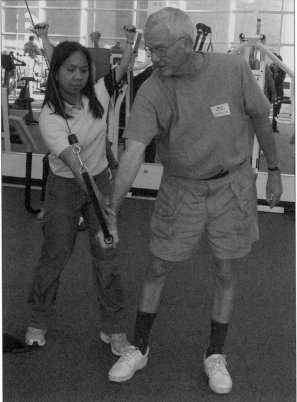

Take care to avoid words or mannerisms that might be misinterpreted as flirtatious.

not work, ask to meet with the participant who is experiencing difficulty privately after other members have left the class. Using demonstration, respectfully explain any changes needed. When the participant makes the desired adjustment, it is important to reward the person with generous approval (e.g., "I knew you could do it!"). Remember, whether a group requires instruction, correction, or praise, as discussed in chapter 19, you should convey honesty, tact, respect, and a positive tone when providing feedback (Clark, 2003).

Gender, Ethnic, and Cultural Sensitivity

Your recognition of the diversity of a group can be crucial for program effectiveness. It is very important to be sensitive to individual differences. Avoid making assumptions about what people like or need. Following are suggestions and recommendations by Ward (1997) to communicate respect and acceptance of the individuality of all participants.

- Be sensitive to the possibility that certain exercises or directions may embarrass some participants, especially in coed classes. For example, "Open the legs" might be better rephrased as "Feet should be about shoulder-width apart."

- Take care to avoid words or mannerisms that might be misinterpreted as flirtatious. Consider practicing in advance how to handle unwanted comments or behavior from participants. Likewise, wear conservative clothing; people from a number of cultural backgrounds find revealing dress offensive.

- When language is a potential barrier, use nonverbal forms of communication, such as gestures and facial expressions. Provide directional cues with hand and arm signals. Avoid lengthy instructions, favoring single word cues and simple phrases instead. Make direct eye contact, nod your head, and smile often. Seek ways to show participants that you value their cultural heritage. For example, play music of different ethnic groups, and acknowledge the religious and cultural holidays observed by your members.

- Resist any tendency to form stereotypical assumptions about a person based on gender, ethnicity, or country of origin.

- Try to gain a greater understanding and appreciation of others by reading about issues related to diversity, by traveling abroad, or by forming friendships with people from various cultural backgrounds. In communicating with any participant, express friendliness, caring, and compassion for that individual.

- Acknowledge the diversity of your clients: play culturally diverse music during the class; post pictures of ethnically diverse people on a bulletin board; celebrate your clients' holidays and special events, such as Cinco de Mayo, Octoberfest, Chinese New Year, and Hanukkah.

Injury Prevention

In addition to the injury prevention strategies that are discussed in chapter 21, a couple of precautions are related specifically to group exercise classes. Floor surface is an important issue in creating a safe exercise environment for older adults. Slippery or hard tile flooring is potentially dangerous, especially when accompanied by poor lighting (Schroeder, 1995; Van Norman, 1998). Vinyl or linoleum flooring may be satisfactory, depending on certain factors: (1) the floor covering's texture (slick or sticky areas can cause falls), (2) the underlying surface (in the best case, a suspended wood floor; in the worst, concrete), and (3) the amount of padding between the covering and the underlying surface. Thicker coverings absorb more shock and transmit less shock to the joints. If too thick, however, padded flooring becomes problematic for clients with balance problems or sensation loss in the feet. Similar considerations apply to carpet, which in addition may tend to catch participants' shoes during lateral steps and moves that involve sliding the foot across the floor. Also, to avoid bumps and collisions, it is important to make sure that clients have enough space for a given exercise routine.

Additional Group Management Considerations

A useful method for strengthening self-confidence and, in turn, improving performance and promoting long-term adherence is to use **empowerment techniques** (i.e., measures that foster the participant's ability to succeed at a given task). In a group setting, this often involves helping the lowest achievers keep up without holding back the highest achievers. Figure 20.2 provides practical steps for serving participants at different ability levels during a group class.

Empowerment can be sustained by maintaining a noncompetitive atmosphere. This applies not only to physical competition but also to the amount of attention and time each group member receives from the instructor. Physical activity instructors should take care to avoid any appearance of favoritism, instead serving all participants fairly and equally.

The use of empowerment techniques helps each class participant feel like a welcome and productive member in good standing. This increases

- Design workouts that each participant can perform at his or her own pace.
- Offer frequent, optional rest and water breaks.
- Provide expert cuing for transitions.
- Include exercises that can use progressive levels of resistance (e.g., dumbbells of different weights or exercise bands of various degrees of tension).
- Include choreography that can be followed with simple movements or intensified by the addition of more demanding or complex dance steps.

FIGURE 20.2   Steps for training groups of individuals at different levels.

cohesion, that sense of oneness within a group that promotes exercise adherence among older adults (Annesi & Zimmerman, 2001). Instructors can do much to solidify group cohesion, such as provide members with opportunities to mix and mingle. To this end, consider conducting periodic health education activities or hosting informal social periods with simple refreshments. Have participants sign get-well cards when a member is absent due to illness. Some groups create a class directory; in others members choose to exchange addresses and telephone numbers with each other directly (Clark, 2002). Reinforce a sense of team purpose in the day-to-day management of your group exercise program. In numerous ways, you can employ group dynamics for the benefit of your participants.

Making Group Activity Fun

According to the **pleasure principle,** human beings tend to pursue activity experienced as enjoyable and satisfying. Perhaps we are programmed to do so for reasons related to the survival of our species; after all, eating and reproductive activity are vital to the future of humanity (Sharkey, 2002). Many older adults have realized the pleasures of regular physical activity through group conditioning programs. One of the physical activity instructor's primary responsibilities is to blend exercise and enjoyment.

Leadership Style

As discussed in chapter 19, an instructor's leadership style is important for making an exercise environment enjoyable for participants. In a group class, the instructor's leadership style sets a mood that spreads like a ripple throughout the room. Indeed, the enjoyment of older adult clients appears to be directly related to the instructor's enthusiasm: The more enthusiastic their instructor, the more older adults enjoy their exercise classes. Their experience is all the more agreeable when the instructor expresses care, compassion, and support for each individual group member. Also, an atmosphere characterized by patience, courtesy, optimism, and *humor* is highly prized by older adult exercise participants (Clark, 2003).

Creativity

One of the most effective ways to add energy to any group conditioning class is through the use of music. Many older adults enjoy exercising to the rhythms of swing music, Broadway hits, the classics, old standards, and light disco or pop tunes. Clearly, the best way to determine appropriate types of music for your class is simply to ask the participants for input. Keep in mind previously noted precautions regarding volume, work at a comfortable tempo, and encourage your participants to have fun (Clark, 1998; Thompson & Hoekenga, 1998).

Another means of enhancing the group exercise experience is fitness accessories. Accessorizing can be beneficial from both a physical and an artistic standpoint. Popular accessories include hand weights, beanbags, exercise bands, wooden dowels, putty or clay, balls of various sizes and weights, balloons, peacock feathers, handkerchiefs, pillows, cones, shakers, towels, and even aluminum pie pans. Conducting occasional special activities also can help to keep a group exercise program fresh and interesting. Consider hosting a wellness fair or inviting an expert health educator to speak to your group. Other creative possibilities include holiday parties, nature walks, group volunteer projects, and a "Grandkids Day" for intergenerational movement activities and socializing (Clark, 2003).

Variety

A well-rounded group class format typically calls for a warm-up followed by an aerobic workout, a postaerobic cool-down, balance and mobility training, strength conditioning, and a final cool-down stretch. Refer to figure 20.3 for a sample lesson plan. However, participants might enjoy varying the sequence occasionally (e.g., performing their strength conditioning activities before the aerobic section; when doing this, repeat a few minutes of active warm-up exercise, such as low-intensity walking, immediately before introducing aerobic activities). Even if the sequence remains constant, you can still introduce variety through new music, different exercises, interesting fitness accessories, and minor changes in the routine (e.g., replacing seated or floor exercises with ballet barre activities every now and then).

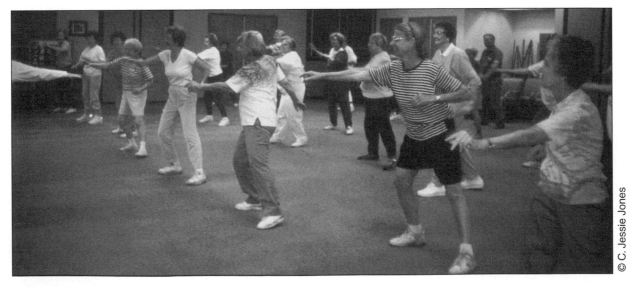

© C. Jessie Jones

Making group exercise fun with dance steps.

The following total-body workout is practical for a group class for older adults. Total exercise time should be approximately one hour or slightly longer. Play slow music with a tempo of 100 to 120 beats per minute (BPM) or slower while warming up and cooling down, medium tempos from 110 to 130 BPM for muscle work, and upbeat rhythms from 120 to 140 BPM during aerobic activity. For details on specific training components (e.g., warm-up and cool-down, aerobics, resistance training, and balance and flexibility exercise), refer to the chapters in parts III and IV that address them at length.

Warm-up: At least 10 to 15 minutes

1. Begin with limbering movements (5 to 7 minutes). Good activity choices include easy-paced walking and marching (in place or moving about), small kicks, and alternate toe touches to the floor at front, back, and sides. Low-intensity work on treadmills and stationary cycles, if available, can also be done.

2. Perform additional nonstrenuous rhythmical exercise (4 to 6 minutes). Older adults' backs are better prepared to undertake spinal rotation and lateral spinal flexion if warmed up first by less-demanding activity that does not require the spine to twist or bend toward the side. Therefore, one good way to begin is with rhythmical shoulder shrugs. Then gently move both shoulders forward and backward. To follow, place hands on front of thighs, and then alternate rounding and extending the back conservatively. Now the back is ready for gentle rotation or lateral flexion (with the torso supported by placing one hand on the outer thigh). Also include shoulder circles, elbow bends, arm reaches in various directions, heel raises, and low knee lifts.

3. Conclude with light dynamic stretching (1 to 2 minutes). Very mild stretches of the calves, hamstrings, back, and other body parts can be included toward the end of the warm-up. However, the warm-up should be devoted primarily to continuous, low-level movement, and more intensive static stretching should be saved for the final cool-down.

Aerobic work: Approximately 15 to 20 minutes

Undertake continuous, rhythmic activity using large muscle groups (e.g., legs). For safety reasons, perform low-impact (joint-sparing) movements, in which one foot maintains contact with the exercise surface, rather than high-impact moves such as running, jogging, or jumping jacks. Activity during the aerobics segment should be more vigorous and energetic than that of the preceding warm-up. Monitor participants to ensure that they exercise at a safe and beneficial intensity. Provide reminders on proper breathing and pacing.

Active postaerobic cool-down: At least 5 to 10 minutes

This segment should feature slow movements that allow the heart rate to gradually decrease. For this purpose, the rhythmical, limbering techniques used in the warm-up can be repeated. Perform the active postaerobic cool-down in a standing position, and keep participants' heads above heart level to prevent dizziness. Continue cool-down activity until ratings of perceived exertion (RPE) return to pre-aerobic levels (i.e., below 12 RPE) and heart rates slow to under 100 beats per minute. (Refer to chapter 13 for more information about the use of RPE during the aerobic exercise.)

Brief stretching: Approximately 5 minutes

Spend a short time statically stretching the calves, hamstrings, and other muscle groups just exercised. The back and other body parts can also be gently stretched at this time. Refer to chapter 11 for examples of appropriate flexibility exercises.

Balance and mobility training: Approximately 10 minutes

Following the guidelines in chapter 14, conduct a series of exercises to enhance balance and mobility.

Resistance training: Approximately 15 minutes

Following the guidelines in chapter 12, complete a series of resistance exercises to condition all the major muscle groups of the body.

Note: If *intensive* strength training is conducted, it should be followed by a few minutes of gentle, active cool-down activity (such as walking or stationary cycling) before commencing the final cool-down and stretch period described next.

Final cool-down and stretch: At least 5 to 10 minutes, longer if time permits

Now is the time for relaxed and sustained static stretching. Following the guidelines in chapter 11, choose a series of flexibility exercises to engage all the major joints and muscle groups of the body. The final cool-down and stretch period also provides an excellent opportunity for breathing and relaxation activities and other mind–body activities (see chapter 15 for sample activities).

FIGURE 20.3 Group lesson plan.

Aerobic Training

The imaginative physical activity instructor can introduce a great deal of variety and fun during the aerobic section of a group exercise class. (Refer to figure 20.4 for sample aerobic routines of gradually increasing intensity level.) Precede the aerobic session with a thorough warm-up period. After aerobic work, perform active cool-down exercises. Monitor intensity level responses during the workout, and provide participants with periodic reminders to slow down as needed. Encourage continuous breathing, and emphasize the use of low-impact techniques (e.g., kick without hopping). Provide further joint protection by varying moves and angles (e.g., leg curls after knee lifts, arm reaches in different directions). Alternate moving activities with stationary work. Balance your directional changes (e.g., forward-and-backward movements with side-to-side movements). During steps like the Charleston that call for one leg to work more than the other, reverse the lead foot midway through the sequence. Avoid quick turns and abrupt changes that might compromise equilibrium.

Help your participants follow their aerobic workout successfully by beginning with basic steps. Teach leg movements before adding the arms, and always

---

The following sample routines provide simple aerobic choreography to assist the novice instructor. With practice and experience, you will be able to build on the movements described here, successfully leading more complex combinations of moves and adding new steps as well. However, avoid being a perfectionist regarding precision dance choreography. Older adult class members may not always move in synchrony with you or with each other, so adopt a flexible, fun-oriented approach in your instruction. In these aerobic exercise routines, energy demand gradually increases, reaching a peak at about the midpoint, after which it begins to decrease. The session includes five routines running approximately four minutes each.

Routine 1

Suggested music: Broadway hit tune
Suggested tempo: 120 beats per minute

1. Begin by walking in place briskly with hands on hips.
2. Continue walking in place while extending relaxed arms down at sides and then swinging them naturally but energetically.
3. Walk in place while finger-snapping, then while clapping, and finally while alternating snaps and claps.
4. Walk in place while performing a variety of arm reaches: with both arms reaching to the front at once, both at once to the sides, both alternately to the front and sides; then with alternating arm reaches (right arm, left arm, etc.) to the front and then to the sides. Continue repeating for as long as desired.
5. Next, walk in place using any or all of the arm moves and patterns already described while facing the front for 16 steps, right for 16 steps, back for 16 steps, and left for 16 steps; repeat as desired.
6. Walk briskly (incorporating any arm moves and patterns) in individual circles and then single-file in large circular laps. After a time, change direction.

Routine 2

Suggested music: Patriotic march performed by an orchestra
Suggested tempo: 130 beats per minute

1. Begin by marching in place briskly with hands on hips.
2. Continue marching in place with arms down at sides and elbows bent, then while swinging bent arms naturally but energetically.
3. March in place while repeating any or all of the arm moves and patterns used during routine 1. Add arm reaches overhead as well as to the front and sides.
4. March in place while substituting pushes for reaches.
5. March in place with active arms while facing different directions, as in routine 1, but for only eight steps per side.

FIGURE 20.4   Group aerobic routines.

6. Using any arm motions performed so far, march four steps forward, four in place, four backward, four in place, and continue repeating as desired.

7. Perform side-stepping: Face front with hands on hips, and starting with right foot, take three side-steps to the right, then touch left toe to the floor beside right foot. To return, starting with left foot, take three side-steps to the left, then touch right toe to the floor beside left foot. Integrate pushes (using both arms at once) to the front, sides, or overhead. Repeat as desired.

8. While marching and swinging bent arms naturally but energetically, form a large circle facing center; march forward (inward) until all participants are close together, then backward (outward) again, and repeat as desired.

Routine 3

Suggested music: Light disco
Suggested tempo: 140 beats per minute

1. Along with any previously used arm motions, perform vigorous knee lifts in place (alternating one lift per side); then proceed to alternate leg curls in place. If desired, add low but wide arm sweeps across the front (arms together) during these lifts and curls.

2. Perform alternate kicks in place while making loose-fisted punches to the front, sides, and overhead.

3. Perform alternate kicks along with arm scissors (cross extended arms low in front; repeat, alternating arms, while gradually raising arms upward till overhead and then down again). Repeat as desired.

4. Perform double knee lifts, leg curls, and kicks (two raises per leg) along with various arm reaches, pushes, and punches.

Routine 4

Suggested music: "Golden oldie" pop rock
Suggested tempo: 130 beats per minute

1. Have some fun with this aerobics number! Include any familiar dance steps you know well enough to lead: the twist, cha-cha, Charleston, pony, monkey, freddie, hustle, or swim (the crawl, breast stroke, and dog paddle).

2. If desired, partner up for square dance moves, or form a group conga line.

Routine 5

Suggested music: Smooth jazz
Suggested tempo: 120 beats per minute

1. Repeat your initial aerobic moves from routine 1.

FIGURE 20.4   *(continued)*

return to a neutral starting position (e.g., kicking in place) before making substantive changes. Facilitate transitions by providing advance verbal notice, and employ both arm and hand gestures to indicate upcoming directional changes. One simple way to handle potentially tricky transitions (e.g., changing lead foot) is to have participants march in place between moves while you describe the next step.

Circuit Training

Circuit training is another means of infusing group conditioning programs with variety. **Circuit training** involves working briskly through a series of carefully selected exercise stations that make up an effective physical workout. Although less efficient at producing major gains in cardiovascular endurance and muscular strength than sustained aerobic activity and intensive strength training, respectively, circuit training nonetheless can result in significant cardiovascular and muscular improvements (Haennel, Quinney, & Kappagoda, 1991; Kaikkonen, Yrjama, Siljander, Byman, & Laukkanen, 2000; Marx et al., 2001). The exercises included in a circuit should reflect the functional fitness level of the participants. One popular circuit format alternates aerobic movement stations with resistance stations featuring dumbbells, exercise bands, strength machines, or calisthenics using body weight for resistance; alternatively, conventional circuit designs include resistance stations only. Each participant works at one station for approximately 45 to 60 seconds before everyone is signaled to move on to the next station. To ensure the smooth progress of participants through a circuit routine, the instructor should provide advance instruction regarding the exercise to be performed at each station. With imagination, circuits can also

be developed to incorporate stretches, simple mind–body activities (e.g., tai chi, qigong, yoga), aquatic exercises, outdoor fitness trail activities, and techniques for improving balance, coordination, power, and agility. Figure 20.5 describes a basic circuit-training routine.

The simple circuit plan presented in figure 20.5 alternates aerobic movement with resistance activity. Precede the circuit-training routine with a group warm-up session; follow it first with postaerobic cool-down activities and then with a final

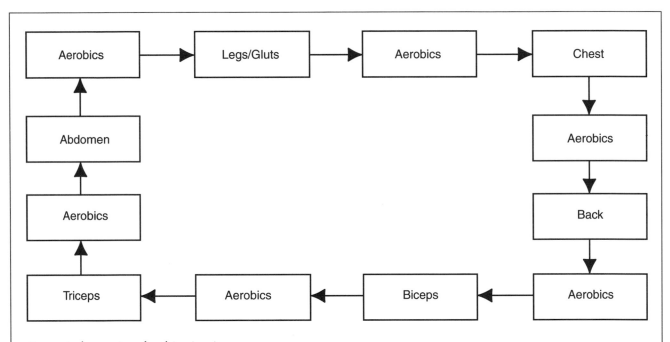

Suggested exercises for this circuit:

1. Quadriceps, hamstrings, gluteals—Squats using body weight or dumbbells for resistance. Do not lower buttocks below knee level.

2. Chest, upper body—Chest presses using resistive tubing or dumbbells. Starting with elbows at sides, slowly push both arms to front, extending the elbows, and then slowly flex the elbows to return to starting position.

3. Back—Scapular retraction using resistive tubing or dumbbells. Move shoulders back, bringing the shoulder blades close together, and then return to starting position.

4. Biceps—Biceps curls using resistive tubing or dumbbells.

5. Triceps—Triceps extensions using resistive tubing or dumbbells.

6. Abdomen—Abdominal contractions, held for approximately three seconds apiece, using no resistive equipment. To increase the workload, during each contraction lift one knee, extend the leg, pause, and then bend the leg and return it to the starting position; alternate sides. Avoid breath holding, and discontinue any exercise that causes pain in the lower back.

7. Aerobic movement—Do not use resistive tubing or dumbbells. This activity can be as simple as marching in place energetically at each aerobic exercise station. For greater variety, incorporate various moves that your group has mastered in previous aerobic sessions, or use aerobic training equipment such as treadmills and stationary cycles.

FIGURE 20.5   Basic circuit design.

cool-down and stretch period. Since all of the exercises can be performed while standing, older adult participants have no need to move quickly between floor and standing exercise positions, which can cause dizziness. Since the resistance activity imposes a modest workload, participants can start the circuit at any station (whereas intensive strength training requires working larger muscle groups first), thereby allowing a group of up to 12 participants to begin and finish their circuit at the same time. For 13 to 18 members, place two aerobic stations between each resistance station. For more members, include additional resistance exercises along with corresponding aerobic stations.

When implementing a circuit, one minute per station allows participants time for comfortably paced station-to-station transitions, including brief rest breaks if necessary. It also eliminates the need to rush resistance work, which should be performed with control and good form for as many repetitions as possible per station (usually between 10 and 20 repetitions, depending on the specific exercise and the individual's ability). Most participants can build up to completing a 12-station circuit two or three times.

Certain practical steps enable your circuit-training classes to run smoothly and safely. Before starting, have the group practice resistance exercises first without and then with resistive devices. Advise participants to slow down and pace themselves as needed while at any exercise station. Have seating nearby in case anyone requires it. Throughout the circuit, assist participants with technique as necessary. Monitor participants to ensure that they work at appropriate intensity levels. Keep in mind that low-fit beginners may not need to use resistive devices and that optimal resistance levels differ among other members. To this end, each resistance station can be equipped with a rack of tubing or dumbbells that provide various degrees of resistance (e.g., tubing of light and moderate tension; small dumbbells of one, three, and five pounds, or one-half, one, and two kilograms). Clearly denote intensity (e.g., by color), and teach participants always to return equipment to its rack after use to prevent falls. Stations might also feature

> Circuit training involves working briskly through a series of stations that make up an effective physical workout.

exercise cards or posters displaying instructions and illustrations. Consider enlisting experienced class members to assist newcomers in moving through the circuit.

Additional Training Options

For variety, instructors may also consider additional group training options. Examples include indoor gym or mall walking, outdoor walking, and routines that incorporate various forms of dance such as tap, clogging, line dancing, square dancing, ballet, ballroom dancing, or old favorites such as the jitterbug and Charleston. Remember that exercise adherence is closely associated with making group activity fun. To keep your group's interest high, provide each participant with a successful and enjoyable exercise experience.

Records Management

To serve its purpose, the paperwork completed by each participant in your class must be filed and maintained in an organized manner. You should always be able to locate desired forms or documents quickly and easily. Without effective organization, the records of a group (or worse, a number of groups) can quickly become unwieldy, making the task of group management more time-consuming and less constructive.

Preexercise Records

The recruitment of new class participants generates certain tangible records, for example, contact information, written medical clearance, health and activity screening data, initial functional performance test results, and perhaps laboratory-based physiological assessment reports. Additionally, an early interview process is recommended to establish realistic and measurable short- and long-term goals for clients. That record, too, should be preserved for ready reference and regular follow-up.

The material accumulated through these procedures forms a participant's *base file*. More information can be added to the base file over the course of an individual's participation in the exercise program. The base file provides a secure repository for important records and, over time, will present a clear picture of the participant's progress. A manageable method for housing such information is to prepare a separate folder for each participant and store the folders in alphabetical order in a file cabinet that can be locked. Alternatively, the documents can be scanned or otherwise converted for input into a computerized database.

Ongoing and Follow-Up Records

Attendance can be recorded at every class by the participants themselves, either by computerized means, by entering their names on a sign-in sheet, or by indicating attendance on individual index cards organized alphabetically in a file box. The group leader can transfer this attendance data to the participants' base files at predetermined intervals (e.g., daily, weekly, or monthly). Attendance records can be useful in evaluating the participants' progress toward their personal fitness goals.

Certain procedures, such as functional performance testing and progress analysis, must be repeated periodically. In a group setting, individual

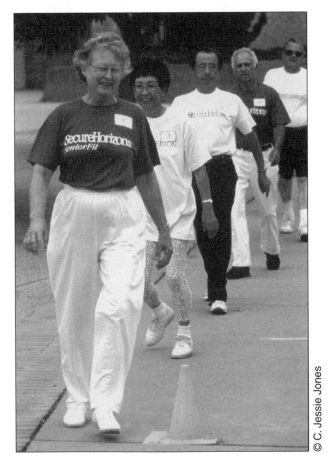

© C. Jessie Jones

Follow-up testing in a group class, such as this six-minute walk test, should be repeated periodically.

participants are likely to require follow-up testing at different times. To conduct such tasks on schedule, the physical activity instructor needs a time-sensitive memo system. A computer program can be employed to apprise the instructor of imminent tasks. Otherwise, important dates and reminders can be marked on a calendar or in an appointment book. Results of recent testing should be retained in the participant's base file for future reference.

Participant Feedback Records

One method of encouraging long-term exercise adherence in a group setting involves **participant feedback** (which may include questions, opinions, or suggestions from participants). Since some participants may be reticent about voicing their opinions and suggestions, a simple form can be designed to solicit information that can aid the instructor in accommodating the group's needs, interests, and preferences. This feedback should be filed separately, *not* in participants' folders, as feedback forms should offer anonymity to those who complete them. Be sure to provide a container in which the completed forms can be submitted privately. While it is always good practice to invite informal feedback on a day-to-day basis, conducting periodic written surveys (perhaps once or twice per year) may prove particularly elucidating. A sample participant feedback form is provided in figure 20.6.

Participant feedback can be useful in several ways. If a numerical ranking system is used (e.g., a scale of 1 to 5), the averages provide quick insight into the majority's view of the program. If only one or two elements are rated poor, that provides a clear direction for how best to improve the program. Over time, a comparison of periodic survey results will indicate whether the program has achieved or maintained high quality in the eyes of its participants. By including at least one open-ended question (e.g., "Any additional comments or suggestions?"), a survey can elicit responses that can completely surprise you and may inspire much-appreciated changes or additions to a program (e.g., "Can our dogs come to walking class?"). Keep in mind that although universal accord might not always be attainable concerning every aspect of a group class, knowing the consensus of members can help you formulate well-received policies.

Participant Survey

Rate each statement on a scale of 1 to 5, with 1 being *not at all* and 5 being *extremely*.

	Not at all				Extremely
Exercise Environment					
The facility is neat and clean.	1	2	3	4	5
The facility's equipment is safe.	1	2	3	4	5
The lighting is satisfactory.	1	2	3	4	5
Room temperature is comfortable.	1	2	3	4	5
The humidity is comfortable.	1	2	3	4	5
Air ventilation is satisfactory.	1	2	3	4	5
The sound system works well.	1	2	3	4	5
The instructor's voice is easy to hear and understand during class.	1	2	3	4	5
The instructor can be seen clearly during class.	1	2	3	4	5
Instructor Characteristics					
Music volume is set at the right level.	1	2	3	4	5
The music selection is enjoyable.	1	2	3	4	5
The instructor's exercise demonstrations are helpful and easy to follow.	1	2	3	4	5
The instructor gives clear, early cues before changing moves.	1	2	3	4	5
The instructor provides useful feedback to participants during class.	1	2	3	4	5
The instructor seems well-organized.	1	2	3	4	5
The instructor is friendly and enthusiastic.	1	2	3	4	5
The instructor is courteous and respectful.	1	2	3	4	5
The instructor is caring and supportive.	1	2	3	4	5
The instructor has a sense of humor.	1	2	3	4	5
The instructor encourages members to enjoy one another's company.	1	2	3	4	5
Program Content					
The exercise class requires an appropriate level of physical exertion.	1	2	3	4	5
The exercise class includes sufficient variety.	1	2	3	4	5
The exercise class is enjoyable.	1	2	3	4	5
I would recommend this class to my friends.	1	2	3	4	5
Any additional comments or suggestions? _____					

FIGURE 20.6   Group participant feedback form.

Reprinted from "Senior fitness instructor training manual," 2002, by the American Senior Fitness Association.

Marketing Considerations

The last component of successfully managing group exercise classes is promoting the program. Most physical activity instructors have to budget their marketing dollars carefully, but many effective promotional strategies are quite inexpensive. One such strategy is community outreach. The following marketing options may prove productive not only for the promotion of group classes but also for the promotion of other types of programming as well.

Community Resources

One economical way to advertise your services is to leave program literature (e.g., leaflets and fliers) at local businesses, agencies, and organizations that serve older adults (Clark, 2002). Group instructors should be sure to approach residential complexes for older adults, civic groups, houses of worship, and clubs devoted to specific hobbies or other special interests. Often they are amenable to starting a group exercise class on their own premises for their members. Figure 20.7 provides a listing of sites where instructors can distribute promotional materials targeting the local older adult population.

Print materials should feature large fonts (at least 14-point), high contrast (e.g., dark lettering on a light background), economy of words, and simple and straightforward art. Wordiness, complicated graphics, or elaborate color schemes could render your message illegible to its target audience as a result of age-associated changes in visual acuity, depth perception, and the ability to distinguish among colors (Valenzuela, 2002). Program description is equally important. When designing ads and fliers, certainly it is appropriate to cite the instructor's professional credentials, note the facility's state-of-the-art features, and point out the economic value of the program's membership terms. However, most of the space and care should be devoted to describing the benefits that potential members stand to gain by joining. Promotional materials can stress social benefits (e.g., "Join our friendly fitness family! We're having fun shaping up together!"). Potential clients prefer

Health-related sales and services	Community service	Recreational outlets	Retail services	Miscellaneous
• Chiropractors • Doctors' offices • Hearing aid sales and service establishments • Massage therapists • Mental health agencies and practices • Optical care practices • Eyeglass sales and service centers • Orthopedic aids sales and service establishments • Smoking cessation clinics • Social service agencies • Weight loss clinics • Wheelchair sales and service centers	• Specialized transportation services and agencies • Meal programs for older adults • Public libraries • Civic organizations	• Bingo parlors • Bowling alleys and leagues • Bridge (and other card or game) clubs • Country clubs • Garden clubs • Golf courses • Shuffleboard leagues • Tennis clubs • Yacht or boating clubs	• All businesses that cater to older clientele • Banks • Barber shops • Bookstores • Clothing retailers • Craft and hobby supply stores • Gardening shops • Restaurants • Salons (e.g., hairdressers, manicurists) • Sport shops (e.g., golf, tennis)	• Places of worship • Residential complexes for older adults • Mobile home parks

FIGURE 20.7   Potential marketing outlets.

Reprinted from "Senior fitness instructor training manual," 2002, by the American Senior Fitness Association.

classes that can offer such benefits as increased energy, weight loss, stress reduction, greater ease of movement, relief from arthritis symptoms, or a better golf swing (Clark, 2002). The stronger the connection you make between exercise benefits and your clients' quality of life (including the ability to perform activities of daily living), the more new, retained, and referred clients you will gain (Valenzuela, 2002).

The media—print, radio, and television—provide an outlet for free publicity as well as paid advertising. Notify local stations and newspapers when your group is planning an interesting activity (e.g., a charity walk-a-thon). As a result, your current members can enjoy a pleasurable experience while inspiring others to join your group. Be sure to use this marketing strategy in moderation. Call on the press too often, and reporters will come to disdain your news; contact them from time to time about stories of interest to the general community, and you can get valuable coverage featuring photographs of your participants (Clark, 2003). Also, consider offering older adult fitness segments to local television stations and columns to area newspapers. Although you may provide this service for free, it can pay off handsomely in terms of advertising. Along the same lines, you can increase your visibility to the older adult community by conducting free lectures and fitness appraisals at local events such as home expositions and philanthropic fund-raisers. Other good locations include shopping malls, supermarkets, senior centers, assisted living facilities, and retirement communities (Valenzuela, 2002).

Underused Marketing Vehicles

Thoughtful program development can attract participants to group conditioning classes. Consider offering specialty exercise programs to address the unique needs of niche markets within the community. Group classes are ideal for bringing together participants with common interests while permitting the economical use of an instructor's valuable time. Here are some examples:

- Classes for people with a particular medical disorder (e.g., diabetes, arthritis, Parkinson's disease)
- Weight loss and stress management courses
- Sport-specific conditioning programs (e.g., golf, tennis, skiing)

Another option is offering small-group sessions for several neighbors or friends at one of their homes. This approach can overcome transportation-related barriers to exercise and can prove economical for older adults since expenses are shared among the group—all while providing the social benefits of group exercise (Valenzuela, 2002).

Hosting certain types of promotional events also can be effective for boosting program membership. These are two practical examples:

- Health fairs—Services can include free blood pressure measurement, vision testing, body mass index calculation, simple pulmonary function testing, and selected functional performance assessments.
- Older adult wellness celebrations—The festivities might include exercise demonstrations, the opportunity to meet instructors, cooking demonstrations, health promotion presentations, and wholesome refreshments.

Of course, at both events all guests should be provided with well-designed advertising literature describing your older adult exercise services (Clark, 2002).

Competitive fee schedules and senior discounts can be practical sales tools. Likewise, group discounts can be profitable, especially when you are proposing to launch group classes on an organization's premises for its members. National compensation statistics provide little guidance to instructors in setting financial terms because fees vary so widely: from gratis to more than $65 per hour for group exercise instruction (Clark, 2002; IDEA Health and Fitness Association, 1999) and from $15 per half-hour session to $80 per hour for individual programming (Valenzuela, 2002). Analyzing your area's overall older adult population, their average income, and their prevalence within specific economic categories can help you to establish realistic rates (Van Norman, 1998). Good sources for such data include the local chamber of commerce and community library. Also, take into account competitors' rates and local practices regarding instructor compensation, both of which you can ascertain by conducting your own informal survey. Keep in mind that offering discounted rates to older adults (and even further savings for classes during slow periods such as late morning and midafternoon) can help you to build and maintain a stable clientele (Valenzuela, 2002).

Other Marketing Tools

The role of office and clerical staff in the success or failure of a group exercise class should not be underestimated. Uninterested front-office personnel can estrange prospective clients, but enthusiastic staff members instill confidence and encourage sign-ups. The people who answer the telephone and greet the public are an instructor's front line in the mission to attract new members. Therefore, instructors should always take the time to inform and enthuse front-desk workers about their physical activity programs (Clark, 2002).

Possibly more than any other form of sales promotion, word of mouth can increase group participation. Be aware that a group setting supplies many people to spread the word about your services. Members who are well satisfied with their exercise program recommend it to their friends and acquaintances. With members' positive word of mouth, your group can grow exponentially! For this reason, among others, you must make certain that your program delivers those valuable participant benefits promised by your advertising copy. Many instructors find it productive to offer incentives to their members for bringing a friend to class. Over the long term, a happy group is a growing group (Clark, 2002).

Summary

Effective group management requires the instructor to wear many hats. For instance, it is essential to manage participants' records well. Important principles of group dynamics must also be understood and applied, including promoting feelings of team purpose, employing empowerment techniques, and most importantly, making your participants feel welcome. You also need a strong commitment to making exercise fun. Useful tools at your disposal include establishing an upbeat atmosphere and being creative, for example, by providing variety in training. Finally, you may be obliged to develop productive marketing skills. Marketing options range from traditional advertising to special promotional events such as health fairs. When all the necessary facets are properly combined, the result is a successful group exercise program that is highly rewarding to both the instructor and the program participants.

Key Terms

Recommended Reading

American Senior Fitness Association. (2002). *Senior fitness instructor training manual* (4th ed.). New Smyrna Beach, FL: Author.

Study Questions

1. Which of the following features should not be present in older adult exercise environments?
   a. dim lighting
   b. wall mirrors
   c. a platform for the instructor
   d. the use of a microphone by the instructor

2. Cohesion is defined as
   a. long-term adherence to a program of regular physical exercise
   b. the constructive use of participant feedback
   c. the feeling of oneness within a group
   d. the efficient management of participant records

3. In group classes, participant enjoyment is most closely linked to which of the following factors?
   a. effectiveness of the workout
   b. music selection
   c. instructor enthusiasm
   d. variety of exercise movements

4. Which of the following statements is true of circuit training?
   a. It is advisable only for highly fit exercise participants.
   b. It works well in personal training venues but is impractical for group classes.
   c. It requires the use of strength-training machines.
   d. It can be undertaken successfully indoors or outdoors.

5. For optimal marketing results, the main emphasis of promotional materials should be
   a. credentials, qualifications, and experience of the instructor
   b. benefits to the participant
   c. high value for low price
   d. state-of-the-art equipment and facilities

Application Activities

1. If you presently teach a class, rate your classroom's safety and comfort level point by point. (If you are not currently teaching, plan a safe and comfortable classroom by listing the features it should have.)

2. Using a mirror (and tape recorder, if one is available), observe yourself demonstrating how you typically communicate during three key phases of group class: the greeting, a sample movement instruction, and class dismissal. Honestly assess your voice, facial expressions, mannerisms, and choice of words. If your teaching delivery is uninspired, practice conveying additional sincere enthusiasm.

3. Design a circuit routine that includes 10 stations featuring different types of exercises.

4. Design an effective promotional flier to market your existing (or future) exercise class.

21

Exercise Considerations for Medical Conditions

James H. Rimmer

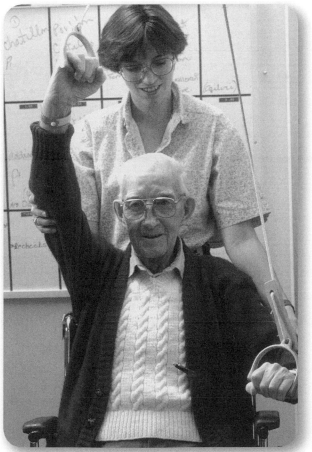

With advances in emergency medicine, rehabilitation science and technology, public health, and consumer education, older people with disabilities and chronic health conditions are living longer (Campbell, Sheets, & Strong, 1999). Bypass surgeries are becoming more common among older adults, replacement parts such as knees and hips are lasting longer, and portable breathing devices are allowing people with chronic lung diseases to lead more active lives. These and other technologies have resulted in a growing number of elderly people with disabilities who, in many instances, need physical activity more than their healthier older counterparts in order to maintain their narrower margin of health (Ostir et al., 1999).

It is not uncommon for older adults with one or more disabilities to lose a significant amount of mobility and physical independence after a minor illness, injury, or exacerbation of their condition (Rimmer, 2001). Older adults with disabilities who are physically active are more likely to maintain their independence for a longer portion of their life and can often improve their health in a substantial way by engaging in low to moderate levels of physical activity (Miller, Rejeski, Reboussin, Ten Have, & Ettinger, 2000).

The purpose of this chapter is to provide physical activity instructors with a general understanding of various exercise modifications and safety-related guidelines that can allow older adults with disabilities and chronic health conditions to participate successfully in various types of exercise programs. Common health conditions affecting older adults in their later years include coronary heart disease, hypertension, stroke, pulmonary disorders, diabetes, osteoporosis, arthritis, Parkinson's disease, and Alzheimer's disease, which are each discussed in this chapter. While it is difficult to ascertain the cumulative toll on health care costs and personal burden, having one or more of these conditions significantly affects the lives of many older individuals. This chapter serves only as a primer for understanding how to work with people with these conditions. For a more complete overview of each disorder, refer to the recommended readings at the end of this chapter.

Cardiovascular Conditions

Cardiovascular disease is a major cause of death and disability in the United States. Older individuals with coronary heart disease have a high rate of functional limitations and disability (Aggarwal & Ades, 2001). Exercise can have a substantial positive impact on cardiovascular health.

Coronary Heart Disease

Coronary heart disease (CHD) is a condition in which one or more of the coronary arteries are narrowed by atherosclerotic plaque or vascular spasm (*Merck Manual of Geriatrics,* 1995). The prevalence of CHD increases with age and peaks between the sixth and seventh decades of life. By the eighth decade, the prevalence of CHD is approximately 60 percent in both sexes (*Merck Manual of Geriatrics,* 1995). CHD is considered a multifaceted disorder with a great deal of heterogeneity (Shapira et al., 1995). Some individuals with CHD are greatly limited physically, while others are able to maintain their usual daily activities. Approximately one quarter of individuals over the age of 65 have symptoms of CHD, and older adults in this age group account for more than two thirds of all acute myocardial infarctions (Aggarwal & Ades, 2001). Symptoms

Approximately 60 percent of adults 80 years and older have coronary heart disease.

often include chest pain, dizziness, arrhythmias, and breathlessness with mild exertion (Groer & Shekleton, 1989).

Since the purpose of this chapter is to discuss conditions that physical activity professionals are likely to encounter in an exercise facility such as a YMCA or private fitness center, advanced CHD is not discussed in this chapter. Cardiac rehabilitation or medically supervised exercise programs that are associated with many hospitals are more appropriate for individuals with advanced CHD.

Exercise is effective in maintaining the integrity of the cardiovascular system and should be prescribed to older individuals whether or not they have been diagnosed with CHD (Aronow, 2001). A primary goal of the physical activity instructor should be to avoid high-intensity exercise, which has a greater likelihood of precipitating a coronary event, and to know the warning signs for stopping exercise. The exercise program for people with known CHD should include a longer warm-up period consisting of low-intensity exercise such as light walking or riding a stationary bike with little or no resistance; several different stretching exercises, particularly in the chest region if a person has had open-heart surgery; and some mild breathing exercises, which could be part of a yoga or postural relaxation section of the class. A longer warm-up can reveal any chest discomfort or dizziness before initiating higher-intensity exercise. The longer warm-up can include various stretching exercises, starting in a chair, then standing, and finally on the floor if possible for the client. Many excellent yoga and stretching videotapes developed for older adults can also be used during the warm-up.

Resistance training is a useful intervention strategy for older people with coronary heart disease (Aggarwal & Ades, 2001). Since many older adults with CHD grow increasingly sedentary, loss of skeletal muscle mass and strength can lead to a loss in physical function and can compromise the person's ability to perform common activities such as walking up a flight of stairs or lifting a bag of groceries (Aggarwal & Ades, 2001). In medically unsupervised settings where there is no input or guidance from a physician, the physical activity

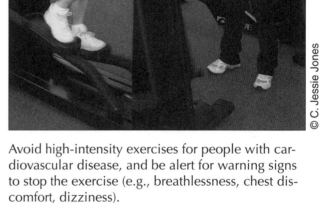

© C. Jessie Jones

Avoid high-intensity exercises for people with cardiovascular disease, and be alert for warning signs to stop the exercise (e.g., breathlessness, chest discomfort, dizziness).

professional should develop a low-intensity resistance-training program based on the client's rating of perceived exertion (RPE). Blood pressure and vital signs should be monitored carefully to ensure that the program is not too strenuous for the individual. You should always consult with the client's physician if you become aware of any symptoms (e.g., breathlessness, chest discomfort, dizziness) related to the exercise program.

Hypertension

Hypertension is a rise in systolic or diastolic blood pressure above normal values. Most research indicates that resting blood pressure increases with age and that elevated blood pressure is a major cardiovascular disease risk factor in the elderly (Hurley & Roth, 2000). The Joint National Committee on Prevention, Detection, Evaluation, and Treatment of High Blood Pressure (1997) categorizes hypertension into three stages (see figure 21.1). Exercise training has been shown to have substantial benefits for older individuals with hypertension (Hagberg, Park, & Brown, 2000; Ohkubo et al., 2001).

Stage 1: Systolic blood pressure of 140 to 159 mmHg or a diastolic blood pressure of 90 to 99 mmHg

Stage 2: Systolic blood pressure of 160 to 179 mmHg or a diastolic blood pressure of 100 to 109 mmHg

Stage 3: Systolic blood pressure of 180 mmHg or greater or a diastolic blood pressure of 110 mmHg or greater.

FIGURE 21.1   Hypertension criteria established by the Joint National Committee on Prevention, Detection, Evaluation, and Treatment of High Blood Pressure (1997).

The most important precaution is to ensure that the person's hypertension is being well controlled with medication and that the exercise program is not causing abnormal fluctuations in blood pressure. Monitor blood pressure more frequently in older clients with hypertension, particularly during the early stages of the program. You should invest in a good blood pressure monitor and stethoscope and take refresher courses on how to accurately measure blood pressure.

Medications used to treat hypertension include beta-blockers, calcium channel blockers, and diuretics. For people who are on beta-blockers, which are heart medications that blunt the heart rate response to exercise, rating of perceived exertion (RPE) is recommended for gauging exercise intensity. It may be necessary, however, to first teach the client how to measure RPE to ensure its accuracy (see chapter 7 for instructions on teaching your older adult clients how to rate their perceived exertion).

Thiazide diuretics are also used to treat hypertension. These drugs decrease blood pressure by increasing urine output. A complication that may arise in people taking these medications is that plasma lipids, with the exception of HDL cholesterol, can increase (Rosenstock, 2001). Clients taking diuretics may avoid drinking fluids so that they do not have to use the bathroom as often. This unfortunately increases the risk of dehydration. It is important to explain to the client that exercise causes a loss of body fluids through perspiration, and if the client does not ingest fluids during and after exercise to compensate for this loss, there is a

Intensity of exercise for people with COPD should be based on RPE because it is a more reliable indicator than heart rate.

greater likelihood of dehydration and other secondary complications.

Occasionally, antihypertensive medications may predispose a person to **postexercise hypotension** (a drop in blood pressure after exercise) resulting from the reduction of total peripheral resistance, which affects blood flow to the extremities (Gordon, 1997). To avoid this, you should require a longer cool-down period, gradually restoring heart rate and blood pressure to resting levels. It has also been noted that exercise training at lower intensities (i.e., 40 to 50 percent of maximal oxygen consumption) appears to lower blood pressure as much as exercise at higher intensities in people with hypertension (Gordon, 1997). Therefore, for older clients who have hypertension, lower-intensity exercises may be safer and yet achieve the same benefit as higher-intensity exercise in terms of reducing blood pressure.

Stroke

Stroke is a sudden, severe decrease in cerebral circulation caused by either a thrombus (blood clot) or a hemorrhage (leaking or ruptured blood vessel) that results in a cerebral infarct (interrupted blood flow in a cerebral artery). It is the third leading cause of death and disability in the United States (Kohl & McKenzie, 1994). Strokes are classified as *hemorrhagic* or *ischemic* (reduced blood flow to brain). Hemorrhagic strokes constitute approximately 10 percent of all strokes, while ischemic strokes make up the vast remainder (Stewart, 1999). Most people who have had a stroke experience a significant improvement during the first six months after the stroke, while others take up to a year or longer to experience significant improvement (Lockette & Keys, 1994). The goal of exercise training for those who have had a stroke is to maximize recovery and sustain and improve fitness and mobility throughout life. All types of activities should be used to improve health and function among individuals with stroke, including endurance activities, resistance training, flexibility exercises, and balance and mobility activities.

Aerobic endurance training for stroke survivors requires adequate supervision. Individuals who have survived a stroke often vary widely in age, severity of disability, motivational level, and number and severity of comorbidities, secondary conditions, and other associated conditions. Appropriate cardiovascular exercise may reduce these associated conditions and improve functional capacity. Aerobic exercise training can improve tolerance to activities of daily living and allow more physical activity to occur at a lower submaximal threshold, thus reducing myocardial oxygen demand (Potempa, Braun, Tinknell, & Popovich, 1996).

Examples of cardiovascular training modalities for stroke survivors include stationary cycling (recumbent and upright), over-ground walking or walking on a treadmill (provided that the clients have adequate balance, are closely supervised, and do not exhibit joint pain), and recumbent stepping (especially useful for clients with severe hemiplegia). Stair stepping in a vertical position may elicit higher heart rates and spikes in blood pressure and may therefore be contraindicated for some stroke survivors (Rimmer, Riley, Creviston, & Nicola, 2000). This is a higher-intensity activity because the exerciser must repeatedly lift his or her own body weight. Participants should be given the opportunity to select their own mode of exercise as long as it is considered safe and does not cause excessive increases in blood pressure or in heart rate, musculoskeletal pain, or injury.

Resistance training is also very important for stroke survivors (Rimmer, 2001). A major determinant of training volume is the amount of muscle mass that is still functional. People with **paralysis** (loss of sensory and motor control), **hemiplegia** (paralysis or weakness on the right or left side of the body), impaired motor control, or limited joint mobility have less **functional muscle mass** (muscle groups that contain nerve innervation and can respond to training) and therefore tolerate a lower training volume. For individuals who cannot lift the minimal weight on certain resistance machines, resistance bands or cuff weights are recommended. If bands and cuff weights are too difficult, use the person's own body weight as the initial resistance. For example, lifting an arm or leg against gravity for 5 to 10 seconds may be the initial starting point for clients with very low strength levels. Another alternative for clients with very little strength is exercises that eliminate or minimize the resistance from gravity, such as horizontal movements, aquatic exercises, and isometrics (Rimmer & Nicola, 2002).

Participants who have survived a stroke should be taught a variety of stretching exercises targeting both upper- and lower-body muscle groups. Participants should stretch at the beginning of each exercise session, at the end of the cardiovascular exercise session, between strength exercises, and at the end of the exercise session. Stretches should be held for 15 to 30 seconds. Emphasize stretches for the tight (spastic) muscle groups on the hemiparetic side, which include the finger and wrist flexors, elbow flexors, shoulder adductors, hip flexors, knee flexors, and ankle plantar flexors.

Balance and mobility training is also important for clients who have had a stroke. The hemiparesis that often occurs after a stroke causes sensory loss on that side of the body along with a loss in strength and range of motion. Lack of sensation on one side of the body can result in a higher risk of falls because the person is unaware of where the center of gravity lies relative to the affected side. The loss in strength and flexibility may exacerbate the problem. Therefore, balance and mobility exercises are important for greater stability and function and to reduce the incidence of falls. If you feel uncomfortable prescribing balance and mobility training exercises, consult with a physical therapist for specific recommendations for your client.

Pulmonary Disorders

Pulmonary disorders are increasing in prevalence in the United States (Cooper, 2001a). These conditions manifest themselves as shortness of breath and, in severe cases, as major limitations in physical function and independence. The primary pulmonary disorders include asthma, chronic bronchitis, and emphysema.

Asthma

Asthma is a respiratory condition characterized by reversible (in most cases) airway obstruction, airway inflammation, and increased airway responsiveness to a variety of stimuli (McFadden & Gilbert, 1992). It appears to be a relatively common health condition in older adults (Interiano & Guntupalli,

> The majority of people with exercise-induced asthma have a reduction in breathing capacity during and, more commonly, after exercise.

1996). In the United States approximately 14.6 million people have asthma (Cooper, 2001a). At an advanced age, asthma can be very disabling. The diagnosis of asthma in older adults is often difficult because the condition is often masked by other problems that simulate asthma, such as emphysema or congestive heart failure (Interiano & Guntupalli, 1996). The majority of people with asthma have a reduction in breathing capacity during and, more commonly, after exercise (Rimmer, 1994). This is called **exercise-induced asthma.** In addition to exercise, other conditions that may trigger an asthma attack are cold, stress, and air pollution (Blumenthal, 1990). Exercise is very beneficial for people with asthma, provided that the program is tailored to the individual's needs (Emtner, Herala, & Stalenheim, 1996).

It is important that the exercise program is coordinated with the timing of asthma medication. Based on input from the client's physician, you must know when the medicine has to be taken to avoid an asthma episode during exercise. This depends on the type of medication that is prescribed. Medicines used in inhalers work within a few minutes, while medicines in oral form may take up to 30 minutes before they reach full effect.

Encourage the client to use a **peak flow meter** to monitor the flow of air through the lungs. Figure 21.2 illustrates an instructor measuring a client's peak flow before an exercise session. A peak flow meter is a simple plastic device that is helpful in evaluating if an asthma episode might occur during or after exercise. The person simply blows into the meter and records the score. When peak flow drops more than 20 percent below its normal value, activity should be reduced on that day (Rimmer, 1994). There is little reliable information on predicted peak flow values for older adults (Gregg & Nunn, 1989), and therefore the baseline measurement for each client on a normal day when airflow is good for that person should be used for day-to-day comparisons. Low-intensity warm-ups may be very helpful in reducing the risk of an asthma attack. The client should perform light cardiovascular activity below 50 percent of target heart rate for 5 to 10 minutes.

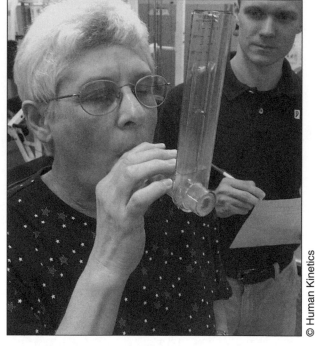

© Human Kinetics

FIGURE 21.2   The peak flow meter can help to determine if an asthma attack is likely to happen during or shortly after exercise.

Some older individuals may experience greater difficulty exercising at a moderate intensity because of the severity of their asthma. The appropriate intensity needs to be determined individually and should take into account the person's health status and difficulty performing aerobic exercise (Cooper, 2001b). Use the RPE scale and peak flow readings along with heart rate to monitor the intensity of the exercise.

People with exercise-induced asthma should *always* carry their inhalers with them. If asthma symptoms occur, a beta-adrenergic agent (used in inhalers) is the only way to reverse the symptoms of a full-blown attack. The physical activity instructor should make sure that a person with asthma has an inhaler at all times. Since cold air is a major trigger of asthma attacks, when exercising outdoors, it may be wise to advise the client to wear a scarf or surgical mask over the nose and mouth to warm the inspired air and reduce heat loss. After a cold or the flu, people with asthma are even more susceptible to breathing problems during exercise. These clients should be monitored closely after an illness and should be encouraged to start back slowly with exercise of reduced duration and intensity.

Chronic Obstructive Pulmonary Disease

Chronic obstructive pulmonary disease (COPD) refers to a group of conditions characterized by airway obstruction. The term *COPD* usually refers to **bronchitis** (inflammation of the bronchial passageways in the lungs) or **emphysema** (destruction of alveoli, where the exchange of oxygen and carbon dioxide occurs) but can also include other respiratory conditions such as asthma and cystic fibrosis (Reid & Samrai, 1995). In this chapter the term *COPD* is used to describe a combination of chronic bronchitis and emphysema. Conditions that characterize COPD include impaired respiratory muscle function due to respiratory muscle weakness, more labored breathing due to pathologic changes in the lungs, and inefficiency of the inspiratory muscles due to hyperinflation. The fatality rate for COPD is more than two times as high in men as in women between the ages of 65 and 74 and three times as high between the ages of 75 and 84. This is probably related to the higher incidence of smoking among men. Symptoms of COPD include **dyspnea** (difficulty breathing), coughing, sputum (mucus) production,

weight loss, and fatigue (Lueckenotte, 1996).

Exercise is considered an essential component of treatment for people with bronchitis and emphysema (Cooper, 2001a). The primary aim of the exercise program is to improve breathing efficiency and exercise tolerance. Exercise intensity should be based on RPE, which seems to be a more reliable indicator than heart rate in this clientele (O'Donnell, Webb, & McGuire, 1993). Individuals who are in the advanced stages of emphysema may require supplemental oxygen during exercise. If you do not feel comfortable working with these clients, you should refer them to a respiratory therapist or physical therapist. The more impaired an older adult with COPD is, the greater the emphasis should be on interval training techniques (see chapter 13 for a discussion of interval training). Some individuals with very low exercise tolerance may find it necessary to exercise for 30 to 60 seconds and then rest for 30 to 60 seconds. As the person's fitness improves, the ratio of work to rest can be altered for a higher intensity.

In addition to improving breathing efficiency and exercise tolerance, the exercise program for older adults with COPD should also address their interests and capabilities with aerobic endurance

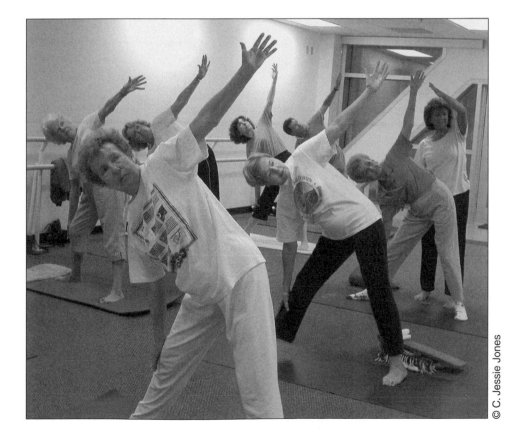

© C. Jessie Jones

Yoga exercises may help some clients with COPD increase the amount of air they can take into their lungs.

activities that vary little in oxygen cost. A relatively constant intensity may help prevent dyspnea, which is the number one problem associated with exercise for those with COPD. Examples of low-variability exercises include walking, recumbent stepping, and stationary cycling. High-variability exercises that should be avoided are calisthenics, dancing, and sports such as basketball and racket sports. Low-intensity weight training is also relatively safe for people with COPD. The client should feel comfortable lifting the weight and should not hyperventilate or become breathless. Avoid large increases in breathing rate by making sure that the weight is not too heavy and that the client is not holding his or her breath.

Although warm-up and cool-down activities are important components of exercise programs for all individuals, they are particularly important for people with COPD. The goal of the warm-up is to gradually increase heart rate so that the lungs can slowly adjust to the increased workload. If strenuous exercise is started too quickly, there is a higher likelihood of respiratory distress. In addition, make sure the cool-down includes exercises of decreasing intensity (e.g., walking or cycling at a progressively slower rate). Refer to figure 21.3 for exercise guidelines when working with a client with COPD.

Teach clients to decrease their breathing frequency and to increase the amount of air they take into their lungs with each breath. Many clients with COPD take shallow breaths and therefore do not get enough oxygen into the pulmonary system,

which ultimately leads to increased breathlessness and fatigue. Yoga is an excellent activity for teaching clients appropriate breathing techniques. Specific breathing exercises are also presented in chapter 15.

Diabetes

Diabetes is a metabolic disorder that results in impaired glucose metabolism. It is a common disorder in older adults. Approximately 50 percent of all people known to have type 2 diabetes are older than 65 years (Rosenstock, 2001). The condition can progressively worsen over time, leading to many other health problems, including loss of vision, heart disease, amputations, stroke, and renal failure (Weir & Singer, 1995). Approximately two thirds of all medical costs related to diabetes are attributable to the elderly (American Diabetes Association, 1998).

The two major forms of diabetes, type 1 and type 2, have similar consequences, but people with type 1 diabetes usually experience an earlier onset. Type 1 diabetes is caused by a destruction of pancreatic cells that produce the body's insulin, whereas type 2 diabetes results from insulin resistance combined with defective insulin secretion.

Eighty to 90 percent of people with type 2 diabetes are also overweight or obese (Rimmer, 1994). Exercise can have a significant effect on lowering blood glucose and is an essential component of treatment for people with type 1 and type 2 diabetes. Exercise is a central component of diabetes treatment and can have a significant positive impact on body weight, glycemic control, and cardiac risk reduction (Hill & Poirier, 1995).

Because glucose is needed to perform exercise, however, people with diabetes can begin to experience difficulties if their baseline blood glucose level is too high (over 250 milligrams per deciliter) or too low (under 100 milligrams per deciliter; Campbell & Colberg, 2000). Most diabetes experts recommend that blood glucose levels be lower than 250 or 300 milligrams per deciliter before exercise is initiated (Albright, 1997). It is important for people with diabetes to maintain the proper balance of food and insulin. High blood glucose values often occur when a person forgets to take his or her insulin or has eaten significantly more calories than usual. As a result, there is not enough insulin available to help

---

1. Modify the program (e.g., use interval training or low-intensity activities) on days when the client has difficulty breathing.

2. Emphasize good diaphragmatic and pursed-lip breathing during various exercise routines and during the warm-up and cool-down sessions.

3. If at all possible, use a pulse oximeter to monitor oxygen saturation.

4. Avoid activities that cause dyspnea or hyperventilation.

5. Emphasize breathing exercises that target increased pulmonary function.

6. Avoid excessively warm or cold environments that may trigger dyspnea.

FIGURE 21.3   Exercise guidelines for clients with COPD.

metabolize the glucose. In clients with poor glycemic control, participation in exercise can worsen **hyperglycemia** (high blood glucose) and increase ketosis, which is a by-product of fat metabolism, resulting from the lack of insulin needed to facilitate the use of glucose. A key precaution for clients who have diabetes is to maintain blood glucose levels in a safe range (100 to 250 milligrams per deciliter). People with diabetes should carry a portable **glucometer** with them. This device is inexpensive and can be used to check blood glucose levels before and after exercise.

Another common problem in people with diabetes is hypoglycemia. **Hypoglycemia** is defined as a blood glucose level less than 60 milligrams per deciliter. Most experts agree that this is an even more dangerous situation than hyperglycemia (high blood glucose) because it can happen very quickly and can lead to an insulin reaction (a medical complication resulting from too much circulating insulin or too little blood glucose). This is often a greater problem in people who have type 1 diabetes (Hill & Poirier, 1995). Signs of hypoglycemia are discussed a little later. Physical activity instructors should always keep rapidly absorbed carbohydrates (e.g., orange juice, fruit drinks, or sport gels) on hand in case of an emergency. Blood glucose should be measured after exercise to make sure that the client does not become hypoglycemic. People with recently diagnosed diabetes may need a few sessions to learn how to maintain a normal balance of glucose and insulin before and after exercise.

The intensity, frequency, and duration of exercise should be based on the client's medical history, taking into consideration other conditions that may affect the exercise prescription. Older adults with type 2 diabetes often have hypertension and joint pain as well, thus challenging the physical activity professional to find activities that are both beneficial and enjoyable but do not require intensities beyond the prescribed training zone.

Since it is difficult to maintain an optimal balance of glucose and insulin, clients with diabetes should exercise daily. This does not necessarily mean that the client has to come to the fitness center on a daily basis. There are many activities that can be performed at home. A client may decide to attend a community-based program three days a week and to walk, garden, or use a stationary cycle the remaining days of the week. The key factor is consistency and regular monitoring of blood glucose levels. Figure 21.4 provides some general guidelines when working with individuals who have diabetes.

Older people with diabetes usually have one or more coexisting conditions, including coronary

1. Regulating blood glucose levels requires optimal timing of exercise periods in relation to meals and insulin dosage.

2. Aim to keep blood glucose levels between 100 and 200 milligrams per deciliter one to two hours after a meal.

3. Exercise can have a significant effect on insulin reduction. Some experts note that insulin may need to be reduced by 10 to 50 percent when starting an exercise program.

4. If blood glucose levels are lower than 100 milligrams per deciliter before exercise, have the person consume a rapidly absorbed carbohydrate to increase blood glucose.

5. If blood glucose is greater than 300 milligrams per deciliter before exercise, make sure that insulin or the oral hypoglycemic agent has been taken. Some doctors recommend that exercise not be initiated when blood glucose is greater than 250 milligrams per deciliter.

6. No client should be allowed to exercise if his or her blood glucose level is not within a safe range before exercise.

7. Teach clients to examine their feet periodically for foot ulcers. If an ulcer is found, have the client consult with a physician immediately for proper treatment. Foot ulcers can worsen and lead to other medical complications if left untreated.

8. Check blood glucose at the end of each exercise session to make sure that the client does not become hypoglycemic. This can happen very quickly, particularly after high-intensity or long-duration activities or if the person does not yet understand how his or her body reacts to exercise.

FIGURE 21.4 Exercise guidelines and safety recommendations for people with diabetes.

artery disease, hyperlipidemia, or hypertension (Rosenstock, 2001). The medications used to treat these conditions can have an adverse effect on blood glucose levels. Thiazide diuretics, used to control hypertension, may induce glucose intolerance by diminishing insulin sensitivity (Rosenstock, 2001).

It is important for older adults participating in exercise programs to maintain good glycemic control. Avoiding hypoglycemia is just as important as avoiding hyperglycemia. The risk for hypoglycemia is a major concern for all individuals with diabetes, but it is a particular concern among the elderly and those beginning new exercise programs. Shorr, Ray, and Daugherty (1997) reported that among adults age 65 and older who used oral hypoglycemic agents or insulin, the incidence of hypoglycemia was 1.23 per 100 person-years. Frail elderly individuals who

used multiple medications were at the greatest risk of drug-associated hypoglycemia. Figure 21.5 lists the major symptoms of hypoglycemia and what to do if a person becomes hypoglycemic.

Musculoskeletal Conditions

Baby boomers are beginning to enter older adulthood, and in a few years the prevalence of arthritis and osteoporosis will rise dramatically. It will be increasingly important therefore that physical activity instructors develop exercise programs that allow individuals with these musculoskeletal conditions to maintain an active lifestyle.

Osteoporosis

One out of every four women over the age of 60 suffers from osteoporosis, and half of all women who have had a hysterectomy will develop the condition (Sato, Grese, Dodge, Bryant, & Turner, 1999). According to the World Health Organization (WHO), the criterion for a diagnosis of osteoporosis is a spinal bone mineral density (BMD) more than 2.5 standard deviations below the mean for young, normal adults of the same sex (Kanis, Melton, Christiansen, Jonston, & Khalaev, 1994).

In the early stages of osteoporosis, there are often no symptoms. However, as a person reaches his or her 60s and 70s, signs of osteoporosis may develop. As the bones in the spine lose their mineral content, **kyphosis** often occurs, a vertebral disorder in the thoracic region of the spine that causes hunching of the spine. This is often accompanied by pain and psychological distress.

It is not entirely clear how much exercise can improve bone density in postmenopausal women and older individuals. Sato and colleagues (1999) reported that although exercise has been shown to improve bone mass during the growth years, only modest increases in bone mass can occur in adulthood. The authors note, however, that exercise has other significant benefits, including improved balance and stability thus decreased risk of falling. Postmenopausal women and older adults need to increase their physical activity levels to at least slow or delay the onset of osteoporosis and possibly make modest improvements in bone mass.

Weight-bearing activities seem to have the most benefit in terms of preventing or slowing osteoporosis. It is wise for physical activity instructors to obtain prior approval from the client's physician for

Early symptoms
- Anxiety, uneasiness
- Irritability
- Extreme hunger
- Confusion
- Headaches

Treatment
1. Stop the activity immediately.
2. Have the client sit down and check blood glucose level.
3. Have the client drink orange juice or ingest some other rapidly absorbed carbohydrate.
4. Allow the client to rest, and wait for a response.
5. When the client feels better, check blood glucose level again.
6. If the blood glucose level is above 100 milligrams per deciliter and the client feels better, resume activity. If not, either wait another 5 to 10 minutes and recheck or provide additional food.
7. Check blood glucose level after 15 to 30 minutes to ensure that it is still within a safe range.
8. Check blood glucose at the end of the exercise session to make sure that it is greater than 100 milligrams per deciliter before the client leaves the facility.

FIGURE 21.5 Early symptoms and treatment of hypoglycemia.

a specific resistance exercise program that will be safe and effective for clients diagnosed with osteoporosis. For safety, it is always best to progress slowly using light weights during the first month of the program. Have clients perform one to three sets of 8 to 12 repetitions, depending on their comfort level. Clients with significant osteoporosis (as indicated by their physician) should use resistance bands during the early stages of the program. Some weight machines start at too high a resistance and are difficult to get into and out of for some older frail clients. After two to three months, progress to heavier resistance bands or light weights. Individuals with advanced osteoporosis require more time to adapt to a resistance-training program and must progress at a much slower rate to avoid injury than healthy older adults.

Resistance exercises should be performed two to three days a week. If the client has pain, avoid exercises near or over the spine such as back extension and flexion exercises, bent-over rowing, overhead presses, or weight-training machines that require extensive spinal flexion (e.g., abdominal machines) or extension (e.g., back extension machines). If the client does not have pain, target the muscles in the back with shoulder retraction exercises and shoulder raises. Make sure that the client performs the movements slowly and that they do not cause pain. These exercises also improve posture (many older adults become round-shouldered as they age) and load the vertebrae, potentially maintaining or hypothetically increasing bone density.

Older people with osteoporosis may have difficulty performing repetitive exercises using the same muscle groups for extended periods of time. Therefore, circuit-training programs that require short periods of work using various muscle groups are recommended. In addition to circuit training, interval training activities that require brief periods of work followed by a rest interval may also be beneficial for deconditioned clientele with advanced osteoporosis. For example, riding a stationary bike for one minute followed by a 30-second rest interval may delay fatigue and allow the client to sustain longer periods of activity.

Other cardiovascular activities can be used to improve functional performance, provided they do not incur pain or result in premature fatigue. Although swimming and aquatic exercises are excellent modalities for improving cardiovascular endurance, they are not recommended for maintaining or improving bone density. Water is a non-weight-bearing environment and does not seem to place a sufficient stress load on bone tissue to increase its mass (Bravo, Gauthier, Roy, Payette, & Gaulin, 1997).

Flexibility exercises are safe for people with osteoporosis, unless they are experiencing pain in a region of the body that is prone to fracture (e.g., hip, spine, wrist). Avoid flexibility exercises that cause pain in any of these areas. Although flexibility exercises do not cause increments in bone mass, they are very important for improving posture, relieving muscle tightness, and maintaining good mobility. People with osteoporosis often become very inflexible in the chest and neck muscles as a result of stooped posture. Avoid exercises such as the bench press that promote forward head and shoulder position and shorten chest musculature, and instead use exercises that open the chest by retracting the scapula (e.g., pectoral stretch performed on a gym ball). Modifying the grip and exercise technique of certain exercises can also facilitate better posture and alignment (e.g., have the client adopt a supinated hand position and avoid front pull-down movements except for lat pull-downs on a machine). The hip flexors should also be stretched, since these muscles become tight in older adults from sitting for long periods and walking with a stooped posture. Figure 21.6 provides some general guidelines for working with older adults with osteoporosis.

1. Know the visible signs of osteoporosis (e.g., kyphosis, recent fracture), and develop an appropriate strength and flexibility regimen for affected areas with physician input.

2. Physician input and approval are important when developing a new exercise program for a client in the advanced stages of osteoporosis.

3. Avoid jarring and high-load exercises for clients with osteoporosis.

4. When older clients who have a high risk of falls or fractures perform standing exercises, make sure they have something to hold on to at all times (e.g., ballet barre, parallel bars, chair).

5. Reevaluate the program if the client experiences any pain or fatigue during or after an exercise session in the osteoporosis zones (hips, back, or wrists).

FIGURE 21.6 Exercise guidelines for people with osteoporosis.

Arthritis

The two major types of arthritis are osteoarthritis and rheumatoid arthritis. **Osteoarthritis,** previously referred to as degenerative joint disease, is the most prevalent form of arthritis in the United States (Hochberg et al., 1995). It results in a thinning of the articular cartilage on the outside of bones in diarthrodial joints. Symptoms of osteoarthritis include pain, morning stiffness, and decreased range of motion in the affected joints. **Rheumatoid arthritis** is more common in women than men. It may begin early or later in life. Symptoms include chronic inflammation in the affected joints, pain, morning stiffness (lasting longer than osteoarthritis), and swelling in the affected joints (Marino & McDonald, 1991). Osteoarthritis is a "wear and tear" disorder, while rheumatoid arthritis is a whole-body autoimmune disease, in which the body's own immune system attacks healthy tissue. Both disease types have joint-destroying properties and similar treatment strategies, including exercise (Hurley & Roth, 2000). Most people with arthritis can benefit from an exercise program in a number of ways, including reduced pain and fatigue, improved fitness, and increased ability to perform various physical tasks independently (Ettinger et al., 1997; O'Grady, Fletcher, & Ortiz, 2000; Van Den Ende, Vlieland, Munneke, & Hazes, 1998).

A major emphasis of the exercise program for people with arthritis is to mitigate pain during activity. The program must not place excessive loads around damaged joints. For people who have been sedentary for a long while, starting slowly is very important. Low-impact, non-weight-bearing activities are recommended. The client may have to learn to tolerate some pain or discomfort. However, pain should be minimized in every way possible, including the use of braces or straps, ice or heat before and after exercise, isolating the damaged joint during exercise, water-based exercises, and avoiding overuse of the damaged joint. You should consult with a physical therapist to learn more about pain management during physical activity.

Exercise machines that allow the use of all four limbs simultaneously seem to have the most benefit for people with arthritis, since the load is evenly distributed through all the limbs. Examples of machines that involve all four limbs include the NuStep recumbent stepper, which is used in a seated position; the Schwinn AirDyne stationary bike, which is also used while sitting; and the elliptical cross-trainer machine, which is used while standing. General exercise guidelines for people with arthritis are listed in figure 21.7.

1. Discontinue any exercise that causes pain during exercise, shortly after exercise (i.e., two hours), or 24 to 48 hours after an exercise session.

2. Find alternative ways to exercise muscles around painful joints. For example, straight-leg exercises are a good way to strengthen the leg muscles around a painful knee.

3. Warm-up and cool-down sessions are essential aspects of all exercise programs but are especially important for people with arthritis because of their joint stiffness.

4. Resistance training should be done, but exercises that cause pain to a particular joint should be replaced with isometric strength exercises.

5. For aquatic exercise, try to maintain water temperature between 85 and 90 degrees Fahrenheit (29-32 degrees Celsius).

6. Use smooth, repetitive motions in all activities.

7. Keep the exercise intensity below the discomfort threshold.

8. Be aware that people with rheumatoid arthritis can experience acute flare-ups. Exercise may not be advisable until the flare-up subsides.

9. Clients with osteoarthritis often perform better in the morning, whereas clients with rheumatoid arthritis may be better off exercising several hours after awakening.

10. Use cross-training to avoid overuse of certain joints.

FIGURE 21.7   Exercise guidelines for people with arthritis.

Hip and Knee Replacements

Many older adults have a hip or knee replacement after living with arthritis for several decades. Joint replacement is one option when the chronic pain cannot be controlled through medication, assistive aids, or exercise and when the pain and decreased range of motion in the affected joint interfere with the person's ability to ambulate (Lueckenotte, 1996). After the client completes physical therapy,

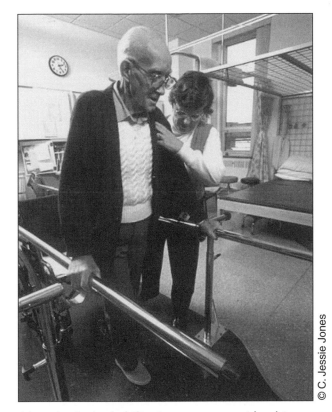

After physical rehabilitation, a person with a hip or knee replacement needs to further improve strength and range of motion when they return home.

exercises to improve strength and range of motion are important.

The exercise protocol can follow a plan similar to that described for arthritis. The only difference is that more attention should be devoted to strength and range-of-motion exercises for strengthening and stretching the muscles supporting the affected joints, in accordance with the physical therapy plan prescribed for the individual. It is important that you maintain an active dialogue with the client's physical therapist or physician to ensure that the treatment plan is progressing smoothly.

Neurological and Cognitive Conditions

Two of the most common neurological conditions in older adults are Parkinson's and Alzheimer's diseases. Both of these conditions are progressive and often result in declining physical and cognitive function. The course and rate of progression of these disorders vary by individual.

Parkinson's Disease

Parkinson's disease is a progressive neurological disorder that affects approximately one million individuals in the United States, with approximately 50,000 new cases reported each year (*Merck Manual of Geriatrics*, 1995). Individuals with Parkinson's disease often experience the following symptoms: **bradykinesia** (slowness of movement), muscle rigidity, resting tremor, postural instability, and impaired balance control (Stanley & Protas, 2002).

One of the hallmark signs of Parkinson's disease is an abnormal gait pattern of increasingly short but quicker steps. This is sometimes referred to as *festinating gait* (Stacy & Jankovic, 1992). The gait pattern makes it appear as if the person is trying to catch up with someone in front of him or her, but he or she does so by leaning forward at the waist first before taking any steps. Once movement does occur, short, shuffling steps are taken. This condition is associated with dysequilibrium, which is the inability to readjust the center of gravity quickly enough to prevent a fall. As a result, many individuals with Parkinson's disease are susceptible to falling, and it is important to protect the individual from falls during class (Schenkman et al., 1998).

Ways to prevent falls include having the client perform exercises while seated in a chair, having the client hold on to a ballet barre or wall rail during standing activities, and supervising the client closely during exercises that require him or her to move around the facility or transfer between different exercise machines. Activities for clients with Parkinson's disease should include slow, controlled movements through various ranges of motion while lying, sitting, standing, and walking. Caution must be taken with aerobic exercise on a treadmill. If a treadmill is prescribed for aerobic exercise, the client should be supervised at all times or wear a harness to avoid falling. Aerobic activities performed in a sitting position, such as stationary cycling, recumbent stepping, or arm cycling, are usually safer modalities for this clientele.

Alzheimer's Disease

Alzheimer's disease (AD) is a progressive neurological disorder resulting in impaired mental function. It affects approximately four million Americans in the United States (*Merck Manual of Geriatrics*, 1995) and increases in prevalence as individuals get progressively older. It is the most common cause of dementia among older adults (Rimmer, 1997). Individuals with AD often experience severe declines in cognition and may also experience moderate to severe balance impairments. AD is marked by progressive, irreversible declines in memory, performance of routine tasks, temporal and spatial orientation, language and communication skills, and abstract thinking and by personality changes and impairment of judgment.

Implementing an exercise training program for individuals with AD poses three major challenges: (1) addressing problems arising from the declining physical and mental health of the participant, (2) accommodating behavioral changes that may cause the client to become agitated with the exercise program or in the exercise setting, and (3) dealing with a caregiver's unwillingness to continue bringing the client to the exercise program as the disease progresses.

The cornerstone of an exercise program for this population is consistency and patience. The physical activity professional must constantly provide verbal encouragement and support to maintain the client's interest in the program. Many people with Alzheimer's disease are uncomfortable participating in new activities; therefore, it is important for the exercise leader to use behavioral modification techniques to increase compliance. (See chapter 8 for a discussion of behavioral management techniques.) It may also be necessary to have the client's spouse or caregiver attend the program to present a familiar face.

Summary

When designing exercise programs for older adults with disabilities, the same general guidelines for programs for older adults without disabilities apply. However, in addition to these, disability-specific exercise guidelines and precautions must be followed to ensure a safe and effective program. It is important to understand the general underlying mechanisms associated with each disabling condition and to consult with rehabilitation professionals, such as physical and occupational therapists, about concerns regarding specific disabling conditions. Moreover, do not hesitate to contact the client's physician if you have questions about a client's condition.

Perhaps your single most important task when working with clients with physical or cognitive disabilities is to thoroughly familiarize yourself with their specific functional abilities and limitations and understand how their health condition may limit their ability to perform certain exercises. Many older clients have multiple disabilities that often interact with each other (e.g., depression, osteoporosis, heart disease), and each of these conditions and their interaction must be taken into consideration when developing an exercise prescription.

Key Terms

Recommended Readings

American College of Sports Medicine. (2002). *ACSM's resources for clinical exercise physiology: Musculoskeletal, neuromuscular, neoplastic, immunologic, and hematologic conditions.* Philadelphia: Lippincott Williams & Wilkins.

American College of Sports Medicine. (2003). *ACSM's exercise management for persons with chronic diseases and disabilities.* Champaign, IL: Human Kinetics.

National Center on Physical Activity and Disability. http://www.NCPAD.org.

Study Questions

1. The third leading cause of death and disability in the United States is
   a. heart disease
   b. stroke
   c. multiple sclerosis
   d. cancer

2. A primary symptom characteristic of Parkinson's disease is
   a. postural hypotension
   b. bradykinesia
   c. irregular breathing
   d. impaired vision

3. Hypoglycemia occurs when blood glucose falls below
   a. 60 milligrams per deciliter
   b. 80 milligrams per deciliter
   c. 100 milligrams per deciliter
   d. 120 milligrams per deciliter

4. A longer warm-up phase is recommended for clients who have
   a. Alzheimer's disease
   b. osteoporosis
   c. coronary heart disease
   d. Parkinson's disease

5. When peak flow drops more than _____ below its normal value on any given day, activity should be reduced in intensity and duration.
   a. 10 percent
   b. 20 percent
   c. 35 percent
   d. 50 percent

6. According to the World Health Organization, the criterion for a diagnosis of osteoporosis is a spinal bone mineral density of more than ___ standard deviations below the mean for young, normal adults of the same sex.
   a. 1.5
   b. 2.5
   c. 3.5
   d. 4

7. Clients who are taking _____ often avoid ingesting fluids during exercise because of the increased need to void their bladders.
   a. beta-blockers
   b. calcium channel blockers
   c. benzodiazepine
   d. diuretics

Application Activities

1. Diabetes is very prevalent among older adults. Prepare a five-minute presentation about the benefits of exercise for people with diabetes to deliver in the community to recruit more participants into your program.

2. Clients with arthritis often have pain during movement. List specific activities or treatments you should use to mitigate pain and help the client have a more successful exercise experience.

22

Legal Standards, Risk Management, and Professional Ethics

Joan Virginia Allen

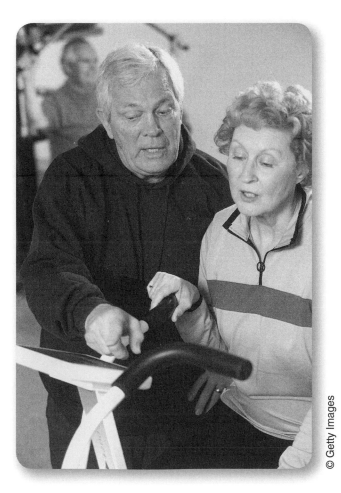

In the 1980s, a lady named Ann sued a fitness club and one of its instructors for injuries suffered as a result of a training session. Ann was a private secretary and engaged in minimal physical activity. She joined the club because it advertised special expertise with adults over the age of 40 years and new to exercise. The first day, her instructor had her complete a series of strength-training exercises on various pieces of equipment. While working on one of the machines, she felt a pain in her neck and upper back. She told the instructor, who replied, "No pain, no gain," and had her continue exercising. When Ann got home, she was in great pain, to the point that she was unable to go to work the next day. Her doctor's examination revealed that she had suffered a significant injury to her neck and upper back, which he attributed to the incident at the club the day before. Ann was required to wear a cervical collar and was told to stay home from work for at least 10 days. Does Ann have grounds for a lawsuit against the fitness club and instructor?

The purpose of this chapter is to provide physical activity instructors of older adults with the necessary knowledge to minimize the risk of injuries to their clients and to help them avoid being part of a scenario like the one just described, thereby minimizing the risk of becoming involved in a lawsuit. The first section of this chapter defines a number of important legal terms associated with a lawsuit and the important elements of a negligence case. Other topics covered in this chapter include the components of a risk management plan (facility standards and guidelines, injury and medical emergency prevention, responding to emergency situations) and professional ethics for personal trainers and group instructors.

The Law and the Physical Activity Instructor

In a lawsuit, the injured party bringing the action is the **plaintiff,** and the party accused of having caused the injury is the **defendant.** In the event of an injury resulting from fitness training, the most common case is brought by the client against the physical activity instructor, the fitness facility, or both for **negligence.** If a piece of equipment is involved, the client may also bring a case against the product manufacturer for products liability, alleging (claiming) that injury was caused by a defect in the manufacture or design of the equipment or a failure to warn of risks, which makes the equipment unreasonably dangerous. **Defenses** (legal reasons for limiting a defendant's liability) that may be viable include **assumption of risk** (the client knowingly and voluntarily assumed the risk inherent to the activity) and **comparative negligence** (the client's actions were part of the cause of the damages so that liability is distributed in proper shares to the parties to the action).

To win a negligence case, the plaintiff must prove four elements: The defendant owed a **duty** to the plaintiff to use reasonable care to avoid risk of injury, that duty was **breached,** the breach caused the injury **(causation),** and the breach resulted in legally recognized **damages** to the plaintiff. In

Ann's case, the fitness facility and the instructor both owed Ann a duty to use reasonable care to avoid risk of injury. That duty was breached when they failed to meet the standard of care. The specific breaches of each defendant are discussed later in this chapter when we revisit Ann's case.

Standard of Care

As a physical activity instructor, your duty to use reasonable care is based on a legal **standard of care.** That standard is based on a reasonably prudent physical activity instructor, which means you must have the knowledge, training, skill, and education (ability and competence) of an ordinary member of your profession in good standing. That is, you must know what is expected of a physical activity instructor of older adults in good standing. It would not be appropriate, for example, to advise clients on such topics as family problems, nutrition, or medications unless you have additional credentials (licensed counselor, dietitian, physician, etc.).

A number of nationally published guidelines and standards are available and should be carefully reviewed by physical activity instructors (see the recommended readings at the end of the chapter). It is important to understand the difference between guidelines and standards. **Guidelines** are usually recommendations or suggestions, while **standards** are required procedures that may indicate a legal duty. In a lawsuit, nationally published standards may be introduced as evidence to establish the standard of care to which you or a fitness facility may be held.

Examples of a breach of your standard of care might include the following (American College of Sports Medicine, 1997):

- Designing a program that contains inappropriate exercises or an unsatisfactory progression of exercises
- Inappropriate equipment
- Inadequate instruction or supervision
- Failure to screen a client before he or she begins an exercise program
- Training a client without the required expertise

Examples of a breach of a health or fitness facility's standard of care include these:

- Inadequate maintenance of equipment by the facility

> The *standard of care* to which you are held is that of a reasonably prudent physical activity instructor, which means that you must have the knowledge, training, skill, and education (ability and competence) of an ordinary member of your profession in good standing.

- Inadequate precautions taken by the employees of the facility to ensure client safety, such as unsafe equipment layout, traffic patterns, and security
- Lack of a risk management plan
- Inadequate staff training
- Employment of unqualified staff
- False or misleading advertising
- Not having an emergency plan in place

If the plaintiff fails to prove that the breach of duty caused legally recognized damages, one of the essential elements of negligence is missing and the case will not be successful.

Minimizing Risk of Exposure to Legal Problems

To minimize your risk of exposure to legal problems, you must work within your personal bounds of competence. In other words, you must offer or perform services that fall within the scope of your expertise. Therefore, your education, training, experience, and skill determine the standard of care to which you are held. You are responsible for knowing and adhering to the guidelines and standards established for your profession. Remember, the key in a negligence case is whether you acted *reasonably* to protect your client from risk of injury under the circumstances, based on your expertise. If you fail to follow procedures that you are reasonably expected to know and follow as a physical activity instructor, you are exposing yourself to the possibility of legal problems.

The following sections offer several suggestions to help physical activity instructors and personal trainers avoid litigation if a client sustains an injury or dies. These suggestions are based on published standards and guidelines from the American College of Sports Medicine (Tharrett & Peterson, 1997) and the National Strength and Conditioning Association (NSCA Professional Standards & Guidelines Task Force, 2001), and my experience as an attorney and a physical activity instructor. Several of these suggestions also help you provide a safe and effective environment for your clients. A more detailed discussion of injury and medical emergency prevention is discussed later in the chapter.

Facility and Equipment

Here are two suggestions to provide safe equipment for your facility:

- Be sure that equipment is properly set up and regularly inspected and maintained and that safety signage is clearly visible where appropriate.

- Either develop a written risk management plan or make sure one is available and posted in the facility. This topic is discussed in more detail later in the chapter.

Instructor

Listed below are several ways to reduce your risk of liability as an instructor of physical activity with older adults:

- Be sure you are adequately and properly educated, certified, and experienced to train within the sphere of expertise in which you are practicing. If you do not know something, admit it, and refer to someone who does know or do the research.

- Obtain and keep current your training and certification in cardiopulmonary resuscitation (CPR) and first aid.

- Continue your education. Stay current with what is going on in your profession, and keep your certifications current.

- Have a written emergency response plan readily available, and practice responding to different types of emergency situations.

- Keep a written training record of each session and a permanent client file for each client. The file should contain the client's health history, a consent form, a copy of the client's training record, documentation of any changes in medical conditions or medications, and written notes of any conversations with the client or his or her physician. Any other client information should be included and treated as confidential unless you have written permission to share the information. This information may later be used as evidence in a lawsuit. It is important never to disclose a client's personal information without written

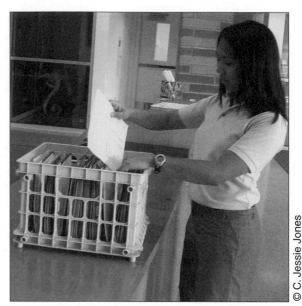

This instructor has lowered her risk for liability because she keeps permanent records on each client.

permission, and keep client files confidential at all times and filed in a locked cabinet.

- Instruct your clients in the proper use of equipment or techniques for any exercise, warn them of inherent risks, and provide continuous supervision.

- Be aware of potential conflicts of interest. As a physical activity instructor, you are building a relationship of trust with your clients. Your recommendations regarding supplements, diet, and weight loss or gain may be seriously considered by your client. Using your position of trust to market or sell products or other services (insurance, financial planning, etc.) may be contrary to your responsibility to watch out for the best interests of your clients. If you engage in another activity resulting in financial gain to you or your employer, disclose the potential conflict in writing and have the client sign that they have been so notified.

- Avoid any appearance of sexual harassment. When teaching a new exercise, either demonstrate it, or ask permission first before touching the client. Also avoid saying anything that can be construed as inappropriate (such as jokes or innuendos). Do not assume because your client is the same sex as you that a risqué comment or joke is OK.

- Do not tolerate sexual harassment by a client. Never assume that age precludes sexual harassment. Reaching a certain chronological age does not necessarily mean that a person has lost interest in sex or an understanding of sexual overtones. You, as the instructor, must establish what is acceptable behavior for both you and your clients. If a client is acting or dressing inappropriately, first try talking with the client. If that fails, be prepared to withdraw as the instructor. If this occurs in a group situation in a facility and talking to the client does not help, discuss the matter with your supervisor before proceeding. You may also want to discuss it with your attorney. It may be necessary to ask the client, in private, to drop the class. A follow-up letter may also be needed. If so, keep a copy in the client file, along with a written record of the dates, circumstances, and any witnesses to the sexual harassment.

• Carry malpractice insurance. Some organizations offer professional trainer liability policies. Ask your certifying agency for a recommendation. Carefully read the policy to understand what is covered and what is excluded. A policy may provide an *aggregate* coverage of $1.5 million, with *each occurrence* covered up to $500,000. Discuss these limits with your insurance agent so that you understand them.

• Consult with an attorney. If you have questions about potential liability related to training older adults, consult with an attorney before a problem occurs. An ounce of prevention is definitely worth a pound of cure.

• Never photograph or videotape a client without first providing full disclosure of how the client's likeness will be used and obtaining his or her written consent.

Participant

As discussed in chapter 5, it is important that you interview your clients individually and have them complete a health history and consent form before the start of the program. Have the clients read, sign, and date the consent form, and make it part of their permanent base file. The health history should disclose any physical limitations, problems, illnesses, diseases, and medications. This information forms the basis of your program design. The consent form should include an agreement that the client will immediately let you know if he or she is feeling any pain or discomfort, and a warning about the potential risks inherent in an exercise program. If you need to talk to the client's physician, be sure to obtain written authorization from the client.

Negligence Case Example

Let us now return to the case study presented in the beginning of the chapter involving Ann and her

lawsuit for negligence against the instructor and the fitness facility. Ann's case alleged negligence on the part of the fitness club for failing to meet the standard of care of a reasonably prudent fitness facility. This was evidenced by the following:

- Hiring unqualified staff
- Inadequate staff instruction on equipment and in working with special populations
- Not having a risk management plan
- Not having requirements for continuing education of staff
- False and misleading advertising

In this case, the instructor had no credentials to work as a fitness trainer. When hired, she claimed that she had previously taught group aerobics at a community college. Knowing that, the club gave her only superficial instruction on the weight-lifting equipment, provided no training on how to deal with special populations (i.e., sedentary adults over 40 years of age), failed to have a plan in place or to provide instruction on how to respond to complaints of pain from a client, and had falsely advertised special expertise with adults over 40 and new to exercise.

The **allegations** (assertions or claims of a party to a lawsuit) against the fitness instructor evidencing her failure to meet the standard of care included the following:

- Not requiring the client to complete a health history questionnaire, waiver, and assumption of risk form before starting the training program
- Not being properly trained to work with this client
- Not being current in her education yet representing herself as a fully qualified strength and conditioning instructor
- Not recommending appropriate exercises for the age and physical condition of the client
- Not choosing appropriate exercise equipment

Before the case went to trial, it was settled. This was in the 1980s. The standard of care was not as clear as it is today because there were fewer published standards and guidelines, certifying agencies, and educational opportunities for professionals interested in working with adults in physical activity settings. Now there is virtually no excuse for a case like Ann's to happen. If you ignore the standards and

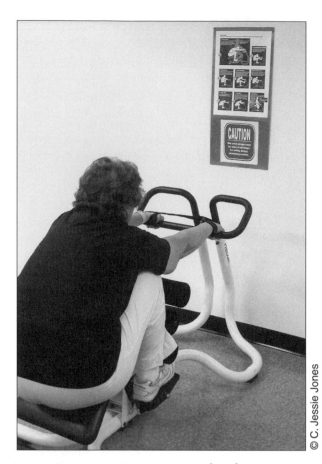

Instructions on equipment use are key for injury prevention.

guidelines that have been established for health and fitness facilities, forgo the education necessary, or work outside your personal bounds of competence, you may find yourself involved in legal action.

A Risk Management Plan

No matter how well trained you are as a physical activity instructor of older adults, an injury or health-related emergency is bound to happen if you teach long enough, especially when your clients are frail older adults. Unfortunately, many fitness and wellness facilities do not have a comprehensive risk management plan. Such a plan can help you to promote a safer exercise environment for your clients, more effectively respond to emergency situations, and minimize your risk for legal ramifications. If the facility where you work does not have a risk management plan, you should recommend that the facility purchase the *ACSM's Health/Fitness Facility Standards and Guidelines* (Tharrett & Peterson, 1997). This section of the chapter pro-

vides some resources to help you develop your own risk management plan, including some basic injury and medical emergency prevention and response procedures.

Health and Fitness Facility Standards and Guidelines

The *ACSM's Health/Fitness Facility Standards and Guidelines* (Tharrett & Peterson, 1997) contains six standards that represent the standard of care that must be followed by all health and fitness facilities; it also contains more than 500 guidelines. It is important to meet five of the six standards that apply specifically to providing a safe exercise environment for your older adult clients; courts allow these standards to be introduced as evidence of the standard of care (i.e., legal duties) in negligence cases (Eickhoff-Shemek, 2001). Facilities offering physical activity classes for older adults can develop a comprehensive risk management plan by referring to this publication.

The five ACSM standards that apply to working with older adults are as follows:

1. Be able to respond in a timely manner to any emergency event, and post a written emergency response plan that is known to all personnel and that includes periodic emergency response drills for all staff. More on this topic is given later in the chapter.

2. Offer preactivity screening to each participant to ensure safe programs. Chapter 5 provides detailed information on this topic.

3. Require instructors to demonstrate professional competence, including current CPR and first aid certification.

4. Post instructions on how to use equipment, and post warnings of any relevant risks.

5. Follow all relevant laws, regulations, and published standards.

Facilities can also minimize equipment-related injuries and subsequent liability by installing equipment in accordance with the manufacturers' or sellers' instructions, inspecting equipment prior to installation, providing initial and ongoing user instruction and supervision, establishing a regular schedule for the inspection and maintenance of equipment, and having a set of procedures in place for the prompt removal of defective and potentially dangerous equipment (Eickhoff-Shemek & Deja, 2002).

If you ignore standards that have been established for health and fitness facilities, forgo necessary education, or work outside your personal bounds of competence, you may find yourself involved in legal action.

Injury and Medical Emergency Prevention

A comprehensive risk management plan should also address injury and medical emergency procedures. Chapter 21 discussed safety precautions and strategies for adapting exercises for older adults with chronic medical problems. The following additional 10 strategies are provided to help you design a safe and effective exercise environment that minimizes clients' risk of injury or medical emergency:

• Conduct a preactivity screening of all participants. Preactivity screenings help determine which clients (1) would be well served by your class, (2) would be better in a different exercise setting, or (3) should be referred to their physicians for additional testing and clearance for exercise.

• If you accept moderate- to high-risk cardiac clients in your exercise program, blood pressure and heart rate should be recorded before exercise and, if necessary, several times during the exercise session. It is also recommended that participants with heart conditions wear heart rate monitors that signal when the exercise intensity exceeds the target heart rate range.

• People with diabetes should bring their own portable glucometers to the fitness center and measure blood glucose before and after each exercise session. Orange juice and other high-carbohydrate snacks should be available for those participants who become hypoglycemic (glucose level below 60 milligrams per deciliter).

• An infectious waste container for blood specimens should be available for clients who must check their blood glucose levels. Blood specimens should be obtained in a clean setting, away from equipment and high-volume traffic areas. Floors where blood specimens are taken should be washed daily with bleach and water.

• Make every effort to avoid causing your clients prolonged or unusual fatigue or delayed-onset muscle soreness. Although this is a common side effect of participation in any new exercise program, soreness and fatigue can prevent older adults from completing their normal activities of daily living.

• Be observant of warning signs of heart distress (e.g., chest pain, irregular pulse, difficulty breathing, and dizziness). If any of these symptoms occur, exercise should be stopped immediately and the client's doctor notified.

• To protect clients from heat-related medical problems, a thermostat should be installed, if not already available, to monitor room temperature.

• Class participants should wear properly fitted athletic shoes with sturdy arch support and soles that provide ample cushioning (although thickly cushioned shoes are contraindicated for older adults with balance problems and sensation loss in the feet). For outdoor exercise, clients should be encouraged to wear protective sunscreen, sunglasses, and hats or visors.

• Encourage participants to wear multiple layers of lightweight clothing that can be removed as body temperature rises during exercise and then replaced as the body cools.

• Participants should be taught how to rate their own perceived exertion, use equipment safely, and understand the warning signs for when to stop exercising. These warning signs, listed in the consent form in chapter 5, should be reviewed with all participants, but especially those who have a diagnosis of coronary heart disease. Once the participant understands these warning signs and can repeat them back to the instructor, both parties should sign the form. This ensures that the client has a basic understanding of how to watch for these warning signs.

Creating a Safe Environment

Physical activity instructors who teach groups of older adults are especially challenged to provide safe environments when their participants have a variety of medical problems. It can be even more difficult to provide a safe and effective exercise environment for clients who are visually or hearing impaired. Clients with visual impairments must exercise in a safe environment that protects them from falls and related injuries.

Following are safety guidelines for establishing a safe instructional environment for older adults with visual and hearing problems:

• Two major obstacles for sight-challenged participants are glare and dim lighting (Martini & Botenhagen, 2003). With proper lighting, mirrored walls may help participants see the instructor's movement demonstrations. In large classes, teaching from a raised platform can help participants more easily follow the workout.

• Participants with visual or hearing impairments should never be in the back row. Positioning participants with visual problems toward the front of the class maximizes their view of the instructor's movements. Also, review clients' health histories to determine the exact nature of their visual impairments for a better understanding of what they can and cannot see.

• People who are visually impaired often do not see objects in their path and can easily trip over equipment that is not stored properly. Make sure that all equipment is stored after use and that no obstacles are left along travel routes.

• Use specific directional signs around the facility, and mark the routes to different areas with bright colors to make them easier to follow.

• Speak slowly and clearly, and try to make verbal instructions easy to understand.

• Any written materials that you distribute should be typed in large print for individuals who have difficulty reading standard-size print or recorded on audiotape for individuals who are blind.

Hearing impairments are common among older adults. It is imperative that all clients understand the proper way to exercise, signs and symptoms of overexertion, and any other instructions necessary for a safe and effective environment. Here is a list of things you can do to provide a safer environment for older adults with hearing problems:

• Use visual cues when giving instructions (e.g., pictures of the exercises, demonstrations).

• Project your voice, but without a simultaneous rise in pitch.

• Make sure that you face the client so that he or she has a clear view of your face. Some clients with limited hearing may be able to read lips or interpret facial expressions and thus be able to understand your spoken directions.

• Find out if the person has better hearing in one ear and speak to the client on the side with better hearing. Background noises can be very distracting. If a person is having difficulty understanding something you are trying to explain, it may be a good idea to move to a quiet area where there is no background noise.

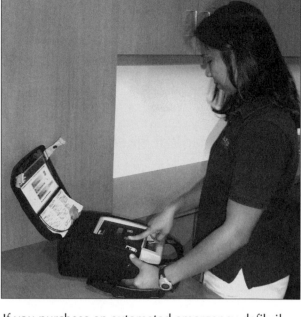

If you purchase an automated emergency defibrillator, it is important to periodically check the batteries to make sure it is ready for use in case of an emergency.

• Speak slowly and clearly; enunciate your words, but do not overexaggerate them. Speaking too fast or slurring words can also make it difficult for an older person with hearing loss to understand you. It may be necessary to repeat instructions. Do not shout at the client. Shouting distorts the sound and makes it even more difficult to understand instructions.

• For participants who use hearing aids, excessive volume is the main ingredient in an unpleasant cacophony of competing sounds. In fact, loud music hinders most participants' ability to follow verbal instructions. To determine the optimal music volume, ask for participants' feedback while simultaneously observing their performance. Some participants may prefer instrumental tunes because the instructor's voice does not have to compete with music lyrics.

Responding to an Emergency Situation

An essential part of a risk management plan is having policies and response procedures for handling emergencies. In your capacity as a physical activity instructor, the standard of care as a reasonably prudent instructor may include the following:

- Current certification in CPR
- Knowing how to administer basic first aid
- Obtaining a complete health history from your client so that you know what health problems he or she has
- Consulting with the client's physician if you have questions about the safety of a program you have designed
- Knowing the signs and symptoms of a particular health problem
- Knowing the response needed for a particular problem (e.g., if your client is diabetic, what to do if he or she feels faint)
- Knowing the location of the nearest telephone for contacting emergency personnel

Following are some policies and procedures to respond to an emergency situation.

- Having a written emergency plan is essential. Figure 22.1 provides an example of an emergency plan. If you work for a facility that does

---

In the event of an emergency when no medical personnel are present, these guidelines should be followed:

1. A staff person trained in CPR should identify himself or herself. This helps to reassure the victim and bystanders. If the victim is conscious, legally we must ask permission to assist the victim. (The law assumes that an unconscious person would give consent.) A senior staff person should stay with the individual at all times. The staff person should attempt to reassure the victim and protect him or her from personal bodily harm. The senior staff person should assume control of the situation and issue further orders as needed.

2. A second staff member should call 9-1-1. (Please review specific emergency procedures and directions posted above the phones in the main office.)

3. The victim should be monitored at all times:

   A. Check heart rate, noting the regularity and strength of each heart beat.

   B. Monitor and record blood pressure.

   C. Observe skin color and breathing pattern.

   D. Maintain an open airway.

   E. Establish unresponsiveness and initiate CPR when appropriate.

   F. Before the individual is transported (if unconscious), give the emergency medical technicians (EMTs) as much information as possible regarding the individual:

   - Name
   - Age
   - Medical considerations
   - Home phone number
   - Emergency phone numbers
   - Physician

   G. Ask EMTs the hospital to which the member will be transported.

4. Once the individual is transported, the senior staff person in charge should do the following:

   A. Notify codirectors and request that they contact the participant's emergency contacts.

   B. Assume responsibility for the individual's personal belongings and valuables. Please remember that it is important to respect the individual's privacy. Be as brief as possible when disclosing information pertinent to the event.

   C. Immediately fill out an accident report, and file one copy in the member's folder and one copy with the center's codirectors.

FIGURE 22.1 Emergency plan.

Centers for Disease Control and Prevention (2002). Promoting active lifestyles among older adults. National center for chronic disease prevention and health promotion. Nutrition and Physical activity. http://www.cdc.gov/nccdphp/dnpa/physical/lifestyles.htm

not have emergency procedures in place, it places you at risk for being liable.

- You should have immediate access to each client's permanent file, which includes his or her medical history and who to contact in case of an emergency.

- An emergency contact number and directions to the facility should be posted by the nearest phone in the facility. An example is provided in figure 22.2.

- After an emergency or injury, be sure to complete an accident form similar to the one provided in figure 22.3. Completing such a form documents what procedures were taken during the incident or injury and helps to protect you in a liability case.

- At this time a growing concern for health and fitness facilities is whether to purchase and use an **automated emergency defibrillator (AED).** In facilities where older adults exercise, an AED is recommended, even if a heart attack is a rare occurrence. An AED works by giving the heart a controlled electric shock, forcing all the heart muscles to contract at once and, hopefully, jolting it back into a regular rhythm. The AED is simple to use, and you can receive training at your local Red Cross. It is very important for the instructor to check the batteries on a regular basis to ensure that the AED is ready to work in case of an emergency.

Ethical Guidelines for the Physical Activity Instructor

Failure to adhere to the ethical guidelines associated with your profession probably will not result in legal action. However, ethics deal with very important issues, such as the quality of your relationship with your client, your level of professionalism, and how you represent the industry of physical activity instructors of older adults. Ethical behavior involves keeping the best interests of your clients in mind, being truthful and fair, and being guided by professional integrity in your decisions. The IDEA Health and Fitness Association has published excellent codes of ethics for both personal fitness trainers and group fitness instructors (see appendixes B and C).

Emergency Procedures and Directions

Fitness Center

Emergency procedures

- Dial 9-1-1.
- The 9-1-1 dispatcher will need to know
    (1) **WHERE** the emergency is
    (2) **WHAT** the emergency is and **HOW MANY** people are involved
    (3) **PHONE NUMBER** from which you are calling
    (4) What is currently being done?

IMPORTANT: Stay on the phone. Do not hang up until dispatcher instructs you to do so.

- Send someone out to flag down the emergency medical technicians and direct them to the scene.

Directions to the Fitness Center

- Go south on State College Road.
- Turn left onto the campus on Gym Drive.
- Go through the first stop sign.
- The Kinesiology and Health Science building is on the right side of the street.
- Someone will meet you next to the back entrance of the building to guide you to the scene.

FIGURE 22.2   Emergency procedures and directions.
Used with permission from the Center for Successful Aging, Cal State University, Fullerton)

Date of injury _____ Time _____ ☐ a.m. ☐ p.m.

             Date/Month/Year   Hour:Minutes

Name of injured person _____ Sex _____ Age _____

Address _____ _____
               Street   City   State   ZIP code   Area code and phone number

Check suspected cause of injury or illness

__ Fall   __ Overexposure __ Hyperflexion   __ Other: _____

__ Blunt trauma   __ Overexertion   __ Hyperextension

Nature of injury/illness in detail (Did it happen before, during, or after exercise? How?) _____

_____

_____

Check site of injury/illness

__ None	__ Chest/ribs	__ Hand	__ Nose	__ Other: _____
__ Abdomen	__ Ear	__ Head	__ Shoulder/collar bone	
__ Ankle	__ Elbow	__ Knee	__ Stomach	
__ Arm	__ Face	__ Leg	__ Teeth	
__ Back (upper)	__ Fingers/thumb	__ Mouth	__ Toes	
__ Back (lower)	__ Foot	__ Neck/throat	__ Wrist	

Check sign or symptom

__ Abrasion	__ Discoloration	__ Loss of function	__ Pain	__ Visual involvement
__ Contusion	__ Fracture	__ Lung involvement	__ Shock	__ Other: _____
__ Cut	__ Heart involvement	__ Nausea/vomiting	__ Sprain/strain	
__ Dislocation	__ Internal injury	__ Numbness	__ Swelling	

What was done for the injured person? _____ By whom? _____

_____

Was the injured person sent to a hospital?   __ Yes __ No   To a physician? __ Yes __ No

To whom was the injured released? __ Self __ Relative __ Other: _____

Signature of person filling out form _____ Date _____

Witness signature _____ Date _____

Witness address _____

Witness phone number _____

FIGURE 22.3   Accident report form.

In addition to the IDEA codes of ethics, the following suggestions are provided to assist you with maintaining the highest professional ethics:

- Do not guarantee results. Let your clients know that each individual responds differently to an exercise or nutrition program.

- Discuss fees up front. More important, have a written agreement setting forth services to be performed and fees to be paid. You and your client should date and sign it, and you should include it in the client's permanent file.

- Charge fees uniformly. Do not charge one client one fee and someone else another unless there is a logical basis for doing so. Keep payment records.

- Be on time. One of the hallmarks of a professional is being on time. Always assume your clients' time is valuable because to them it is, even if they are retired. Being on time is a sign of respect. If you are going to be late, call to let them know or to see if the session can be rescheduled.

- Give full measure. If you are paid for a one-hour training session, be sure you give an hour's worth of time.

- Give advance notice of sessions that you will miss. Part of your written agreement may ask clients to give 24 hours' notice if they are going to have to cancel a session.

- Do what you say you will do in a timely fashion. If you offer to do something for the client, do it in a timely fashion. Otherwise, don't offer.

- Maintain confidentiality. It is important to establish a relationship of trust with a client that encourages the client to freely discuss the exercise program and related questions. To gain a client's confidence and to keep it, do not talk about one client with another. Client communications should be confidential. If you want to discuss a client with his or her medical professional, get the client's written permission and keep it in his or her file.

- Establish good client relations. Develop a caring attitude and genuine interest in the goals of your clients, their progress, and their concerns. In other words, *listen to your clients*. This is particularly important with older adults, because listening is how you

can learn about challenges that may have to be addressed in an exercise program. Keep in mind that people are less likely to sue someone they like.

Summary

A number of health and fitness organizations and associations publish standards and guidelines for health and fitness facilities and for physical activity instructors. The best way to provide a safe physical activity environment for older adults and avoid legal problems is to know the standard of care to which you are held: the degree of care a reasonable and prudent physical activity instructor would exercise under the same or similar circumstances.

This chapter summarized components of a risk management plan, including health and fitness facility standards and guidelines, prevention of injuries and medical emergencies, and responding to emergency situations. It also provided information regarding professional ethics for personal trainers and group instructors. In the future, more specific standards and guidelines for physical activity instructors of older adults will be published and recognized by the leading associations in the industry. You should stay abreast of these developments by being involved as a member in your professional organization and by attending conferences and training workshops to update your knowledge and hone your skills as an instructor.

Key Terms

Recommended Readings

NSCA Professional Standards & Guidelines Task Force. (2001, May). *Strength & conditioning professional standards & guidelines.* Colorado Springs, CO: National Strength & Conditioning Association.

Tharrett, S.J., & Peterson, J.A. (Eds.). (1997). *ACSM's health/fitness facility standards and guidelines* (2nd ed.). Champaign, IL: Human Kinetics.

Study Questions

1. In legal terms, the party accused of having caused an injury resulting from fitness training is referred to as the:
   a. plaintiff
   b. defendant
   c. defense team
   d. plaintiff team

2. The *standard of care* to which you are held is that of
   a. a reasonably prudent physical activity instructor of older adults
   b. an expert physical activity instructor of older adults
   c. a college degree physical activity instructor of older adults
   d. a certified physical activity instructor of older adults

3. You can reduce your risk of liability as an instructor of physical activity with older adults if you:
   a. tolerate sexual harassment
   b. keep medical and emergency information on each client posted up on the wall for easy access
   c. have a written emergency response plan readily available
   d. don't let on to your clients that you made a mistake

4. When working with older adults with hearing problems you should NOT
   a. use visual cues
   b. project your voice and raise the pitch
   c. face your clients when talking
   d. project your voice, but don't raise the pitch

5. Which of the following will help you design a safe and effective exercise environment that minimizes client's risk of injury or medical emergency:
   a. ask your diabetic clients to bring their own portable glucometers to the fitness class
   b. monitor the room temperature during exercise
   c. observe for warning signs of heart distress
   d. all of the above

Application Activities

1. An 80-year-old woman contacts you to start a program of exercise. She says her health is good, although she appears about 50 pounds (23 kilograms) overweight. She says her doctor has approved an exercise program. Set up a file for this fictitious potential client, and list all the paperwork you feel you should have before designing and starting a program for her.

(continued)

2. An 85-year-old man you have been training for several weeks in his home seems to be flirting with you. He takes every opportunity to touch your arm or shoulder, stands too close, wears workout clothes that are inappropriate, and tells suggestive jokes. You have tried to discuss your discomfort with his behavior tactfully with him but to no avail. Write a letter to this client setting forth the problem and proposing a solution that will work for you.

3. You teach group exercise classes for older adults at a facility that does not have a risk management plan. Develop your own emergency response plan.

International Curriculum Guidelines for Preparing Physical Activity Instructors of Older Adults

In collaboration With the Aging Life Course, World Health Organization

Executive Summary

Nancy A. Ecclestone, Canada
C. Jessie Jones, United States

The recognized value of physical activity in preserving functional capacity and reducing physical frailty in later years, combined with the support of the medical community, has resulted in numerous senior fitness and physical activity classes springing up in various facilities (e.g., senior centers, hospitals, recreation departments, health and fitness clubs, churches, YMCAs, community centers, retirement communities, long-term care facilities) throughout the world. Because of the lack of licensure or endorsement of training guidelines for preparing physical activity instructors of older adults, facility directors can hire whom they want, regardless of the instructors' educational backgrounds. People receiving little or no specialized training can advertise themselves as senior fitness instructors. Most older adults lack the knowledge and experience to determine whether the physical activity program in which they are participating is safe and effective. Experts in the field have argued that because of the range of medical conditions and functional abilities of the 65-and-older population, physical activity instructors of older adults require more knowledge, skills, and experience than instructors of younger adults. Unfortunately, because of the lack of endorsed curriculum training guidelines to prepare physical activity instructors of older adults, some training programs have not required instructors to attain essential knowledge and skills for instructing older adults in a safe and effective way.

Historical Background

Historically, the development of the *International Curriculum Guidelines for Preparing Physical Activity Instructors of Older Adults* began at the 1996 World International Congress on Physical Activity, Aging and Sport held in Heidelberg, Germany. Delegates from several countries met and developed a draft document; however, the guidelines were never published. Subsequently, Canada developed national guidelines in 2003 (appendix A) under the leadership of the Canadian Centre for Activity and Aging and with the support of Health Canada. In the United States, representatives from six national organizations developed and published national standards in 1998 (appendix B).

In 2003, the two separate documents from the United States (national standards) and Canada (national guidelines) were condensed into one document and titled the *International Curriculum Guidelines for Preparing Physical Activity Instructors of Older Adults*. Then, a coalition of members from 13 countries and a committee from the United States (appendix C) agreed to review and make recommendations for this document. These international guidelines were then presented at the 6th World

Congress on Aging and Physical Activity held in London, Ontario, Canada (August 3 to 7, 2004) by the cochairs of this initiative, Nancy Ecclestone (Canada) and C. Jessie Jones (United States).

The *International Curriculum Guidelines for Preparing Physical Activity Instructors of Older Adults* is a consensus document that outlines each of the major content areas that experts recommend should be included in any entry-level training program with the goal of preparing physical activity instructors to work with older adults. The principles and perspectives of the World Health Organization (WHO) Active Ageing Policy Framework are reflected in this document. Organizations and coalitions currently endorsing the guidelines are listed in appendix D.

These guidelines can be applied to older adults across the continuum from healthy, independent older adults in community settings to functionally dependent older adults in long-term care. Advanced training would be necessary for instructors interested in working with older adults with severe disabilities or cognitive impairment in rehabilitation settings or managing and directing facilities, especially ones providing insurance reimbursement and those that serve a more frail older adult population.

Because of the complexity of the fitness industry and the differences in state and national requirements throughout the world, we believe that it is the responsibility of individual associations and organizations to develop the details of each major content area within each curriculum module, to develop appropriate areas of emphasis, and to develop performance standards that indicate the level of achievement expected of their students. Because of the varied functional ability levels of older adults, it is important to be aware of the target population (community-dwelling, able older adults versus homebound or institutionalized frail older adults) and to develop the content to meet the specific needs of that population.

Purposes and Delimitations

The purpose of the *International Curriculum Guidelines for Preparing Physical Activity Instructors of Older Adults* is to (1) ensure safe, effective, and accessible physical activity and fitness programs for older adults; (2) develop competent physical activity instructors of older adults; (3) provide more consistency among instructor training programs preparing physical activity instructors of older adults; (4) inform administrators, physical activity

instructors, and others about the minimum training guidelines recommended by the profession when recruiting physical activity instructors of older adults; (5) clarify the definition and role of a physical activity instructor for older adults; and (6) establish the level of expertise required to help protect instructors and other facility staff from litigation (lawsuits). *These curriculum guidelines are not being developed to promote one certification or licensing body of physical activity instructors of older adults, but rather to provide curriculum guidelines to encourage more consistency among instructor training programs throughout the world.*

These guidelines do not include recommendations for (1) qualifications and experience of trainers and course tutors, (2) methods of curriculum delivery, (3) assessment requirements for students, or (4) requirements of the training providers.

Definitions of Terms

The following terms are commonly used when discussing training modules.

instructor—A physical activity instructor is broadly defined as a professional who teaches, educates, and trains people to do physical activities.

physical activity—An encompassing term to mean any body movement produced by a skeletal muscle that results in energy expenditure.

exercise—A subset of physical activity. It is planned and repetitive body movement, which improves or maintains one or more components of physical fitness (e.g., cardiovascular endurance, muscular strength, balance, flexibility).

Training Module 1: Overview of Aging and Physical Activity

Recommended areas of study include general background information about the aging process and the benefits of an active lifestyle.

Suggested Topics

1. Demographic considerations (e.g., ethnicity, culture, gender) as they relate to individual participation in physical activity programs
2. Various definitions of aging (including pathological, usual, and successful aging)
3. The difference between the terms chronological, biological, and functional aging

4. The benefits of physical activity as it relates to the multiple dimensions of wellness (e.g., intellectual, emotional, physical, vocational, social, spiritual) and the prevention of chronic medical conditions, health promotion, and quality of life throughout the lifespan

5. Current research and epidemiology related to health and physical activity

Training Module 2: Psychological, Sociocultural, and Physiological Aspects of Physical Activity and Older Adults

Recommended areas of study include psychological, sociocultural, and physiological aspects of physical activity in order to develop safe and effective physical activity and exercise programs for older adults.

Suggested Topics

1. Exercise science: Basic anatomy, physiology, neurology, motor learning and control, and exercise psychology

2. Myths, stereotypes, and barriers associated with aging and physical activity participation in later life

3. Predictors of successful aging (e.g., biological, psychological, and sociological theories of aging, environmental factors, and lifestyle choices)

4. The relationship between physical activity and psychosocial well-being

5. Age-associated physiological and biomechanical changes in multiple body systems (e.g., cardiovascular and respiratory systems, musculoskeletal system, and central nervous system) and how these changes affect functional mobility and independence

Training Module 3: Screening, Assessment, and Goal Setting

Recommended areas of study include information on selection, administration, and interpretation of preexercise health and activity screening and fitness and mobility assessments appropriate for older adults. This information will provide the basis for exercise program design and appropriate referrals to other health professionals.

Suggested Topics

1. Guidelines and procedures for the selection, administration, and interpretation of screening tools to determine the health, physical activity, and disability status of older adult participants

2. Health, activity, and other lifestyle appraisals, including identification risk factors for falls and cardiovascular complications

3. How and when to make appropriate referrals to, or seek advice from, physicians and other qualified allied health and fitness professionals

4. Physiological and functional fitness assessments (e.g., heart rate, blood pressure, body mass index, and field tests for strength, flexibility, submaximal endurance, and functional mobility such as balance, agility, gait, coordination, and power)

5. Psychological (e.g., self-efficacy, depression) and sociological (e.g., social support) assessments

6. For homebound or institutionalized older adults, assessments of functional abilities (e.g., mobility, grooming, dressing, toileting) with input from caregivers

It is further recommended that training programs include information on establishing, with client input, realistic and measurable short-term, medium-term, and long-term goals.

Suggested Topics

1. Factors influencing physical activity participation among older adults, including barriers, motivators, regular involvement in physical activity, and behavior modification

2. Developing, monitoring, and modifying short-term and long-term activity goals based on results from screening and assessments and input from the participants and caregivers if appropriate

3. Importance of encouraging lifetime leisure physical activities (e.g., dancing, gardening, hiking, tennis, swimming) in addition to structured exercise programs

Training Module 4: Program Design and Management

Recommended areas of study include information about using results from screening, assessment, and client goals to make appropriate decisions regarding individual and group physical activity and exercise program design and management.

Suggested Topics

1. Interpretation of prescreening and assessment data, and consideration of client goals, for effective program development

2. Exercise variables (e.g., mode, frequency, duration, intensity) and principles (i.e., overload, functional relevance, challenge, accommodation) for program design in both individual and group settings

3. Exercise training components and methods, including warm-up and cool-down, flexibility, resistance, aerobic endurance, balance and mobility, mind–body exercise, and aquatics for program design in both individual and group settings

4. Applied movement analysis for proper selection and implementation of specific exercises

5. Training formats and session designs for various functional abilities and individual and group exercise sequencing for exercise programming

6. Economic considerations and consequent options for equipment (e.g., quality for cost, safety, and age-friendliness)

7. Importance of making healthy lifestyle choices (e.g., proper nutrition, stress management, and smoking cessation)

8. An organizational system for participant recruitment, tracking exercise compliance, and maintaining other client information

9. Methods for client reassessment and program evaluation

Training Module 5: Program Design for Older Adults With Stable Medical Conditions

Recommended areas of study include information on common medical conditions of older adults, signs and symptoms associated with medication-related negative interactions during activity and how to adapt exercise for clients with varying fitness levels, and stable medical conditions to help prevent injury and other emergency situations.

Suggested Topics

1. Age-related medical conditions (e.g., cardiovascular disease, stroke, hypertension, respiratory disorders, obesity, arthritis, osteoporosis, back pain, diabetes, balance and motor control deficits, visual and hearing disorders, dementia, and urinary incontinence)

2. How to adapt group and individual exercise programs to accommodate for age-related medical conditions and for people who have experienced falls, operations, and illness

3. How to adapt group and individual exercise programs to accommodate for prosthetics (e.g., artificial hips, knees, legs)

4. How to design programs for preventive health (e.g., exercises to reduce risk of falling, control diabetes, heart disease)

5. Recognizing signs and symptoms associated with medication-related negative interactions during physical activity (e.g. postural hypotension, arrhythmias, fatigue, weakness, dizziness, balance and coordination problems, altered depth perception, depression, confusion, dehydration, and urinary incontinence) and refer back to health professional

Training Module 6: Teaching Skills

Recommended areas of study include information about motor learning principles that guide the selection and delivery of effective individualized and group exercises and physical activities, and the construction of safe and effective practice environments.

Suggested Topics

1. Application of motor learning principles for proper client instruction, verbal cues, feedback, and reinforcement

2. Structure of the learning environment to facilitate optimal learning of motor skills

3. Development of safe, friendly, and fun exercise and physical activity environments (e.g., appropriate use of humor, special equipment, creative movements, music, novelty, and props)

4. Issues facing older adults that may affect motivation (e.g., depression, social isolation, learned helplessness, low self-efficacy)

5. Development of lesson plans and elements of instruction

6. Methods for self-evaluation of teaching effectiveness

7. Monitoring and adjustment of exercise variables (e.g., frequency, intensity, duration, mode)

Training Module 7: Leadership, Communication, and Marketing Skills

Recommended areas of study include information on incorporating effective motivational, communication, and leadership skills related to teaching individual and group exercise classes as well as professional leadership skills, and how to create effective marketing tools for program and self.

Suggested Topics

1. Principles of individual and group dynamics in structured exercise settings

2. Translation of technical terminology into client-friendly language

3. Incorporating leadership skills into personal training and group physical activity classes to enhance teaching effectiveness and client satisfaction

4. Application of positive interpersonal interaction behaviors to work with a heterogeneous older adult population (e.g., gender, ethnicity, education level) in both group and individual exercise settings

5. Listening skills and reception to participants' feedback

6. Development of social support strategies (e.g., buddy system, telephone support)

7. Development of effective, age-friendly marketing strategies and tools of program and

self, and methods of delivering the "right" message

Training Module 8: Client Safety and First Aid

Recommended areas of study include information on developing a risk-management plan to promote a safe exercise environment and respond to emergency situations.

Suggested Topics

1. Signs that indicate need for immediate exercise cessation or immediate medical consultation

2. Appropriate response to emergency situations such as would be covered in standard first-aid and CPR classes (e.g., cardiac arrest; airway obstruction; emergencies requiring rescue breathing; heat- and cold-related injuries; musculoskeletal injuries including strains, sprains, and fractures; diabetic emergencies; bleeding; falls; seizures; and shock)

3. Establishment of an emergency action plan

4. Identification of a safe and age-friendly exercise environment (e.g., working conditions of equipment, accessibility, ventilation, lighting, floor surfaces, proper footwear, access to water and washroom facilities) and precautions for environmental extremes (e.g., high or low temperatures and excessive humidity)

Training Module 9: Ethics and Professional Conduct

Recommended areas of study include information on legal, ethical, and professional conduct.

Suggested Topics

1. Legal issues related to delivering physical activity programs to older adults, including legal concepts and terminology

2. Issues related to lawsuits, including scope of practice, industry standards, and negligence and types of applicable insurance coverage

3. Ethical standards and personal conduct and scope of practice for physical activity instructors of older adults

4. Accessing resources for the enhancement of professional skills (e.g., position stands, ethical practices, professional practice guidelines consistent with the standards of care)

5. Methods of continuing education to enhance one's professional skills

Appendix A Canadian Guidelines

Canadian Guidelines for Leaders of Physical Activity Programs for Older Adults in Long-Term Care, Home Care and the Community (2003) can be found on the Web site of the Canadian Centre for Activity and Aging at www.uwo.ca/actage.

These guidelines were produced as a result of the release, in the International Year of Older Persons (1999), of the following:

- *Canada's Physical Activity Guide to Healthy Active Living* (endorsed by more than 56 organizations)

- *Blueprint for Action for Active Living and Older Adults: Moving Through the Years* (contributors: La Fondation en adaptation motrice [FAM], Active Living Coalition for Older Adults [ALCOA], Canadian Centre for Activity and Aging [CCAA], and Health Canada)

- Recommendations from the *Roundtable of Leaders in Physical Activity and Aging* (1998)* and the *ALCOA National Forum—Older Adults and Active Living* (1999). ★Both events were hosted by the Canadian Centre for Activity and Aging.

Several delegates representing a cross-section of health-related perspectives were instrumental in contributing to the development of the Canadian Guidelines. These contributions were solicited on the basis of their expertise and not necessarily their affiliations. Delegates (66) to the forums ([1]Long-Term Care Forum, [2]Home Care and Community Forum) that contributed to the Canadian guidelines include the following:

Newfoundland

Elsie McMillan, St. John's Nursing Home Board, St. John's[1]

Janet O'Dea, Memorial University of Newfoundland, Health Sciences Centre, St. John's[1]

Fran Cook, Memorial University Recreation Complex, St. John's[2]

Moira Hennessey, Department of Health and Community Services, St. John's[2]

Patricia Nugent, Health and Community Services, St. John's Region, St. John's[2]

Prince Edward Island

Marilyn Kennedy, Acute and Continuing Care, Department of Health and Social Services, Charlottetown[1]

Pat Malone, Senior Services Liaison—Acute and Continuing Care, Department of Health and Social Services, Charlottetown[1]

Lona Penny, Dr. John Gillis Memorial Lodge, Belfast[1]

Sharon Claybourne, Island Fitness Council, Charlottetown[2]

Nova Scotia

Denise Dreimanis, Nova Scotia Fitness & Lifestyle Leaders Association, ALCOA Speakers Bureau Dartmouth[1]

Debra Leigh, Continuing Care Association of Nova Scotia, Halifax[1]

Lygia Figueirado, Continuing Care, Government of Nova Scotia, Halifax[2]

Andrea Leonard, Home Support Association of Nova Scotia, Halifax[2]

New Brunswick

Flora Dell, Active Living Coalition for Older Adults (ALCOA), Fredericton[1]

Vicky Knight, Fredericton[1]

Ron Davis, Camden Park Terrace, Moncton[2]

Québec

Phillipe Markon, Ste-Famille, Ile d'Orleans[1]

Jaques Renaud, Association des Etablissments Prives Conventionnes, Montreal[1]

Clermont Simard, DEP-PEPS, Université Laval, Sainte-Foy[2]

Ontario

Jane Boudreau-Bailey, Chelsey Park Nursing Home, London[1]

Liz Cyarto, Canadian Centre for Activity and Aging, London[1,2]

Nancy Ecclestone, Canadian Centre for Activity and Aging, London[1,2]

Clara Fitzgerald, Canadian Centre for Activity and Aging, London[1,2]

Janice Hutton, Canadian Association of Fitness Professionals, Markham[1]

Marita Kloseck, Division of Geriatric Medicine, Parkwood Hospital, London[1]

Jody Kyle, YMCA St. Catherines, St. Catherines[1]

Darien Lazowski, Canadian Centre for Activity and Aging, London[1]

Stephanie Luxton, Canadian Centre for Activity and Aging, London[1,2]

Karen Macdonald, Canadian Red Cross Link to Health Program, Mississauga

Sandra Mallett, Allendale Long Term Care, Milton[1]

Colleen Sonnenberg, Ministry of Health and Long-Term Care, Toronto[1]

Sue Veitch, Kingston[1]

Gabriel Blouin, Institute for Positive Health for Seniors, ALCOA, Ottawa[2]

Lynne Briggs, Advocacy Committee, Older Adult Centres Association of Ontario, Evergreen Seniors Centre, Guelph[2]

Carol Butler, PSW Program, Fanshawe College, London[2]

Trish Fitzpatrick, Client Services and Program Development, CCAC Oxford County, Woodstock[2]

Hania Goforth, Recreation Services, Lifestyle Retirement Communities, Mississauga[2]

John Griffin, George Brown College, Toronto[2]

Joan Hunter, Link to Health, Canadian Red Cross, Toronto[2]

Janice Hutton, Canadian Association of Fitness Professionals, Markham[2]

Jane Miller, Ontario Fitness Council, Toronto[2]

Don Paterson, University of Western Ontario, Canadian Centre for Activity and Aging, London[1,2]

Sheila Schuehlein, VON Canada, Kitchener[2]

Nancy Stelpstra, Ontario Fitness Council, Guelph[2]

Bert Taylor, University of Western Ontario, London[1]

Bruce Taylor, Health Canada, Ottawa[2]

Sue Thorning, Ontario Community Support Association, Toronto[2]

Manitoba

Cindy Greenlay-Brown, West St. Paul[1]

Jim Hamilton, Manitoba Seniors Directorate, Winnipeg[1,2]

Hope Mattus, Health Accountability Policy and Planning, Seniors and Persons With Disabilities, Manitoba Health, Winnipeg[1,2]

Russell Thorne, Manitoba Fitness Council, University of Manitoba, Winnipeg[2]

Saskatchewan

Angela Nunweiler, Community Care Branch, Saskatchewan Health, Regina[1]

Bob Lidington, Saskatoon Home Support Services, Ltd, Saskatoon[2]

Alberta

Jennifer Dechaine, Alberta Centre for Active Living, Edmonton[1]

Timothy Fairbank, Capital Health Authority ADL/CRP, Edmonton[2]

Debbie Lee, Calgary Regional Health Authority, Calgary[2]

Debbie Ponich, Alberta Fitness Leadership Certification Association, Provincial Fitness Unit[2] Faculty of Physical Education & Recreation, University of Alberta, Edmonton[2]

British Columbia

Carol Hansen, Kwantlan University College, Surrey[1, 2]

Linda Mae Ross, Continuing Care Renewal Regional Programs, Victoria[1]

Catherine Rutter, McIntosh Lodge, Chilliwack[1]

Barbara Harwood, NLTI Project Advisory Committee, Speakers Bureau ALCOA, North Saanich[2]

Cheryl Hedgecock, British Columbia Parks and Recreation, Richmond[2]

Yukon

Willy Shippey, Yukon Health and Social Services, Thompson Centre, Whitehorse[1,2]

Northwest Territory

Marjorie Sandercock, Yellowknife[1]

Nunavut

Jason Collins, Recreation and Leadership Division, Government of Nunavut, Igloolik[2]

Federal

Health Canada

Appendix B U.S. Standards

The *National Standards for Preparing Senior Fitness Instructors* were published by Jones, C.J. & Clark, J. (1998). National standards for preparing senior fitness instructors. *Journal of Aging and Physical Activity,* 6, 207-221.

Coalition Members

Chair: C. Jessie Jones, Council on Aging and Adult Development, American Association for Active Lifestyles and Fitness

Members

Janie Clark, American Senior Fitness Association

Richard Cotton, American Council on Exercise

Laura Gladwin, Aerobics and Fitness Association of America

Gwen Hyatt, Desert Southwest Fitness, Inc.

Lee Morgan, Cooper Institute of Aerobic Research

Kay Van Norman, Council on Aging and Adult Development, American Association for Active Lifestyles and Fitness

Appendix C International Recommendations

A coalition of members from 13 countries and a committee from the United States made recommendations for the *International Curriculum Guidelines for Preparing Physical Activity Instructors of Older Adults.*

International Coalition

Cochairs

Nancy Ecclestone, Canada and C. Jessie Jones, United States

Members

Susie Dinan	England
Dorothy Dobson	Scotland
Ellen Freiberger	Germany
Linda Halliday	South Africa
Carol Hansen	Canada
Eino Heikkinen	Finland
Keith Hill	Australia
Marijke Hopman-Rock	The Netherlands
Gareth Jones	Canada
Alexandre Kalache	WHO
Stephanie Luxton	Canada
Michele Porter	Canada
Suely Santos	Brazil
Federico Schena	Italy
Cody Sipe	United States
Kiyoji Tanaka	Japan
Janice Tay	Singapore
Bruce Taylor	Canada
Catrine Tudor-Locke	United States

United States Coalition

Chair: C. Jessie Jones	***American College of Sports Medicine (ACSM)***

Members

Kazuko Aoyagi	World Instructor Training Schools (WITS)
Ken Baldwin	A.H. Ismail Center for Health, Exercise & Nutrition, Purdue University
Grant Clark	American Senior Fitness Association
Janie Clark	American Senior Fitness Association
Wojtek Chodzko-Zajko	National Blueprint on Active Aging
Laura Gladwin	American Fitness and Aerobic Association
Carol Kennedy	Indiana University
Steve Keteyian	ACSM
Rainer Martens	Human Kinetics
Julie McNeney	International Council on Active Aging
Colin Milner	International Council on Active Aging
Tammy Peterson	American Academy of Health and Fitness
Jerry Purvis	American Kinesiotherapy Association

Roberta Rikli	Center for Successful Aging, Cal State University, Fullerton
Debra Rose	Center for Successful Aging, Cal State University, Fullerton
Christine Schnitzer	Healthy Strides, Kisco Senior Living Facilities
Cody Sipe	A.H. Ismail Center for Ilcalth, Excrcisc & Nutrition, Purdue University
Christian Thompson	Council on Adult Development and Aging (CAAD), American Association for Active Lifestyles and Fitness (AAALF)
Mary Visser	CAAD, AAALF
Judy Wright	Human Kinetics

Appendix D Supporting Organizations and Coalitions

Organizations and Coalitions supporting the *International Curriculum Guidelines for Preparing Physical Activity Instructors of Older Adults* as of this printing include the following:

> American Association for Active Lifestyles and Fitness, Council on Adult Development and Aging
>
> American Kinesiotherapy Association
>
> American Fitness and Aerobic Association
>
> American Senior Fitness Association
>
> Dessert Southwest Fitness, Inc.
>
> International Council on Active Aging
>
> National Blueprint: Increasing Physical Activity Among Adults Age 50 and Older
>
> World Instructor Training Schools

Organizations and Coalitions endorsing the *International Curriculum Guidelines for Preparing Physical Activity Instructors of Older Adults* as of this printing include the following:

> Active Living Coalition for Older Adults
>
> Canadian Centre for Activity and Aging
>
> Canadian Society for Exercise Physiology

Personal Fitness Trainers

IDEA Code of Ethics

As a member of IDEA Health & Fitness Association, I will be guided by the best interests of the client and will practice within the scope of my education and knowledge. I will maintain the education and experience necessary to appropriately train clients, will behave in a positive and constructive manner, and will use truth, fairness, and integrity to guide all my professional decisions and relationships.

Ethical Practice Guidelines for Personal Fitness Trainers

1. **Always be guided by the best interests of the client.**

   a. Remember that a personal trainer's primary responsibility is to the client's safety, health, and welfare; never compromise this responsibility for your own self-interest, personal advantage, or monetary gain.

   b. Recommend products or services only if they will benefit the client's health and well-being, not because they will benefit you financially or occupationally.

   c. If recommending products or services will result in financial gain for you or your employer, be aware that disclosure to the client may be appropriate.

   d. Base the number of training sessions on the client's needs, not your financial requirements.

2. **Maintain appropriate professional boundaries.**

   a. Never exploit—sexually, economically, or otherwise—a professional relationship with a supervisor, an employee, a colleague, or a client.

   b. Respect the client's right to privacy. A client's conversations, behavior, results, and—if appropriate—identity should be kept confidential.

   c. Use physical touching appropriately during training sessions, as a means of correcting alignment or focusing a client's concentration on the targeted area. Immediately discontinue the use of touch at a client's request or if the client displays signs of discomfort.

   d. Focus on the business relationship, not the client's personal life, except as appropriate.

   e. When you are unable to maintain appropriate professional boundaries or to work within the legitimate agenda of the training relationship, whether because of your own attitudes and behaviors or those of the client, either terminate the relationship or refer the client to an appropriate professional, such as another trainer, a medical doctor, or a mental health specialist.

   f. Avoid sexually oriented banter and inappropriate physical contact.

3. **Maintain the education and experience necessary to appropriately train clients.**

   a. Continuously strive to keep abreast of the new developments, concepts, and practices essential to providing the highest-quality services to clients.

   b. Recognize your limitations in services and techniques, and engage only in activities that fall within the boundaries of your professional credentials and competencies. Refer clients to other professionals for issues that fall beyond the boundaries of a personal fitness trainer's profession or your current competencies.

   c. For health screening, fitness assessment, prudent progression, and exercise technique, follow the standards outlined by professionals in the fields of medicine and health and fitness.

4. **Use truth, fairness, and integrity to guide all professional decisions and relationships.**

   a. In all professional and business relationships, clearly demonstrate and support honesty, integrity, and trustworthiness.

   b. Accurately represent your qualifications.

(continued)

(continued)

---

    c. In advertising materials, be truthful and fair. When describing personal training services, be guided by the primary obligation of helping the client develop informed judgments, opinions, and codes. Avoid ambiguity, sensationalism, exaggeration, and superficiality.

    d. Make your contract language clear and understandable.

    e. Administer consistent pricing and procedural policies.

    f. Never solicit business from another trainer's client. When interacting with clients of other trainers, be open and honest so those clients cannot interpret the interaction as solicitation of their business.

    g. If you work for a business that finds clients and assigns them to you, recognize that the clients belong to that business.

5. Show respect for clients and fellow professionals.

    a. Act with integrity in your relationships with colleagues, facility owners, and other health professionals to help ensure that each client benefits optimally from all professionals.

    b. Never discriminate based on race, creed, color, gender, age, physical handicap, or nationality.

    c. When disagreements or conflicts occur, focus on behavior, factual evidence, and nonderogatory forms of communication, not on judgmental statements, hearsay, the placing of blame, or other destructive responses.

    d. Present fitness information completely and accurately in order to help the client make informed decisions.

6. Uphold a professional image through conduct and appearance.

    a. Avoid smoking, substance abuse, and unhealthy eating habits.

    b. Speak and dress in a manner that increases the client's comfort level.

Appendix C

Group Fitness Trainers

IDEA Code of Ethics

As a member of IDEA Health & Fitness Association, I will be guided by the best interests of the client and will practice within the scope of my education and knowledge. I will maintain the education and experience necessary to appropriately teach classes, will behave in a positive and constructive manner, and will use truth, fairness, and integrity to guide all my professional decisions and relationships.

Ethical Practice Guidelines for Group Fitness Trainers

1. **Always be guided by the best interests of the group, while acknowledging individuals.**

   a. Remember that a group fitness instructor's primary obligation is to the group as a whole, taking class level and class description into account.

   b. Strive to provide options and realistic goals that take individual variations into account.

   c. Offer modifications for all levels of fitness and experience (i.e., demonstrate easy and more challenging options).

   d. Recommend products or services only if they will benefit a client's health and well-being, not because they will benefit you or your employer financially or occupationally.

2. **Provide a safe exercise environment.**

   a. Prioritize all movement choices by (1) safety, (2) effectiveness, and (3) creativity. Do not allow creativity to compromise safety.

   b. Use good judgment in exercise selection. Assess all class moves according to risk versus reward, making sure rewards and benefits always outweigh risks.

   c. Adhere to safe guidelines for music speed in all classes.

   d. Follow guidelines for maximum music volume. IDEA recommends that "music intensity during group exercise classes should measure no more than 90 decibels (dB). Since the instructor's voice needs to be about 10dB louder than the music in order to be heard, the instructor's voice should measure no more than 100dB."

   e. Consider whether exercises that can be properly monitored in a one-to-one setting are appropriate in a group environment.

3. **Obtain the education and training necessary to lead group exercise.**

   a. Continuously strive to keep abreast of the latest research and exercise techniques essential to providing effective and safe classes.

   b. Maintain certifications and continuing education.

   c. Obtain specific training for teaching specialty classes or instructing special populations. Teach a class such as kickboxing or yoga only after mastering the skill and understanding the important aspects of the class. Instruct a special population, like older adults or perinatal women, only after studying the specific needs of the group.

   d. Work within the scope of your knowledge and skill. When necessary, refer participants to professionals with appropriate training and expertise beyond your realm of knowledge.

4. **Use truth, fairness, and integrity to guide all professional decisions and relationships.**

   a. In all professional and business relationships, clearly demonstrate and support honesty, integrity, and trustworthiness.

   b. Speak in a positive manner about fellow instructors, other staff, participants, and competitive facilities and organizations, or say nothing at all.

(continued)

Reprinted with permission from IDEA Health & Fitness Association, the leading international membership association in the health and fitness industry, (800) 999-4332, www.IDEAfit.com.

(continued)

c. When disagreements or conflicts occur, focus on behavior, factual evidence, and nonderogatory forms of communication, not on judgmental statements, hearsay, the placing of blame, or other destructive responses.

d. Accurately represent your certifications, training, and education.

e. Do not discriminate based on race, creed, color, gender, age, physical handicap, or nationality.

5. **Maintain appropriate professional boundaries.**

a. Never exploit—sexually, economically, or otherwise—a professional relationship with a supervisor, an employee, a colleague, or a client.

b. Use physical touching appropriately during training sessions, as a means of correcting alignment or focusing a client's concentration on the targeted area. Immediately discontinue the use of touch at a client's request or if the client displays signs of discomfort.

c. Avoid sexually oriented banter and inappropriate physical contact.

6. **Uphold a professional image through conduct and appearance.**

a. Model behavior that values physical ability, function, and health over appearance.

b. Demonstrate healthy behaviors and attitudes about bodies (including your own). Avoid smoking, substance abuse, and unhealthy exercise and eating habits.

c. Encourage healthful eating for yourself and others.

d. Dress in a manner that allows you to perform your job while increasing the comfort level of class participants. Be more conservative in dress, decorum, and speech when the class standard is unclear.

e. Establish a mood in class that encourages and supports individual effort and all levels of expertise.

Study Questions Answer Key

Chapter 1
1. d
2. d
3. b
4. a

Chapter 2
1. b
2. a
3. b
4. d
5. b
6. d

Chapter 3
1. c
2. a
3. c
4. d
5. d

Chapter 4
1. d
2. a
3. b
4. d
5. a
6. b
7. c

Chapter 5
1. c
2. d
3. a
4. c

5. b
6. b
7. a
8. c
9. d

Chapter 6
1. c
2. a
3. a
4. b

Chapter 7
1. d
2. c
3. a
4. b
5. a
6. c
7. d

Chapter 8
1. d
2. d
3. b
4. d
5. c
6. a
7. b

Chapter 9
1. c
2. a
3. c
4. d

5. c
6. a

Chapter 10
1. c
2. d
3. b
4. a
5. d
6. d

Chapter 11
1. d
2. b
3. c
4. a
5. c
6. c
7. d

Chapter 12
1. a
2. b
3. d
4. d
5. d

Chapter 13
1. c
2. c
3. c
4. a
5. c
6. b
7. c

Chapter 14
1. d
2. d
3. a
4. d
5. b
6. d
7. d
8. d

Chapter 15
1. b
2. b
3. d
4. a
5. d
6. a

Chapter 16
1. d
2. c
3. b
4. a
5. b
6. a
7. c
8. b

Chapter 17
1. b
2. b
3. a
4. d
5. c
6. d

Chapter 18
1. c
2. d
3. d
4. b
5. a
6. c
7. b
8. b
9. b
10. d

Chapter 19
1. b
2. d
3. a
4. d

Chapter 20
1. a
2. c
3. c
4. d
5. b

Chapter 21
1. b
2. b
3. a
4. c
5. b
6. b
7. d

Chapter 22
1. b
2. a
3. c
4. d
5. d

References

Preface

Ecclestone, N.A., & Jones, C.J. (2004) International curriculum guidelines for preparing physical activity instructors or older adults. *Journal of Aging and Physical Activity, 12,* 5.

Jones, C.J., & Clark, J. (1998). National standards for preparing senior fitness instructors. *Journal of Aging and Physical Activity, 6,* 207-221.

Chapter 1

Centers for Disease Control and Prevention, National Center for Chronic Disease Prevention and Health Promotion, Division of Nutrition and Physical Activity. (2002). *Promoting active lifestyles among older adults.* www.cdc.gov/nccdphp/dnpa/physical/lifestyles.htm.

Fries, J.F., & Crapo, L.M. (1981). *Vitality and aging.* San Francisco: Freeman.

Jones, C.J., & Clark, J. (1998). National standards for preparing senior fitness instructors. *Journal of Aging and Physical Activity, 6,* 207-221.

Jones, C.J., & Rikli, R.E. (1993). The gerontology movement—Is it passing us by? *Journal of Physical Education, Recreation, and Dance, 64,* 17-26.

Jones, C.J., & Rikli, R.E. (1994). The revolution in aging: Implications for curriculum development and professional preparation in physical education. *Journal of Aging and Physical Activity, 2,* 261-272.

Katz, S., Branch, L.G., Branson, M.H., Papsidero, J.A., Beck, J.C., & Greer, D.S. (1983). Active life expectancy. *New England Journal of Medicine, 309,* 1218-1224.

Kinsella, K., & Velkoff, V.A. (2001). *An aging world: 2001* (U.S. Census Bureau Series P95/01-1). Washington, DC: U.S. Government Printing Office.

Nied, R.J., & Franklin, B. (2002). Promoting and prescribing exercise for the elderly. *American Family Physician, 65,* 419-428.

Rowe, J.W., & Kahn, R.L. (1987). Human aging: Usual and successful. *Science, 237,* 143-149.

Shephard, R. (1997). *Aging, physical activity, and health.* Champaign, IL: Human Kinetics.

Spirduso, W.W. (1995). *Physical dimensions of aging.* Champaign, IL: Human Kinetics.

U.S. Department of Health and Human Services. (2000). *Healthy people 2010* (2nd ed.). Washington, DC: U.S. Government Printing Office.

U.S. Department of Health and Human Services. (2001). *Physical activity and good nutrition: Essential elements to prevent chronic diseases and obesity.* Atlanta, GA: Centers for Disease Control and Prevention.

World Health Organization. (2000). *Active aging: From evidence to action.* Geneva: World Health Organization.

Chapter 2

American College of Sports Medicine. (1998). ACSM position stand on exercise and physical activity for older adults. *Medicine and Science in Sports and Exercise, 30,* 992-1008.

Atchley, R.C. (1972). *The social forces in later life: An introduction to social gerontology.* Belmont, CA: Wedsworth.

Baltes, M.M., & Baltes, P.B. (1980). Plasticity and variability in psychological aging: Methodological and theoretical issues. In G.E. Gurski (Ed.), *Determining the effects of aging on the central nervous system* (pp. 41-66). Berlin: Schering.

Baltes, M.M., & Baltes, P.B. (1990). Psychological perspectives on successful aging: The model of selective optimization with compensation. In M.M Baltes & P.B. Baltes (Eds.), *Successful aging: Perspectives from the behavioral sciences.* Cambridge: Cambridge University Press.

Bandura, A. (1997). *Self-efficacy: The exercise of control.* New York: Freeman.

Blair, S.N., Kampert, J.B., Kohl, H.W., III, Barlow, C.E., Macera, C.A., Paffenbarger, R.S., Jr., & Gibbons, L.W. (1996). Influences of cardiorespiratory fitness and other precursors on cardiovascular disease and all-cause mortality in men and women. *Journal of the American Medical Association, 276,* 205-210.

Bouchard, C., Shephard, R.J., & Stephens, T. (Eds.). (1994). *Physical activity, fitness, and health: International proceedings and consensus statement.* Champaign, IL: Human Kinetics.

Chopra, C. (1993). *Ageless body, timeless mind.* Nevada City, CA: Harmony Books.

Crowther, M.R., Parker, M.W., Achenbaum, W.A., Larimore, W.L., & Koenig, H.G. (2002). Rowe and Kahn's model of successful aging revisited: Positive spirituality—the forgotten factor. *Gerontologist, 42,* 613-620.

Deci, E.L., & Ryan, R.M. (Eds.). (2002). *Handbook of self-determination research.* Rochester, NY: University of Rochester Press.

Erikson, E., Erikson, J., & Kivnick. (1986). *Vital involvement in old age.* New York: Norton.

Finch, C.E. (1976). The regulation of physiological changes during mammalian aging. *Quarterly Review of Biology, 51,* 49-83.

Fisher, B.J. (1995). Successful aging, life satisfaction and generativity in later life. *International Journal of Aging and Human Development, 41,* 239-250.

Frolkis, V.V. (1968). Regulatory process in the mechanisms of aging. *Experimental Gerontology, 3,* 113-123.

Harman, D. (1956). Aging: A theory based on free radical and radiation chemistry. *Journal of Gerontology, 11,* 298-300.

Havighurst, R.J. (1961). Successful aging. *Gerontologist, 1,* 8-13.

Hayflick, L. (1961). The limited in vitro lifetime of human diploid cell strains. *Experimental Cell Research, 37,* 614-636.

House, J.S., Landis, K.R., & Umberson, D. (1988). Social relationships and health. *Science, 241,* 540-545.

Leder, D. (1997). *Spiritual passages: Embracing life's sacred journey.* New York: Tarcher/Putnam.

Lemon, B.W., Bengtson, V.L., & Peterson, J.A. (1972). An exploration of the activity theory of aging: Activity types and life expectation among in-movers to a retirement community. *Journal of Gerontology, 27,* 511-523.

Maslow, A. (1943). A theory of human motivation. *Psychological Review, 50,* 370-396.

Maslow, A., & Lowery, R. (Eds.). (1998). *Toward a psychology of being* (3rd ed.). New York: Wiley.

Medvedev, Z.A. (1981). Age changes and the rejuvenation processes related to reproduction. *Mechanisms of Ageing and Development, 17,* 331-349.

Palmore, E.B. (1979). Predictors of successful aging. *Gerontologist, 19,* 427-431.

Pelletier, K.R. (1994). *Sound mind, sound body: A new model for lifelong health.* New York: Simon & Schuster.

Pert, C. (1993). The chemical communicators. In B. Moyers (Ed.), *Healing and the mind.* New York: Doubleday.

Robert Wood Johnson Foundation. (2001). *National blueprint: Increasing physical activity among adults age 50 and older.* Princeton, NJ: Author.

Rowe, J.W., & Kahn, R.L. (1987). Human aging: Usual and successful. *Science, 237,* 143-149.

Rowe, J.W., & Kahn, R.L. (1998). *Successful aging.* New York: Pantheon Books.

Ryan, R.M. (1991). The nature of the self in autonomy and relatedness. In J. Strauss & G.R. Goethals (Eds.), *Multidisciplinary perspectives on the self* (pp. 208-238). New York: Springer-Verlag.

Seaward, B.L. (2001). *Health of the human spirit.* Boston: Allyn and Bacon.

Seeman, T.E., & Crimmins, E. (2001). Social environment effect on health and aging: Integrating epidemiologic and demographic approaches and perspectives. *Annals of the New York Academy of Sciences, 954,* 88-117.

Seeman, Singer, Ryff, Dienberg Love, Levy-Storms (2002). Social relationships, gender, and allostatic load across two age cohorts. *Psychosomatic Medicine, 64,* 395-406.

Stathi, A., Fox, K.R., & McKenna, J. (2002). Physical activity and dimensions of subjective well-being in older adults. *Journal of Aging and Physical Activity, 10,* 76-92.

Sugtswawa, S., Liang, J., & Liu, X. (1994). Social networks, social support and mortality among older people in Japan. *Journals of Gerontology, 49,* S3-S13.

U.S. Department of Health and Human Services. (1996). *Physical activity and health: A report of the Surgeon General.* Washington, DC: U.S. Government Printing Office.

U.S. Department of Health and Human Services. (2000). *Healthy people 2010* (2nd ed.). Washington, DC: U.S. Government Printing Office.

Warner, H., Butler, R.N., Sprott, R.L., & Schneider, E.L. (Eds.). (1987). *Modern biological theories of aging.* New York: Raven.

World Health Organization. (1998). *Growing older—Staying well: Ageing and physical activity in everyday life.* Geneva: Author.

Chapter 3

American College of Sports Medicine. (1998). ACSM position stand on exercise and physical activity for older adults. *Medicine and Science in Sports and Exercise, 30,* 992-1008.

Armstrong, S., et al. (2001). National blueprint: Increasing physical activity among adults age 50 and older [Special supplement]. *Journal of Aging and Physical Activity, 9.*

Bandura, A. (1997). *Self-efficacy: The exercise of control.* New York: Freeman.

Bengtson, V.L., & Schaie, K.W. (Eds.). (1999). *Handbook of the theories of aging.* New York: Springer.

Blair, S.N., Dunn, A.L., Marcus, B.H., Carpenter, R.A., & Jaret, P. (2001). *Active living every day: Twenty weeks to lifelong vitality.* Champaign, IL: Human Kinetics.

Blumenthal, J.A., & Madden, D.J. (1988). Effects of aerobic exercise training, age, and physical fitness on memory-search performance. *Psychology and Aging, 3,* 280-285.

Butler, R.N., & Lewis, M.I. (1982). *Aging and mental health* (3rd ed.). St. Louis, MO: Mosby.

Chodzko-Zajko, W.J. (1990). The influence of general health status on the relationship between chronological age and depressed mood state. *Journal of Geriatric Psychiatry, 23,* 13-22.

Chodzko-Zajko, W.J. (1995). The roots of ageism in contemporary society: An historical and scientific perspective. *Gerontologist, 35,* 105.

Chodzko-Zajko, W.J. (1997). Editorial: World Health Organization issues guidelines for physical activity in older adults. *Journal of Aging and Physical Activity, 5*(1), 1.

Chodzko-Zajko, W.J. (2000). Successful aging in the new millennium—The role of regular physical activity. *Quest, 52,* 333-343.

Chodzko-Zajko, W.J., & Moore, K.A. (1994). Physical fitness and cognitive functioning in aging. *Exercise and Sport Sciences Reviews, 22,* 1995-220.

Colcombe, S., & Kramer, A.F. (2003). Fitness effects on the cognitive function of older adults: A meta-analytic study. *Psychological Science, 14,* 125-130.

Cousins, S.O. (1997). Elderly tomboys? Sources of self-efficacy for physical activity in late life. *Journal of Aging and Physical Activity, 5*(3), 229-243.

Cousins, S.O., & Vertinsky, P.A. (1995). Recapturing the physical activity experiences of the old: A study of three women. *Journal of Aging and Physical Activity, 3*(2), 146-162.

Diener, E. (1984). Subjective well-being. *Psychological Bulletin, 95,* 542-575.

DiPietro, L., Seeman, T.E., Merrill, S.S., & Berkman, L.F. (1996). Physical activity and measures of cognitive function in healthy older adults: The MacArthur Study of Successful Aging. *Journal of Aging and Physical Activity, 4,* 362-376.

Dunn, A.L., Andersen, R.E., & Jakicic, J.M. (1998). Lifestyle physical activity interventions: History, short- and long-tern effects, and recommendations. *American Journal of Preventive Medicine, 15*(4), 398-412.

Dunn, A.L., Garcia, M.E., Marcus, B.H., Kampert, J.B., Kohl, H.W., & Blair, S.N. (1998). Six-month physical activity and fitness changes in Project Active, a randomized trial. *Medicine and Science in Sports and Exercise, 30,* 1076-1083.

Dustman, R.E., Ruhling, R.O., Russell, E.M., Shearer, D.E., William-Bonekat, H., Shigeoka, J.W., et al. (1984). Aerobic exercise training and improved neuropsychological function of older individuals. *Neurobiology of Aging, 5,* 35-42.

Etnier, J.R., Salazar, W., Landers, D.M., Petruzzello, S.J., Han, M., & Nowell, P. (1997). The influence of physical fitness and exercise upon cognitive functioning: A meta-analysis. *Journal of Sport and Exercise Psychology, 19,* 249-277.

Folkins, C.H., & Sime, W.E. (1981). Physical fitness training and mental health. *American Psychologist, 36,* 373-389.

Hawkins, H., Kramer, A.F., & Capaldi, D. (1992). Aging, exercise, and attention. *Psychology and Aging, 7,* 643-653.

Heath, G.W., Hagberg, J.M., Ehasani, A.A., & Holloszy, J.O. (1981). A physiological comparison of young and older endurance athletes during exercise. *Journal of Applied Physiology, 58*(6), 2041-2046.

Hill, R.D., Storandt, M., & Malley, M. (1993). The impact of long-term exercise training on psychological functioning in older adults. *Journal of Gerontology, 48,* 12-17.

King, A.C., Taylor, C.B., & Haskell, W.L. (1993). Effects of differing intensities and formats of 12 months' exercise training on psychological outcomes in older adults. *Health Psychology, 12,* 292-300.

Kramer, A.F., Colcombe, S., Erickson, K., Belopolsky, A., McAuley, E., Cohen, N.J., et al. (2002). Effects of aerobic fitness training on human cortical functioning. *Journal of Molecular Neuroscience, 19,* 227-231.

Kramer, A.F., Hahn, S., Cohen, N.J., Banich, M.T., McAuley, E., Harrison, C.R., et al. (1999). Ageing, fitness and neurocognitive function. *Nature, 400,* 418-419.

McAuley, E., Blissmer, B., Marquez, D.X., Jerome, G., Kramer, A.F., & Katula, J. (2000). Social relations, physical activity, and well-being in older adults. *Preventive Medicine, 31,* 608-617.

McAuley, E., & Katula, J. (1998). Physical activity interventions in the elderly: Influence on physical health and psychological function. In R. Schulz, M.P. Lawton, & G. Maddox (Eds.), *Annual review of gerontology and geriatrics* (Vol. 18, pp. 115-154). New York: Springer.

McAuley, E., & Rudolph, D. (1995). Physical activity, aging, and psychological well-being. *Journal of Aging and Physical Activity, 3*(1), 67-98.

McPherson, B.D. (1990). *Aging as a social process.* Toronto: Butterworths.

McPherson, B.D. (1994). Sociocultural perspectives on aging and physical activity. *Journal of Aging and Physical Activity, 2*(4), 329-353.

Neugarten, B.L., Havighurst, R.J., & Tobin, S.S. (1961). The measurement of life satisfaction. *Journal of Gerontology, 16,* 134-143.

Panton, L.B., Graves, J.E., Pollock, M.L., Hagberg, J.M., & Chen, W. (1990). Effect of aerobic resistance training on fractionated reaction time and speed of movement. *Journal of Gerontology, 45,* 26-31.

Pavot, W., & Diener, E. (1991). *A Manual for the Satisfaction With Life Scale.* Urbana: University of Illinois.

Pollock, M.L., Foster, C., Knapp, D., Rod, J.L., & Schmidt, D.H. (1987). Effect of age and training on aerobic capacity and body composition of masters athletes. *Journal of Applied Physiology, 62,* 725-731.

Rejeski, W.J., & Mihalko, S.L. (2001). Physical activity and quality of life in older adults. *Journal of Gerontology, 56*(A), 23-35.

Rodin, J. (1986). Aging and health: Effects of the sense of control. *Science, 233,* 1271-1276.

Rogers, M.A., Hagberg, J.M., Martin, W.H., & Holloszy, J.O. (1990). Decline in VO₂max with aging in masters athletes and sedentary men. *Journal of Applied Physiology, 68,* 2195-2199.

Scully, D., Kremer, J., Meade, M.M., Graham, R., & Dudgeon, K. (1998). Physical exercise and psychological well being: A critical review. *Journal of Sports Medicine, 32,* 111-120.

Stewart, A.L., King, A.C., & Haskell, W.L. (1993). Endurance exercise and health-related quality of life in 50-65-year-old adults. *Gerontologist, 33,* 782-789.

Tzankoff, S.P., & Norris, A.H. (1978). Longitudinal changes in basal metabolic rate in man. *Journal of Applied Physiology, 33,* 536-539.

U.S. Surgeon General. (1996). *Physical activity and health.* Washington, DC: U.S. Department of Health and Human Services.

Ware, J.E., Kosinski, M., & Keller, S.D. (1994). *SF-36 physical and mental health summary scales: A user's manual.* Boston: Health Assessment Lab.

World Health Organization. (1997). The Heidelberg guidelines for promoting physical activity among older persons. *Journal of Aging and Physical Activity, 5*(1), 2-8.

Chapter 4

Alexander, N. (1994). Postural control in older adults. *Journal of the American Geriatrics Society, 42,* 93-108.

Barbosa, A.R., Santarem, J.M., Filho, W.J., & Marucci, M.de. F. (2002). Effects of resistance training on the sit-and-reach test in elderly women. *Journal of Strength and Conditioning Research, 16,* 14-18.

Billman, G.E. (2001). Aerobic exercise conditioning: A nonpharmocological antiarrhythmic intervention. *Journal of Applied Physiology, 92,* 446-454.

Blanchet, C., Giguere, Y., Prud'homme, D., Dumont, M., Rousseau, F., & Dodin, S. (2002). Association of physical activity and bone influence of vitamin D receptor genotype. *Medicine and Science in Sports and Exercise, 34,* 24-31.

Bougie, J.D. (2001). Osteoporosis. In J.D. Bougie and A.P. Morgenthal (Eds.), *The aging body: Conservative management of common neuromusculoskeletal conditions* (pp. 69-94). New York: McGraw-Hill.

Bouvier, F.B., Saltin, B., Nejat, M., & Jensen-Urstad, M. (2001). Left ventricular function and perfusion in elderly endurance athletes. *Medicine and Science in Sports and Exercise, 33,* 735-740.

Burr, D.B. (1997). Muscle strength, bone mass, and age-related bone loss. *Journal of Bone and Mineral Research, 12,* 1547-1551.

Connelly, D.M. (2000). Resisted exercise training of institutionalized older adults for improved strength and functional mobility: A review. *Topics in Geriatric Rehabilitation, 15,* 6-28.

Daley, M.J., & Spinks, W.L. (2000). Exercise, mobility, and aging. *Sports Medicine, 29,* 1-12.

Drinkwater, B. (1994). Physical activity, fitness, and osteoporosis. In C. Bouchard, R.J. Shephard, & T. Stephens (Eds.), *Physical activity, fitness, and health.* Champaign, IL: Human Kinetics.

Eagan, M.S., & Sedlock, D.A. (2001). Kyphosis in active and sedentary postmenopausal women. *Medicine and Science in Sports and Exercise, 33,* 688-695.

Eskurza, I., Donato, A.J., Moreau, K.L., Seals, D.R., & Tanaka, H. (2002). Changes in maximal aerobic capacity with age in endurance-trained women: 7-yr follow up. *Journal of Applied Physiology, 92,* 2302-2308.

Etnier, J.L., & Berry, M. (2001). Fluid intelligence in an older COPD sample after short- or long-term exercise. *Medicine and Science in Sports and Exercise, 33,* 1620-1628.

Etnier, J.L., & Landers, D.M. (1997). The influence of age and fitness on performance and learning. *Journal of Aging and Physical Activity, 5,* 175-189.

Ettinger, W.H., Burns, R., Messier, S.P., Applegate, W., Rejeski, W.J., Morgan, T., et al. (1997). A randomized trial comparing aerobic exercise and resistance exercise with a health education program in older adults with knee osteoarthritis: The Fitness Arthritis and Seniors Trial (FAST). *Journal of the American Medical Association, 277,* 25-31.

Fagard, R.H. (2001). Exercise characteristics and the blood pressure response to dynamic physical training. *Medicine and Science in Sports and Exercise, 33*(Suppl. 6), S484-S492.

Fatouras, K.G., Taxildaris, K., Tokmakidas, S.P., Kalapotharakos, V., Aggelousis, N., Athanasopoulos, S., et al. (2002). The effects of strength training, cardiovascular training and their combination on flexibility of inactive older adults. *International Journal of Sports Medicine, 23,* 112-119.

Fiatarone Singh, M.A. (2000). *Exercise, nutrition and the older woman.* Boca Raton, FL: CRC.

Fitzgerald, M.D., Tanaka, H., Tran, Z.V., & Seals, D.R. (1997). Age-related declines in maximal aerobic capacity in regularly exercising vs. sedentary women: A meta-analysis. *Journal of Applied Physiology, 83,* 160-165.

Foldvari, M., Clark, M., Laviolette, L.A., Bernstein, M.A., Kaliton, D., Castaneda, C., et al. (2000). Association of muscle power with functional status in community-dwelling elderly women. *Journal of Gerontology, 55A,* M192-M199.

Franklin, B.A. (Ed.). (2000). *ACSM's guidelines for exercise testing and prescription,* 6th ed. Philadelphia: Lippincott Williams & Wilkins.

Gonzales McNeal, M., Zareparsi, S., Camicioli, R., Dame, A., Howieson, D., Quinn, J., et al. (2001). Predictors of healthy brain aging. *Journal of Gerontology: Biological Sciences, 56A,* B294-B301.

Harada, N. (1995). Invited commentary. *Physical Therapy, 75,* 895-896.

Hawkins, S.A., Marcell, T.J., Jaque, S.V., & Wiswell, R.A. (2001). A longitudinal assessment of change in $\dot{V}O_{2max}$ and maximal heart rate in master athletes. *Medicine and Science in Sports and Exercise, 33,* 1744-1750.

Hepple, R.T. (2000). Skeletal muscle: Microcirculatory adaptation to metabolic demand. *Medicine and Science in Sports and Exercise, 32,* 117-123.

Ho, C.W., Beard, J.L., Farrell, A., Minson, C.T., & Kenney, W.L. (1997). Age, fitness, and regional blood flow during exercise in the heat. *Journal of Applied Physiology, 82,* 1126-1135.

Holloszy, J.O. (2001). Cellular adaptations to endurance exercise: Master athletes. *International Journal of Sports Nutrition and Exercise Metabolism, 11,* S186-S188.

Hughes, M.A., Duncan, P., Rose, D., Chandler, J., & Studenski, S.A. (1996). The relationship of postural sway to sensorimotor function, functional performance, and disability in the elderly. *Archives of Physical Medicine and Rehabilitation, 77,* 567-572.

Humphries, B., Newton, R.U., Bronks, R., Marshall, S., McBride, J., Triplett-McBride, T., et al. (2000). Effect of exercise intensity on bone density, strength, and calcium turnover in older women. *Medicine and Science in Sports and Exercise, 32,* 1043-2000.

Hunter, G.R., Wetzstein, C.J., Fields, D.A., Brown, A., & Bamman, M.M. (2000). Resistance training increases total energy expenditure and free-living physical activity in older adults. *Journal of Applied Physiology, 89,* 977-984.

Ishida, K., Sato, Y., Katayama, K., & Miyamura, M. (2000). Initial ventilatory and circulatory response to dynamic exercise are slowed in the elderly. *Journal of Applied Physiology, 89,* 1771-1777.

Kasch, F.W., Boyer, J.L., Schmidt, P.K., Wells, R.H., Wallace, J.P., Verity, L.S., et al. (1999). Ageing of the cardiovascular system during 33 years of aerobic exercise. *Age and Ageing, 28,* 531-536.

Katzman, R., & Terry, R. (1991). Normal aging of the nervous system. In R. Katzman & J.W. Rowe (Eds.), *Principles of geriatric neurology* (pp. 18-58). Philadelphia: Davis.

Kohrt, W.M. (2001). Aging and the osteogenic response to mechanical loading. *International Journal of Sports Nutrition and Exercise Metabolism, 11,* S137-S142.

Kohrt, W.M., Ehsani, A.A., & Birge, S.J., Jr. (1997). Effects of exercise involving predominantly either joint-reaction or ground-reaction forces on bone mineral density in older women. *Journal of Bone and Mineral Research, 12,* 1253-1261.

Krivickas, L.S., Suh, D., Wilkins, J., Hughes, V.A., Robenoff, R., & Frontera, W.A. (2001). Age- and gender-related differences in maximum shortening velocity of skeletal muscle fibers. *American Journal of Physical Medicine and Rehabilitation, 80,* 447-455.

Landers, K.A., Hunter, G.R., Wetzstein, C.J., Bamman, M.M., & Wiensier, R.L. (2001). The interrelationship among muscle mass, strength, and the ability to perform physical tasks of daily living in younger and older women. *Journal of Gerontology: Biological Sciences, 56A,* B443-B448.

Laurin, D., Verreault, R., Lindsay, J., MacPherson, K., & Rockwood, K. (2001). Physical activity and risk of cognitive impairment and dementia in elderly persons. *Archives of Neurology, 58,* 498-504.

Marcus, R. (2001). Role of exercise in preventing and treating osteoporosis. *Rheumatic Disease Clinics of North America, 27,* 131-141.

Masoro, E.J. (2001). Physiology of aging. *International Journal of Sports Nutrition and Exercise Metabolism, 11,* S218-S222.

McCole, S.D., Brown, M.D., Moore, G.E., Zmuda, J.M., Cwynar, J.D., & Hagberg, J.M. (1999). Cardiovascular hemodynamics with increasing exercise intensities in postmenopausal women. *Journal of Applied Physiology, 87,* 2334-2340.

Metcalfe, L., Lohman, T., Going, S., Houtkooper, L., Ferriera, D., Flint-Wagner, H., et al. (2001). Postmenopausal women and exercise for prevention of osteoporosis. *ACSM's Health and Fitness Journal, 5,* 6-14.

Moreau, K.L., Degarmo, R., Langley, J., McMahon, C., Howley, E.T., Bassett, D.R., Jr., et al. (2001). Increased daily walking lowers blood pressure in postmenopausal women. *Medicine and Science in Sports and Exercise, 33,* 1825-1831.

Morgenthal, A.P. (2001). The age-related challenges of posture and balance. In J.D. Bougie & A.P. Morgenthal (Eds.), *The aging body: Conservative management of common neuromusculoskeletal conditions* (pp. 45-68). New York: McGraw-Hill.

Overstall, P.W., & Downton, J.H. (1998). Gait, balance, and falls. In M.S.J. Pathy (Ed.), *Principles and practices of geriatric medicine* (pp. 1121-1132). Chichester, UK: Wiley.

Paterson, D.H., Cunningham, D.A., Koval, J.J., & St. Croix, C.M. (1999). Aerobic fitness in a population of independently living men and women aged 55-86 years. *Medicine and Science in Sports and Exercise, 31,* 1813-1820.

Perini, R., Fisher, N., Veicsteinas, A., & Pendergast, D.L. (2002). Aerobic training and cardiovascular responses at rest and during exercise in older men and women. *Medicine and Science in Sports and Exercise, 34,* 700-708.

Pollock, M.L., Mengelkoch, L.J., Graves, J.E., Lowenthal, D.T., Limacher, M.C., Foster, C., et al. (1997). Twenty-year follow-up of aerobic power and body composition of older track athletes. *Journal of Applied Physiology, 82,* 1508-1516.

Proctor, D.N., Beck, K.C., Shen, P.H., Eickhoff, T.J., Halliwill, J.R., & Joyner, M.J. (1998a). Influence of age and gender on cardiac output–$\dot{V}O_2$ relationships during submaximal cycle ergometry. *Journal of Applied Physiology, 84,* 599-605.

Proctor, D.N., Shen, P.H., Dietz, N., Eickhoff, T.J., Lawler, L.A., Ebersold, E.J., et al. (1998b). Reduced leg blood flow during dynamic exercise in older endurance-trained men. *Journal of Applied Physiology, 85,* 68-75.

Rappaport, L.J., Hanks, R.A., Millis, J.R., & Deshpande, S.A. (1998). Executive functioning and predictors of falls in the rehabilitation setting. *Archives of Physical Medicine and Rehabilitation, 79,* 629-633.

Richardson, R.S., Harms, C.A., Grassi, B., & Hepple, R.T. (2000). Skeletal muscle: Master or slave of the cardiovascular system? *Medicine and Science in Sports and Exercise, 32,* 89-93.

Robbins, S., Waked, E., & McClaran, J. (1995). Proprioception and stability: Foot position awareness as a function of age and footwear. *Age and Ageing, 24,* 67-72.

Roth, S.M., Martell, G.F., Ivey, F.M., Lemmer, J.T., Metter, E.J., Hurley, B.F., et al. (2000). High-volume, heavy-resistance strength training and muscle damage in young and older women. *Journal of Applied Physiology, 88,* 1112-1118.

Scheuermann, B.W., Bell, C., Paterson, D.H., Barstow, T.J., & Kowalchuk, J.M. (2002). Oxygen uptake kinetics for moderate exercise are speeded up in older humans by prior heavy exercise. *Journal of Applied Physiology, 92,* 609-616.

Seals, D.R., Monahan, K.D., Bell, C., Tanaka, H., and Jones, P.P. (2001). The aging cardiovascular system: Changes in autonomic function at rest and in response to exercise. *International Journal of Sports Nutrition and Exercise Metabolism, 11,* S189-S195.

Shephard, R.J. (1997). *Aging, physical activity, and health.* Champaign, IL: Human Kinetics.

Short, K.R., & Nair, K.S. (2001). Muscle protein metabolism and the sarcopenia of aging. *International Journal of Sports Nutrition and Exercise Metabolism, 11,* S119-S127.

Siddiqui, N.A., Shetty, K.R., & Duthie, E.H. (1999). Osteoporosis in older men: Discovering when and how to treat it. *Geriatrics, 54,* 20-30.

Silvestrone, J.M. (2001). Neurologic changes with age. In J.D. Bougie & A.P. Morgenthal (Eds.), *The aging body: Conservative management of common neuromusculoskeletal conditions* (pp. 17-34). New York: McGraw-Hill.

Slade, J.M., Miszko, T.A., Laity, J.H., Agrawal, S.K., and Cress, M.E. (2002). Anaerobic power and physical function in strength-trained and non-strength-trained older adults. *Journal of Gerontology: Medical Sciences, 57A,* M168-M172.

Snow, C.M., Shaw, J.M., Winters, K.M., & Witzke, K.A. (2000). Long-term exercise using weighted vests prevents hip bone loss in postmenopausal women. *Journal of Gerontology: Medical Sciences, 55A,* M489-M491.

Thompson, L.V. (2002). Skeletal muscle adaptations with age, inactivity, and therapeutic exercise. *Journal of Orthopaedic and Sports Physical Therapy, 32,* 44-57.

Timiras, P.S. (1994). *Physiological basis of aging and geriatrics.* Boca Raton, FL: CRC Press.

Van Boxtel, M.P.J., Paas, F.G.W.C., Houx, P.J., Adam, J.J., Teeken, J.L., & Jolles, J. (1997). Aerobic capacity and cognitive performance in a cross-sectional aging study. *Medicine and Science in Sports and Exercise, 29,* 1357-1365.

Vincent, K.R., & Braith, R.W. (2002). Resistance exercise and bone turnover in elderly men and women. *Medicine and Science in Sports and Exercise, 34,* 17-23.

Wiebe, C.G., Gledhill, N., Jamnik, V.K., & Ferguson, S. (1999). Exercise cardiac function in young through elderly endurance trained women. *Medicine and Science in Sports and Exercise, 31,* 684-691.

Wilmore, J.H., & Costill, D.L. (2004). *Physiology of sport and exercise* (3rd ed.). Champaign, IL: Human Kinetics.

Womack, C.J., Ivey, F.M., Gardner, A.W., & Macko, R.F. (2001). Fibrinolytic response to acute exercise in patients with peripheral arterial disease. *Medicine and Science in Sports and Exercise, 33,* 214-219.

Yaffe, K., Barnes, D., Nevitt, M., Lui, L.-Y., & Covinski, K. (2001). A prospective study of physical activity and cognitive decline in elderly women: Women who walk. *Archives of Internal Medicine, 161,* 1703-1708.

Chapter 5

American College of Sports Medicine. (2000). *ACSM's guidelines for exercise testing and prescription* (6th ed.). Philadelphia: Lippincott Williams & Wilkins.

Expert Panel on the Identification, Evaluation, and Treatment of Overweight and Obesity in Adults. (1998). Executive summary of the clinical guidelines on the identification, evaluation, and treatment of overweight and obesity in adults. *Archives of Internal Medicine, 158,* 1855-1867.

Heyward, V.E., & Stolarczyk, L.M. (1996). *Applied body composition assessment.* Champaign, IL: Human Kinetics, 82.

Rikli, R.E., & Jones, C.J. (1998). The reliability and validity of a 6-minute walk test as a measure of physical endurance in older adults. *Journal of Aging and Physical Activity, 6,* 363-375.

Siscovick, D.S., Weiss, N.S., Fletcher, R.H., & Lasky, T. (1984). The incidence of primary cardiac arrest during vigorous exercise. *New England Journal of Medicine, 311,* 874-877.

Chapter 6

Berg, K., Wood-Dauphinee, S.L., & Williams, J.T. (1992). Measuring balance in the elderly: Validation of an instrument. *Canadian Journal of Public Health, 83,* S9-S11.

Berg, K.O., Wood-Dauphinee, S.L., Williams, J.I., & Gayton, D. (1989). Measuring balance in the elderly: Preliminary development of an instrument. *Physiotherapy Canada, 41,* 304-311.

Guralnik, J.M., Ferrucci, L., Pieper, C., et al. (2000). Lower extremity function and subsequent disability: Consistency across studies, predictive models, and value of gait speed alone compared with the short physical performance battery. *Journal of Gerontology: Medical Sciences, 55,* M221-M231.

Rikli, R.E., & Jones, C.J. (1997). Assessing physical performance in independent older adults: Issues and guidelines. *Journal of Aging and Physical Activity, 5,* 244-261.

Rikli, R.E., & Jones, C.J. (1999). Functional fitness normative scores for community-residing older adults, ages 60-94. *Journal of Aging and Physical Activity, 7,* 162-181.

Rikli, R.E., & Jones, C.J. (2001). *Senior fitness test.* Champaign, IL: Human Kinetics.

Rose, D.J. (2003). *FallProof: A comprehensive balance and mobility program.* Champaign, IL: Human Kinetics.

VanSwearingen, J.M., & Brach, J.S. (2001). Making geriatric assessment work: Selecting useful measures. *Physical Therapy, 81,* 1233-1252.

Chapter 7

Enoka, R.M. (2001). *Neuromechanics of human movement* (3rd ed.). Champaign, IL: Human Kinetics.

Franklin, B.A., Whaley, M.H., & Howley, E.T. (2000). *ACSM's guidelines for exercise testing and prescription* (6th ed.). Philadelphia: Lippincott Williams & Wilkins.

Hunter, S., White, M., & Thompson, M. (1998). Techniques to evaluate elderly human muscle function: A physiological basis. *Journal of Gerontology: Biological Sciences, 53A,* B204-B216.

Paterson, D.H., Cunningham, D.A., Koval, J.J., & St. Croix, C.M. (1999). Aerobic fitness in a population of independently living men and women. *Medicine and Science in Sports and Exercise, 31,* 1813-1820.

Patla, A.E., Winter, D.A., Frank, J.S., Walt, S.E., & Prasad, S. (1990). The role of instability in falls among older persons. In P.T. Duncan (Ed.), *Balance: Proceedings of the APTA Forum.* Nashville, TN: American Physical Therapy Association.

Rose, D.J. (2003). *FallProof: A comprehensive balance and mobility program.* Champaign, IL: Human Kinetics.

Sale, D., & MacDougall, D. (1981). Specificity in strength training: A review for the coach and athlete. *Canadian Journal of Applied Sports Sciences, 6,* 87-92.

Chapter 8

Bandura, A. (1977). Self-efficacy: Toward a unifying theory of behavioral change. *Psychological Review, 84,* 191-215.

Bandura, A. (1982). Self-efficacy mechanism in human agency. *American Psychologist, 37,* 122-147.

Boutelle, K.N., & Kirschenbaum, D.S. (1998). Further support for consistent self-monitoring as a vital component of successful weight control. *Obesity Research, 6,* 219-224.

Brawley, L.R., Rejeski, W.J., & Lutes, L. (2000). A group-mediated cognitive-behavioral intervention for increasing adherence to physical activity in older adults. *Journal of Applied Biobehavioral Research, 5,* 47-65.

Brittain, E.L., Jones, C.J., & Rikli, R.E. (2002). Barriers to physical activity in older adults as a function of age, gender, and activity level [Abstract]. *Medicine and Science in Sports and Exercise, 33,* S75.

Ettinger, W.H., Jr., Burns, R., Messier, S.P., Applegate, W., Rejeski, W.J., Morgan, T., et al. (1997). A randomized trial comparing aerobic exercise and resistance exercise with a health education program in older adults with knee osteoarthritis: The Fitness Arthritis and Seniors Trial (FAST). *Journal of the American Medical Association, 277,* 25-31.

Goldstein, A.P., & Higginbotham, H.N. (1991). Relationship-enhancement methods. In F.H. Kanfer & A.P. Goldstein (Eds.), *Helping people change: A textbook of methods* (4th ed., pp. 20-69). New York: Pergamon Press.

Goran, M.I., & Poehlman, E.T. (1992). Endurance training does not enhance total energy expenditure in healthy elderly persons. *American Journal of Physiology, 263,* E950-E957.

Jette, A.M., Lachman, M., Giorgetti, M.M., Assmann, S.F., Harris, B.A., Levenson, C., et al. (1999). Exercise—it's never too late: The strong-for-life program. *American Journal of Public Health, 89,* 66-72.

King, A.C. (2001). Interventions to promote physical activity by older adults. *Journal of Gerontology, 56A,* 36-46.

King, A.C., Castro, C., Wilcox, S., Eyler, A.A., Sallis, J.F., & Brownson, R.C. (2000). Personal and environmental factors associated with physical inactivity among different racial-ethnic groups of U.S. middle-aged and older-aged women. *Health Psychology, 19,* 354-364.

King, A.C., Haskell, W.L., Taylor, C.B., Kraemer, H.C., & DeBusk, R.F. (1991). Group- vs home-based exercise training in healthy older men and women: A community-based clinical trial. *Journal of the American Medical Association, 266,* 1535-1542.

King, A.C., Haskell, W.L., Young, D.R., Oka, R.K., & Stefanick, M.L. (1995). Long-term effects of varying intensities and formats of physical activity on participation rates, fitness, and lipoproteins in men and women aged 50 to 65 years. *Circulation, 91,* 2596-2604.

King, A.C., Pruitt, L.A., Phillips, W., Oka, R., Rodenburg, A., & Haskell, W.L. (2000). Comparative effects of two physical activity programs on measured and perceived physical functioning and other health-related quality of life outcomes in older adults. *Journal of Gerontology, 55A,* M74-M83.

King, A.C., Rejeski, W.J., & Buchner, D.M. (1998). Physical activity interventions targeting older adults: A critical review and recommendations. *American Journal of Preventive Medicine, 15,* 316-333.

Marcus, B.H., & Forsyth, L.H. (2003). *Motivating people to be physically active.* Champaign, IL: Human Kinetics.

Marlatt, G.A., & Gorden, J.R. (1985). *Relapse prevention: Maintenance strategies in the treatment of addictive behaviors.* New York: Guilford Press.

Neale, A.V. (1991). Behavioural contracting as a tool to help patients achieve better health. *Family Practice, 8,* 336-342.

O'Brien, S.J., & Vertinsky, P.A. (1991). Unfit survivors: Exercise as a resource for aging women. *Gerontologist, 31,* 347-357.

Prochaska, J.O., DiClemente, C.C., & Norcross, J.C. (1992). In search of how people change: Applications to addictive behaviors. *American Psychologist, 47,* 1102-1114.

Prochaska, J.O., & Marcus, B.H. (1994). The transtheoretical model: Applications to exercise. In R.K. Dishman (Ed.), *Advances in exercise adherence* (pp. 161-180). Champaign, IL: Human Kinetics.

Robert Wood Johnson Foundation. (2001). *National blueprint: Increasing physical activity among adults age 50 and older.* Princeton, NJ: Author.

Sallis, J.F., & Owen, N. (1999). *Physical activity and behavioral medicine.* Thousand Oaks, CA: Sage.

Stewart, A.L., Mills, K.M., Sepsis, P.G., King, A.C., McLellan, B.Y., Roitz, K., et al. (1997). Evaluation of CHAMPS, a physical activity promotion program for older adults. *Annals of Behavioral Medicine, 19,* 353-361.

Stewart, A.L., Verboncoeur, C.J., McLellan, B.Y., Gillis, D.E., Rush, S., Mills, K.M., et al. (2001). Physical activity outcomes of CHAMPS II: A physical activity promotion program for older adults. *Journal of Gerontology, 56A,* M465-M470.

U.S. Department of Health and Human Services. (1996). *Physical activity and health: A report of the Surgeon General.* Atlanta, GA: National Center for Chronic Disease Prevention and Health Promotion, Centers for Disease Control and Prevention, U.S. Department of Health and Human Services.

Wilcox, S., King, A.C., Brassington, G.S., & Ahn, D.K. (1999). Physical activity preferences of middle-aged and older adults: A community analysis. *Journal of Aging and Physical Activity, 7,* 386-399.

Wilcox, S., Tudor-Locke, C.E., & Ainsworth, B.E. (2002). Physical activity patterns, assessment, and motivation in older adults. In R.J. Shephard (Ed.), *Gender, physical activity, and aging* (pp. 13-39). Boca Raton, FL: CRC Press.

Chapter 9

American College of Sports Medicine. (1998). ACSM position stand on exercise and physical activity for older adults. *Medicine and Science in Sports and Exercise, 30,* 992-1008.

American College of Sports Medicine. (2000). *ACSM's guidelines for exercise testing and prescription* (6th ed.). Philadelphia: Lippincott Williams & Wilkins.

Buchner, D.M. (1997). Preserving mobility in older adults. *Western Journal of Medicine, 167,* 258-264.

Buchner, D.M., Beresford, S.A.A., Larson, E.B., LaCroix, A.Z., & Wagner, E.H. (1992). Effects of physical activity on health status in older adults II: Intervention studies. *Annual Review of Public Health, 13,* 469-488.

Cress, M.E., Buchner, D.M., Questad, K.A., Esselman, P.C., deLateur, B.J., & Schwartz, R.S. (1999). Exercise: Effects on physical functional performance in independent older adults. *Journal of Gerontology: Medical Sciences, 54A,* M242-M248.

Evans, W.J. (1995). What is sarcopenia? *Journals of Gerontology Series A, 50A* (Special issue), 5-8.

Jones, C.J. (2002). Assessment-based exercise prescription for older adults. Paper presented at the metting fo the ACSM: Health and Fitness Summit, Orlando, FL.

Nagi, S.Z. (1976). An epidemiology of disability among adults in the United States. *Milbank Memorial Fund Quarterly, 54,* 439-467.

Nagi, S.Z. (1991). Disability concepts revisited: Implications for prevention. In A.M. Pope & A.R. Tarlov (Eds.), *Disability in America: Toward a national agenda for prevention* (pp. 309-327). Washington, DC: National Academy Press.

National Institute on Aging. (1998). *Exercise: A guide from the National Institute on Aging* (Publication No. NIH 98-4258). Washington, DC: National Institutes of Health.

Ostchega, Y., Harris, T.B., Hirsch, R., Parsons, V.L., & Kington, R. (2000). The prevalence of functional limitations and disability in older persons in the US: Data from the National Health and Nutrition Examination Survey III. *Journal of the American Geriatrics Society, 48,* 1132-1135.

Partnership for Solutions. (2002). *Chronic conditions: Making the case for ongoing care.* Baltimore: Johns Hopkins University.

Pope, A.M., & Tarlov, A.R. (Eds.) (1991). *Disability in America: Toward a national agenda for prevention.* Washington, DC: National Academy Press.

Rikli, R.E., & Jones, C.J. (1999). Development and validation of a functional fitness test for community-residing older adults. *Journal of Aging and Physical Activity, 7,* 129-161.

Rikli, R.E., & Jones, C.J. (2001). *Senior fitness test manual.* Champaign, IL: Human Kinetics.

Rose, D.J. (2003). *FallProof!: A comprehensive balance and mobility program.* Champaign, IL: Human Kinetics.

Schlicht, J., Camaione, D.N., & Owen, S.V. (2001). Effect of intense strength training on standing balance, walking speed, and sit-to-stand performance in older adults. *Journal of Gerontology: Medical Sciences, 56A,* M281-M286.

Shephard, R.J. (1993). Exercise and aging: Extending independence in older adults. *Geriatrics, 48,* 61-64.

Simonsick, E.M., Newman, A.B., Nevitt, M.C., Kritchevsky, S.B., Ferrucci, L., Guralnik, J.M., et al., for the Health ABC Study Group. (2001). Measuring higher level physical function in well-functioning older adults: Expanding familiar approaches in the Health ABC Study. *Journal of Gerontology: Medical Sciences, 56A,* M644-M649.

Stewart, A.L., & Painter, P.L. (1998). A conceptual framework for studying functional decline, disability, and health-related quality of life in exercise studies. *Medicine and Science in Sports and Exercise, 30*(Suppl.), S86.

Stewart, A.L. (2003). Conceptual challenges in linking physical activity and disability research. *American Journal of Preventive Medicine, 25*(Suppl.), 137-140.

Verbrugge, L.M., & Jette, A.M. (1994). The disablement process. *Social Science and Medicine, 38,* 1-14.

Vita, A.J., Terry, R.B., Hubert, H.B., & Fries, J.F. (1998). Aging, health risks, and cumulative disability. *New England Journal of Medicine, 338,* 1035-1041.

Chapter 10

American College of Sports Medicine. (2000). *ACSM's guidelines for exercise testing and prescription* (6th ed.). Philadelphia: Lippincott Williams & Wilkins.

Bandura, A. (1997). *Self-efficacy: The exercise of control.* New York: Freeman.

Borg, G. (1998). *Borg's Perceived Exertion and Pain Scales.* Champaign, IL: Human Kinetics.

DeVries, H.A., & Housh, T.J. (1994). *Physiology of exercise for PE: Athletes and exercise science.* Dubuque, IA: Brown and Benchmark.

Nieman, D.C. (1999). *Exercise testing and prescription: A health-related approach.* Mountain View, CA: Mayfield.

Wise, J.B., & Trunnell, E.P. (2001). The influence of sources of self-efficacy upon efficacy strength. *Journal of Sport and Exercise Psychology, 23,* 268-280.

Chapter 11

Bell, R., & Hoshizaki, T. (1981). Relationships of age and sex with joint range of motion of seventeen joint actions in humans. *Canadian Journal of Applied Sport Sciences, 6,* 202-206.

Brooks, S.V., & Faulkner, J.A. (1996). The magnitude of the initial injury induced by stretches of maximally activated muscle fibres of mice and rats increases in old age. *Journal of Physiology, 497,* 573-580.

Brown, M., & Holloszy, J.O. (1991). Effects of a low intensity exercise program on selected physical performance characteristics of 60- to 71-year-olds. *Aging: Clinical and Experimental Research, 3,* 129-139.

Brown, M., Sinacore, D.R., Ehsani, A.A., Binder, E.F., & Holloszy, J.O. (2000). Low-intensity exercise as a modifier of physical frailty in older adults. *Archives of Physical Medicine and Rehabilitation, 81,* 960-965.

Buckwalter, J.A., Woo, S.L., Goldberg, V.M., Hadley, E.C., Booth, F., Oegema, T.R., et al. (1993). Soft tissue aging and musculoskeletal function. *Journal of Bone and Joint Surgery, 75,* 1533-1548.

Cetta, G., Tenni, R., Zanaboni, G., & Maroudas, A. (1982). Biochemical and morphological modifications in rabbit Achilles tendon during maturation and ageing. *Biomechanics Journal, 204,* 61-67.

Eddinger, T.J., Cassens, R.G., & Moss, R.L. (1986). Mechanical and histochemical characterization of skeletal muscles from senescent rats. *American Journal of Physiology, 251,* C421-C430.

Einkauf, D.K., Gohdes, M.L., Jensen, G.M., & Jewell, M.J. (1987). Changes in spinal mobility with increasing age in women. *Physical Therapy, 67,* 370-375.

Frekany, M.A., & Leslie, D.K. (1975). Effects of an exercise program on selected flexibility measurements of senior citizens. *Gerontologist 15,* 182-183.

Golding, L.A., & Lindsay, A. (1989). Flexibility and age. *Perspective, 15*(6): 28-30.

Holland, G.J., Tanaka, K., Shigematsu, R., & Nakagaichi, M. (2002). Flexibility and physical functions of older adults: A review. *Journal of Aging and Physical Activity, 10,* 169-206.

James, B., & Parker, A.W. (1989). Active and passive mobility of lower limb joints in elderly men and women. *American Journal of Physical Medicine and Rehabilitation, 68,* 162-167.

Lindsay, D.M., Horton, J.F., & Vandervoort, A.A. (2000). A review of injury characteristics, aging factors and prevention programmes for the older golfer. *Sports Medicine, 30,* 89-103.

Lung, M.W., Hartsell, H.D., & Vandervoort, A.A. (1996). Effects of aging on joint stiffness: Implications for exercise. *Physiotherapy Canada, 48,* 96-106.

McHugh, M.P., Connolly, D.A., Eston, R.G., Kremenic, I.J., Nicholas, S.J., & Gleim, G.W. (1999). The role of passive muscle stiffness in symptoms of exercise-induced muscle damage. *American Journal of Sports Medicine, 27,* 594-599.

Misner, J.E., Massey, B.H., Bemben, M., Going, S., & Patrick, J. (1992). Long-term effects of exercise on the range of motion of aging women. *Journal of Orthopedic and Sports Physical Therapy, 16,* 37-42.

Moskowitz, R.W. (1989). Clinical and laboratory findings in osteoarthritis. In D.J. McCarty (Ed.), *Arthritis and allied conditions* (pp. 1605-1630). Philadelphia: Lea & Febiger.

Munns, K. (1981). Effects of exercise on the range of joint motion in elderly subjects. In E.L. Smith & R.C. Serfass (Eds.), *Exercise and aging: The scientific basis* (pp. 167-178). Hillside, NJ: Enslow.

Nigg, B.M., Fisher, V., Allinger, T.L., Ronsky, J.R., & Engsberg, J.R. (1992). Range of motion of the foot as a function of age. *Foot and Ankle, 13,* 336-343.

Noonan, T.J., & Garrett, W.E., Jr. (1999). Muscle strain injury: Diagnosis and treatment. *Journal of American Orthopaedic Surgery, 7,* 262-269.

Ploutz-Snyder, L.L., Giannis, E.L., Formikell, M., & Rosenbaum, A.E. (2001). Resistance training reduces susceptibility to eccentric exercise-induced muscle dysfunction in older women. *Journal of Gerontology: Biological Sciences, 56,* B384-B390.

Raab, D.M., Agre, J.C., McAdam, M., & Smith, E.L. (1988). Light resistance and stretching exercise in elderly women: Effect upon flexibility. *Archives of Physical Medicine and Rehabilitation, 69,* 268-272.

Sjostrom, M., Lexell, J., & Downham, D.Y. (1992). Differences in fiber number and fiber type proportion within fascicles: A quantitative morphological study of whole vastus lateralis muscle from childhood to old age. *Anatomical Records, 234,* 183-189.

Svenningsen, S., Terjesen, T., Auflem, M., & Berg, V. (1989). Hip motion related to age and sex. *Acta Orthopaedica Scandinavia, 60,* 97-10.

Vandervoort, A.A., Chesworth, B.M., Cunningham, D.A., Paterson, D.H., Rechnitzer, P.A., & Koval, J.J. (1992). Age and sex effects on mobility of the human ankle. *Journal of Gerontology: Medical Sciences, 47,* M17-M21.

Walker, J.M., Sue, D., Miles-Elkousy, N., Ford, G., & Trevelyan, H. (1984). Active mobility of the extremities in older subjects. *Physical Therapy, 64,* 919-923.

Wolf, (2002). Moving the body. *IDEA Personal Trainer* (June): 24-31.

Chapter 12

Baechle, T.R., & Earle, R.W. (2000). *Essentials of strength training and conditioning* (2nd ed.). Champaign, IL: Human Kinetics.

Bassey, E.J., Fiatarone, M.A., O'Neill, E.F., Kelly, M., Evans, W.J., & Lipsitz, L.A. (1992). Leg extensor power and functional performance in very old men and women. *Clinical Science (London), 82,* 321-327.

Bendall, M.J., Bassey, E.J., & Pearson, M.B. (1989). Factors affecting walking speed of elderly people. *Age and Ageing, 18,* 327-332.

Charette, S.L., McEvoy, L., Pyka, G., Snow-Harter, C., Guido, D., Wiswell, R.A., et al. (1991). Muscle hypertrophy response to resistance training in older women. *Journal of Applied Physiology, 70,* 1912-1916.

Clyman, B. (2001). Exercise in the treatment of osteoarthritis. *Current Rheumatology Reports, 3,* 520-523.

Ebbeling, C.B., & Clarkson, P.M. (1989). Exercise-induced muscle damage and adaptation. *Sports Medicine, 7,* 207-234.

Evans, W.J. (1996). Reversing sarcopenia: How weight training can build strength and vitality. *Geriatrics, 51,* 46-47, 51-53; quiz 54.

Evans, W.J. (1999). Exercise training guidelines for the elderly. *Medicine and Science in Sports and Exercise, 31,* 12-17.

Faigenbaum, A.D., Skrinar, G.S., Cesare, W.F., Kraemer, W.J., & Thomas, H.E. (1990). Physiologic and symptomatic responses of cardiac patients to resistance exercise. *Archives of Physical Medicine and Rehabilitation, 71,* 395-398.

Feigenbaum, M.S., & Pollock, M.L. (1999). Prescription of resistance training for health and disease. *Medicine and Science in Sports and Exercise, 31,* 38-45.

Fiatarone, M.A., Marks, E.C., Ryan, N.D., Meredith, C.N., Lipsitz, L.A., & Evans, W.J. (1990). High-intensity strength training in nonagenarians: Effects on skeletal muscle. *Journal of the American Medical Association, 263,* 3029-3034.

Fleck, S.J., & Kraemer, W.J. (2004). *Designing resistance training programs* (3rd ed.). Champaign, IL: Human Kinetics.

Gersten, J.W. (1991). Effect of exercise on muscle function decline with aging. *Western Journal of Medicine, 154,* 579-582.

Häkkinen, K., Newton, R.U., Gordon, S.E., McCormick, M., Volek, J.S., Nindl, B.C., et al. (1998). Changes in muscle morphology, electromyographic activity, and force production characteristics during progressive strength training in young and older men. *Journal of Gerontology: Biological Sciences, 53,* B415-B423.

Hather, B.M., Tesch, P.A., Buchanan, P., & Dudley, G.A. (1991). Influence of eccentric actions on skeletal muscle adaptations to resistance training. *Acta Physiologica Scandinavia, 143,* 177-185.

Heitkamp, H.C., Horstmann, T., Mayer, F., Weller, J., & Dickhuth, H.H. (2001). Gain in strength and muscular balance after balance training. *International Journal of Sports Medicine, 22,* 285-290.

Hunter, G.R., & Treuth, M.S. (1995). Relative training intensity and increases in older women. *Journal of Strength and Conditioning Research, 9,* 188-191.

Hurley, B.F., & Roth, S.M. (2000). Strength training in the elderly: Effects on risk factors for age-related diseases. *Sports Medicine, 30,* 249-268.

Kelley, G.A., & Kelley, K.S. (2000). Progressive resistance exercise and resting blood pressure: A meta-analysis of randomized controlled trials. *Hypertension, 35,* 838-843.

Komi, P.V., Kaneko, M., & Aura, O. (1987). EMG activity of the leg extensor muscles with special reference to mechanical efficiency in concentric and eccentric exercise. *International Journal of Sports Medicine, 8*(Suppl. 1), 22-29.

Kraemer, W.J., Adams, K., Cafarelli, E., Dudley, G.A., Dooly, C., Feigenbaum, M.S., et al. (2002). American College of Sports Medicine position stand: Progression models in resistance training for healthy adults. *Medicine and Science in Sports and Exercise, 34,* 364-380.

Kraemer, W.J., & Ratamess, N.A. (2000). Physiology of resistance training: Current issues. *Orthopaedic Physical Therapy Clinics of North America: Exercise Technologies, 9,* 467-513.

Kraemer, W.J., Ratamess, N.A., & French, D.N. (2002). Resistance training for health and performance. *Current Sports Medicine Reports, 1,* 165-171.

Pollock, M.L., Franklin, B.A., Balady, G.J., Chaitman, B.L., Fleg, J.L., Fletcher, B., et al. (2000). Resistance exercise in individuals with and without cardiovascular disease: Benefits, rationale, safety, and prescription. *Circulation, 101,* 828-833.

Rogers, M.A., & Evans, W.J. (1993). Changes in skeletal muscle with aging: Effects of exercise training. *Exercise and Sport Sciences Reviews, 21,* 65-102.

Shaw, C.E., McCully, K.K., & Posner, J.D. (1995). Injuries during the one repetition maximum assessment in the elderly. *Journal of Cardiopulmonary Rehabilitation, 15,* 283-287.

Sipila, S., Elorinne, M., Alen, M., Suominen, H., & Kovanen, V. (1997). Effects of strength and endurance training on muscle fibre characteristics in elderly women. *Clinical Physiology, 17,* 459-474.

Chapter 13

American College of Sports Medicine. (1990). The recommended quantity and quality of exercise for developing and maintaining cardiorespiratory and muscular fitness in healthy adults. *Medicine and Science in Sports and Exercise, 22,* 265-274.

American College of Sports Medicine. (1998). ACSM position stand on exercise and physical activity for older adults. *Medicine and Science in Sports and Exercise, 30,* 992-1008.

American College of Sports Medicine. (2000). *ACSM's guidelines for exercise testing and prescription* (6th ed.). Philadelphia: Lippincott Williams & Wilkins.

Bell, J. (2001). Delivering an exercise prescription for patients with coronary artery disease. In A. Young & M. Harries (Eds.), *Physical activity for patients: An exercise prescription.* (71-81). London: Royal College of Physicians.

Bell, J.M., & Bassey, E.J. (1996). Post exercise heart rates and pulse palpation as a means of determining exercising intensity in an aerobic dance class. *British Journal of Sports Medicine 30,* 48-52.

Bompa, T.O. (1999). *Periodization: Theory and methodology of training.* Champaign, IL: Human Kinetics.

Borg, G., & Hassmen, P. (1999). Physical activity and perceived exertion: Basic knowledge with applications for the elderly. *Advances in Rehabilitation, 1,* 17-34.

Brooks, D.S. (1997). *Program design for personal trainers.* Champaign, IL: Human Kinetics.

Brown, D.R., Wang, Y., Ward, A., Ebbeling, C.B., Fortlage, L., Puleo, E., Benson, H., Rippe, J.M. (1995). Chronic psychological effects of exercise and exercise plus cognitive strategies. *Medicine and Science in Sports and Exercise, 27,* 765-775.

Ceci, R., & Hassmen, P. (1991). Self-monitored exercise at three different RPE intensities in treadmill vs. field running. *Medicine and Science in Sports and Exercise, 23,* 732-738.

Cooper, K.H., Purdy, J.G., White, S.R., & Pollock, M.L. (1977). Age-fitness adjusted maximal heart rates. *Medicine and Sport, 10,* 78-88.

Dinan, S. (2002). Exercise for vulnerable older patients. In A. Young & M. Harries (Eds.), *Physical activity for patients: An exercising prescription.* (53-70). London: Royal College of Physicians.

Dinan, S. (2001). Safety first. In *Alive and kicking.* London: Age Concern Books.

Dinan, S., & Skelton, D. (2000). In J. Bassey & K. Malbut (Eds.), *Department of Health exercise for the prevention of falls and injuries advanced instructor training course manual.* (Manual 2, Section 3). London: Later *Life Training.*

Evans, W.J. (1999). Exercise training guidelines for the elderly. *Medicine and Science in Sports and Exercise, 31,* 12-17.

Fiatarone Singh, M.A. (2000). *Exercise, nutrition and the older woman.* Boca Raton, FL: CRC Press.

Haskell, W.L. (1997). Medical clearance for exercise program participation by older persons: The clinical versus the public health approach. In G. Huber (Ed.), *Healthy aging, activity and sports.* Hamburg: Health Promotion.

Hassmen, P., & Koivula, N. (1997). Mood, physical working capacity and cognitive performance in the elderly as related to physical activity. *Aging (Milano), 9,* 136-142.

Health Education Authority. (1997). *Physical activity "at our age": Qualitative research among people over the age of 50.* Physical Activity Research. London: Health Education Authority.

Heyward, V.H. (1998). *Advanced fitness assessment exercise prescription.* Champaign, IL: Human Kinetics.

Hill, R.D., Storandt, M., & Malley, M. (1993). The impact of long-term exercise training on psychological function in older adults. *Journal of Gerontology, 48,* 12-17.

King, A.C., Rejeski, J., & Buchner, D.M. (1998). Physical activity interventions targeting older adults—A critical review and recommendations. *American Journal of Preventative Medicine, 15,* 316-333.

Kohrt, W.M., Spina, R.J., Holloszy, J.O., & Ehsani, A.A. (1998). Prescribing exercise intensity for older women. *Journal of the American Geriatrics Society, 46,* 129-133.

Koltyn, K.F., & Morgan, W.P. (1992). Efficacy of perceptual versus heart rate monitoring in the development of endurance. *British Journal of Sports Medicine, 26,* 132-134.

Lavie, C.J., & Milani, R.V. (1995). Effects of cardiac rehabilitation programs on exercise capacity, coronary risk factors, behavioral characteristics, and quality of life in a large elderly cohort. *American Journal of Cardiology, 76,* 177-179.

Malbut, K.E., Dinan, S., & Young, A. (2002). Aerobic training in the "oldest old"—The effects of 24 weeks of training. *Age and Ageing, 31,* 255-260.

Malbut-Shennan, K.E., Greig, C., & Young, A. (2000). Aerobic exercise. In A. Young (Ed.), section on "muscle," (Eds.) J.G. Evans, T.F. Williams, B.L. Beattie, J.P. Michel, and G.K. Wilcock, 968-972. *Oxford textbook of geriatric medicine* (2nd ed.). Oxford: Oxford University Press.

Pandolf, K.B. (1982). Differentiated ratings of perceived exertion during physical exercise. *Medicine and Science in Sports and Exercise, 14,* 397-405.

Panton, L.B., Graves, J.E., Pollock, M.L., Garzarella, L., Carroll, J.F., Leggett, S.H., Lowenthal, D.T., Guillen, G.J., et al. (1996). Relative heart rate, heart rate reserve, and VO_2 during submaximal exercise in the elderly. *Journal of Gerontology: Applied Biological Science, Medical Science, 51,* M165-M171.

Pollock, M.L., Wilmore, J.H., & Fox, S.M. (1984). *Exercise in health and disease.* Philadelphia: Saunders.

Puggaard, L., Larsen, J., Stovring, H., & Jeune, B. (2000). Maximal oxygen uptake, muscle strength and walking speed in 85-year-old women: Effects of increased physical activity. *Aging, Clinical and Experimental Research, 12, 180-189.*

Scharff-Olsen, M., Williford, H.N., & Smith, F.H. (1992). The heart rate VO_2 relationship of aerobic dance: A comparison of target heart rate methods. *Journal of Sports Medicine and Physical Fitness 32,* 372-377.

Shephard, R.J. (1984). Management of exercise in the elderly. *Canadian Journal of Applied Sports Science, 9,* 109-120.

Shephard, R.J. (1990). The scientific basis of exercise prescribing for the very old. *Journal of the American Geriatrics Society, 38,* 62-70.

Shephard, R.J. (1991). Exercise prescription for the healthy aged: Testing and programs. *Clinical Journal of Sports Medicine, 1,* 88-99.

Sidney, K.H., & Shephard, R.J. (1977). Perception of exertion in the elderly, effects of aging, mode of exercise and physical training. *Perceptual and Motor Skills, 44,* 999-1010.

Skelton, D.A., & Dinan, S.M. (1999). Exercise for falls management: Rationale for an exercise programme to reduce postural instability. *Physiotherapy: Theory and Practice, 15,* 105-120.

Skelton, D.A., & McLaughlin, A. (1996). Training functional ability in old age. *Physiotherapy, 82,* 159-167.

Skelton, D.A., Young, A., Greig, C.A., & Malbut, K.E. (1995). Effects of resistance training on strength, power and selected functional abilities of women aged 75 and over. *Journal of the American Geriatrics Society, 43,* 1081-1087.

U.S. Department of Health and Human Services. (1996). *Physical activity and health: A report of the Surgeon General.* Atlanta, GA: Centers for Disease Control and Prevention, National Center for Chronic Prevention and Health Promotion, and the President's Council on Physical Fitness and Sports.

Williams, P., & Lord, S.R. (1995). Predictors of adherence to a structured exercise program for older women. *Psychology and Aging, 10,* 617-624.

Yessis, M. (1987). *The secret of Soviet sports fitness and training.* London: Arbour House.

Young, A. (2001). An exercise prescription for a healthier old age. In A. Young & M. Harries (Eds.), *Physical activity for patients: An exercise prescription.* London: Royal College of Physicians.

Young, A., & Dinan, S.M. (2000). Active in later life. In M. Harries, G. McLatchie, C. Williams, & J. King (Eds.), *ABC sports medicine* (2nd ed., pp. 51-56). London: BMJ Books.

Chapter 14

Alexander, N.B. (1994). Postural control in older adults. *Journal of the American Geriatrics Society, 42,* 93-108.

American Geriatrics Society, British Geriatrics Society, and American Academy of Orthopaedic Surgeons Panel on Falls Prevention. (2001). Guideline for the prevention of falls in older persons. *Journal of the American Geriatrics Society, 49,* 664-672.

Brown, L.A., Shumway-Cook, A., & Woollacott, M.H. (1999). Attentional demands and postural recovery: The effects of aging. *Journal of Gerontology: Medical Sciences, 54A,* M165-M171.

Bruce, M.F. (1980). The relation of tactile thresholds to histology in the fingers of the elderly. *Journal of Neurology, Neurosurgery, and Psychiatry, 43,* 730.

Campbell, A.J., Spears, G.F., & Borrie, M.J. (1990). Examination by logistic regression modelling of the variables which increase the relative risk of elderly women falling compared to elderly men. *Journal of Clinical Epidemiology, 43,* 1415-1420.

Frank, J.S., Patla, A.E., & Brown, J.E. (1987). Characteristics of postural control accompanying voluntary arm movement in the elderly. *Society for Neuroscience Abstracts, 13,* 335.

Horak, F.B. (1994). Components of postural dyscontrol in the elderly: A review. *Neurobiology of Aging, 10,* 727-738.

Hu, M., & Woollacott, M.H. (1994). Multisensory training of standing balance in older adults: I. Postural stability and one-leg stance balance. *Journal of Gerontology, 49,* M52-M61.

Inglin, B., & Woollacott, M.H. (1988). Age-related changes in anticipatory postural adjustments associated with arm movements. *Journal of Gerontology, 43,* M105-M113.

Luchies, C.W., Alexander, N.B., Shultz, A.B., & Ashton-Miller, J. (1994). Stepping response of young and old adults to postural disturbances: Kinematics. *Journal of the American Geriatrics Society, 42,* 506-512.

McIlroy, W.E., & Maki, B.E. (1996). Age-related changes in compensatory stepping in response to unpredictable perturbations. *Journal of Gerontology: Medical Sciences, 51A, 6,* M289-M296.

Nashner, L.M., & McCollum, G. (1985). The organization of human postural movements: A formal basis and experimental synthesis. *Behavioral and Brain Sciences, 8,* 135-172.

Paige, G.D. (1991). The aging vestibular-ocular reflex (VOR) and adaptive plasticity. *Acta Otolaryngolica, 481*(Suppl.), 297.

Patla, A.E., & Shumway-Cook, A.S. (1999). Dimensions of mobility: Defining the complexity and difficulty associated with community mobility. *Journal of Aging and Physical Activity, 7*(1), 7-19.

Rose, D.J. (2003). *FallProof!: A comprehensive balance and mobility program.* Champaign, IL: Human Kinetics.

Rubenstein, L.Z., & Josephson, K.R. (2002). The epidemiology of falls and syncope. In R.A. Kenny & D. O'Shea (Eds.), *Clinics in geriatric medicine.* Philadelphia: Saunders.

Shumway-Cook, A., & Woollacott, M.H. (2001). *Motor control: Theory and practical applications* (2nd ed.). Philadelphia: Lippincott Williams & Wilkins.

Shumway-Cook, A., Woollacott, M., Baldwin, M., & Kerns, K. (1997). The effects of cognitive demands on postural control in elderly fallers and non-fallers. *Journal of Gerontology, 52,* M232-M240.

Spirduso, W. (1995). *Physical dimensions of aging.* Champaign, IL: Human Kinetics.

Stelmach, G.E., Phillips, J., DiFabio, J.P., & Teasdale, N. (1989). Age, functional postural reflexes, and voluntary sway. *Journal of Gerontology: Biological Sciences, 44,* B100-B106.

Thelen, D.G., Wojcik, L.A., Schultz, A.B., Ashton-Miller, J.A., & Alexander, N.B. (1997). Age differences in using a rapid step to regain balance during a forward fall. *Journal of Gerontology: Medical Sciences, 52A, 1,* M8-M13.

Wolfson, L. (1997). Balance decrements in older persons: Effects of age and disease. In J.C. Masdeu, L. Sudarsky, & L. Wolfson (Eds.), *Gait disorders of aging: Falls and therapeutic strategies.* Philadelphia: Lippincott-Raven.

Woollacott, M.H., Shumway-Cook, A., & Nashner, L.M. (1986). Aging and postural control: Changes in sensory organization and muscular coordination. *International Journal of Aging and Human Development, 23,* 97-114.

Chapter 15

Berger, B., & Owen, D. (1992). Mood alteration with yoga and swimming: Aerobic exercise may not be necessary. *Perceptual and Motor Skills, 75,* 1331-1343.

DiCarlo, L.J., Sparling, P.B., Hinson, B.T., Snow, T.K., & Rosskopf, L.B. (1995). Cardiovascular, metabolic, and perceptual responses to hatha yoga standing poses. *Medicine, Exercise, Nutrition, and Health, 4,* 107-112.

Garfinkel, M.S. (1994). Evaluation of a yoga-based regimen for treatment of osteoarthritis of the hands. *Journal of Rheumatology, 21,* 2341-2343.

Janakiramaiah, N., Gangaadhar, B.N., Murthy, P.J., Harish, M.G., Subbakrishna, D.K., Vedamurthachar, A., et al. (2000). Antidepressant efficacy of Sudarshan Kriya Yoga (SKY) in melancholia: A randomized comparison with electroconvulsive therapy and imipramine. *Journal of Affective Disorders, 57,* 255-259.

Lasater, J. (1995). *Relax and renew: Restful yoga for stressful times.* Berkeley, CA: Rodmell Press.

Manchanda, S.C. (2000). Retardation of coronary atherosclerosis with yoga lifestyle intervention. *Journal of the Association of Physicians in India, 48,* 687.

Manocha, R., Marks, G.B., Kenchington, P., Peters, D., & Salome. (2002). Sahaja yoga in the management of moderate to severe asthma: Randomized controlled trial. *Thorax, 57,* 110-115.

Murugesan, R., Govindarajulu, N., & Bera, T.K. (2000). Effects of selected yoga practices on hypertension. *Indian Journal of Physiological Pharmacology, 44,* 207-210.

Province, M.A., Halley, E.C., Hornbrook, M.C., Lipsitz, L.A., Miller, J.P., Mulrow, C.D., et al. (1995). The effects of exercise on falls in elderly patients: A preplanned meta-analysis of the FICSIT trials. Frailty and injuries. Cooperative Studies of Intervention Techniques. *Journal of the American Medical Association, 273,* 1341-1347.

Ray, U.S., Mukhopadhyaya, S., Purkayastha, S.S., Asnani, V., Tomer, O.S., Prashad, R., et al. (2001). Effect of yogic exercises on physical and mental health of young fellowship course trainees. *Indian Journal of Physiological Pharmacology, 45,* 37-53.

Savic, K., Pfau, D., Skoric, S., Pfau, J. & Spasojevic, N. (1990). The effect of hatha yoga on poor posture in children and the psychophysiologic condition in adults. *Medicinski Pregled, 43,* 268-276.

Schell, F.J., Allolio, B., & Schonecke, O.W. (1994). Physiological and psychological effects of hatha-yoga exercise in healthy women. *International Journal of Psychosomatics, 41,* 46-52.

Schmidt, T. (1997). Changes in cardiovascular risk factors and hormones during a comprehensive residential three month kriya yoga training program and vegetarian nutrition. *Acta Physiological Scandinavia Supplement, 640,* 158-162.

Sovik, R. (2000). The science of breathing—The yogic view. *Progress in Brain Research, 122,* 491-505.

Telles, S. (2000). Oxygen consumption and respiration following two yoga relaxation techniques. *Applied Psychophysiology and Biofeedback, 25,* 221.

Tse, M. (1995). *Qigong for health and vitality.* New York: St. Martin's Griffin.

Wang, J.S., Lan, C., & Wong, M.K. (2001). Tai chi chuan training to enhance microcirculatory function in healthy elderly subjects. *Archives of Physical Medicine and Rehabilitation, 82,* 1176-1180.

Wolf, S.L., Barnhart, H.X., Kutner, N.G., McNeely E., Coogler, C., & Xu, T. (1996). Reducing frailty and falls in older persons: An investigation of tai chi and computerized balance training. Atlanta FICSIT Group. Frailty and Injuries: Cooperative Studies of Intervention Techniques. *Journal of the American Geriatrics Society, 44,* 489-497.

Chapter 16

Arient, J. (2002). Meniscus injuries. *Aquatic Therapy Journal, 4*(1), 26-29.

Becker, B. (2001, June). Aquatic physical principles. *Aquatic Therapy Journal, 3,* 11-17.

Bravo, G., Gauthier, P., Roy, P.M., Payette, H., & Gaulin, P. (1997). A weight bearing, water-based exercise program for osteopenic women: Its impact on bone, functional fitness and well-being. *Archives of Physical Medicine and Rehabilitation, 78 (12),* 1375-1380.

D'Acquisto, L., D'Acquisto, D., & Renne, D. (2001). Metabolic and cardiovascular responses in older women during shallow-water exercise. *Journal of Strength and Conditioning Research, 15(1),* 12-19.

Davis, B.C., & Harrison, R.A. (1988). *Hydrotherapy in practice.* Edinburgh: Churchill Livingstone.

Hall, J., Skevington, S.M., Maddison, P.J., & Chapman, K. (1996). A randomized and controlled trial of hydrotherapy in rheumatoid arthritis. *Arthritis Care and Research, 9 (3),* 206-215.

Herfert, D. (2000, January). Stay above water with exercise-induced asthma. *Aquatic Therapy Journal, 2,* 5-12.

Hurley, R., & Turner, C. (1991). Neurology and aquatic therapy. *Clinical Management, 11,* 26-29.

Krist, P. (2000, January). Just do it. *AKWA, 13,* 17.

La Forge, R. (1995). Exercise associated mood alterations: A review of neurobiologic mechanisms. *Medicine, Exercise, Nutrition, and Health 4,* 17-32.

Maybeck, J. (2002). Going for the silver. *AKWA, 16,* 9-11.

Nakanishi, Y., Kimura, T., & Yokoo, Y. (1999). Physiological responses to maximal and deep water running in young and middle aged males. *Applied Human Science, 18,* 81-86.

Norton, C. (1997). Effectiveness of aquatic exercise in the treatment of women with osteoarthritis. *Journal of Physical Therapy, 5(3),* 8-15.

Schoedinger, P. (2002). Hydrodynamics and physiological effects of immersion. Aquatic Therapy Symposium.

Suomi, R., & Lindaur, S. (1997). Effectiveness of arthritis foundation program on strength and range of motion in women with arthritis. *Journal of Aging and Physical Activity, 5,* 341-351.

Takeshima, N., Rogers, M.E., Watanabe, E., Brechue, W.F., Okada, A., Yamada, T., Islam, M.M., & Hayano, J. (2002). Water-based exercise improves health-related aspects of fitness in older women. *Medicine & Science in Sports & Exercise, 33 (3),* 544-551.

Templeton, M., Booth, D., & O'Kelly, W. (1996). Effects of aquatic therapy on joint flexibility and functional ability in subjects with rheumatic disease. *Journal of Orthopaedic and Sports Physical Therapy, 23 (6),* 376-81.

Chapter 17

Allen, W.K., Seals, D.R., Hurley, B.F., Ehsani, A.A., & Hagberg, J.M. (1985). Lactate threshold and distance-running performance in young and older endurance athletes. *Journal of Applied Physiology, 58*(4), 1281-1284.

American College of Sports Medicine. (2000). *ACSM's guidelines for exercise testing and prescription* (6th ed.). Philadelphia: Lippincott Williams & Wilkins.

Bompa, T. (1985). *Theory and methodology of training—The key to athletic performance.* Dubuque, IA: Kendall Hunt.

Bortz, W.M., IV, & Bortz, W.M., II. (1996). How fast do we age? Exercise performance over time as a biomarker. *Journal of Gerontology: Medical Sciences, 51A*(5), M223-M225.

Brown, M. (1989). Special considerations during rehabilitation of the aged athlete. *Clinics in Sports Medicine, 8*(4), 893-901.

Carron, A., & Leith, L. (1986). Psychology of the masters athlete: Motivational considerations. In J.R. Sutton & R.M. Brock (Eds.), *Sports medicine for the mature athlete* (pp. 233-239). Indianapolis: Benchmark Press.

Eskurza, I., Donato, A.J., Moreau, K.L., Seals, D.R., & Tanaka, H. (2002). Changes in maximal aerobic capacity with age in endurance-trained women: 7-yr follow-up. *Journal of Applied Physiology, 92,* 2303-2308.

Gambetta, V. (1981). Planning a training program. In V. Gambetta (Ed.), *TAC track and field coaching manual* (pp. 42-45). West Point, NY: Leisure Press.

Gill, T.M., DiPietro, L., & Krumholz, H.M. (2000). Role of exercise stress testing and safety monitoring for older persons starting an exercise program. *Journal of the American Medical Association, 284*(3), 342-349.

Hawkins, S.A., Marcell, T.J., Jaque, S.V., & Wiswell, R.A. (2001). A longitudinal assessment of change in VO_2max and maximal heart rate in master athletes. *Medicine and Science in Sports and Exercise, 33*(10), 1744-1750.

Hopkins, W.G., & Hewson, D.J. (2001). Variability of competitive performance of distance runners. *Medicine and Science in Sports and Exercise, 33*(9), 1588-1592.

Klitgaard, H., Mantoni, M., Schiaffino, S., Ausoni, S., Gorza, L., Laurent-Winter, C., et al. (1990). Function, morphology and protein expression of ageing skeletal muscle: A cross-sectional study of elderly men with different training backgrounds. *Acta Physiologica Scandinavia, 140,* 41-54.

Kohrt, W.M., Spina, R.J., Holloszy, J.O., & Ehsani, A.A. (1998). Prescribing exercise intensity for older women. *Journal of the American Geriatrics Society, 46,* 129-133.

Magee, M., & D'Antonio, M. (2001). *The new face of aging.* New York: Spencer Books.

Maharam, L.G., Bauman, P.A., Kalman, D., Skolnik, H., & Pearle, S.M. (1999). Masters athletes: Factors affecting performance. *Sports Medicine, 28*(4), 273-285.

Meltzer, D.E. (1996). Body-mass dependence of age-related deterioration in human muscular performance. *Journal of Applied Physiology, 80*(4), 1149-1155.

Menard, D., & Stanish, W.D. (1989). The aging athlete. *American Journal of Sports Medicine, 17*(2), 187-196.

Moore, J. (1999, July/August). Overtraining? Listen to your body. *Swim,* pp. 23-25.

Pollock, M.L., Mengelkoch, L.J., Graves, J.E., Lowenthal, D.T., Limacher, M.C., Foster, C., et al. (1997). Twenty-year follow-up of aerobic power and body composition of older track athletes. *Journal of Applied Physiology, 82*(5), 1508-1516.

Rogers, M.A., Hagberg, J.M., Martin, W.H., III, Ehsani, A.A., & Holloszy, J.O. (1990). Decline in VO$_2$max with aging in master athletes and sedentary men. *Journal of Applied Physiology, 68*(5), 2195-2199.

Shephard, R.J., Kavanagh, T., Mertens, D.J., Qureshi, S., & Clark, M. (1995). Personal health benefits of masters athletics competition. *British Journal of Sports Medicine, 29*(1), 35-40.

Sipila, S., Viitasalo, J., Era, P., & Suominen, H. (1991). Muscle strength in male athletes aged 70-81 years and a population sample. *European Journal of Applied Physiology, 63,* 399-403.

Spirduso, W. (1995). *Physical dimensions of aging.* Champaign, IL: Human Kinetics.

Starkes, J.L., Weir, P.L., Singh, P., Hodges, N.J., & Kerr, T. (1999). Aging and the retention of sport expertise. *International Journal of Sport Psychology, 30*(2), 283-301.

Stones, M.J., & Kozma, A. (1981). Adult age trends in record running performances. *Experimental Aging Research, 6,* 407-416.

Tanaka, H., & Seals, D.R. (1997). Age and gender interactions in physiological functional capacity: Insight from swimming performance. *Journal of Applied Physiology, 82*(3), 846-851.

Trappe, S.W., Costill, D.L., Vukovich, M.D., Jones, J., & Melham, T. (1996). Aging among elite distance runners: A 22-yr longitudinal study. *Journal of Applied Physiology, 80*(1), 285-290.

U.S.A. Track & Field (1991). National Coaching Education Program Level II Endurance Events.

Weir, P.L., Kerr, T., Hodges, N.J., McKay, S.M., & Starkes, J.L. (2002). Master swimmers: How are they different from younger elite swimmers? An examination of practice and performance patterns. *Journal of Aging and Physical Activity, 10*(1), 41-63.

Wiswell, R.A., Hawkins, S.A., Jaque, S.V., Hyslop, D., Constantino, N., Tarpenning, K., et al. (2001). Relationship between physiological loss, performance decrements, and age in master athletes. *Journal of Gerontology: Medical Sciences, 56A*(10), M618-M626.

Wiswell, R.A., Jaque, S.V., Marcell, T.J., Hawkins, S.A., Tarpenning, K.M., Constantino, N., et al. (2000). Maximal aerobic power, lactate threshold, and running performance in male and female master athletes. *Medicine and Science in Sports and Exercise, 32*(6), 1165-1170.

Chapter 18

Brady, F. (1998). A theoretical and empirical review of the contextual interference effect and the learning of motor skills. *Quest, 50,* 266-293.

Gentile, A.M. (1972). A working model of skill acquisition with application to teaching [Monograph]. *Quest, 17,* 3-23.

Gentile, A.M. (2000). Skill acquisition: Action, movement, and neuromotor processes. In J.H. Carr & R.B. Shephard (Eds.), *Movement science: Foundations for physical therapy* (2nd ed., pp. 111-187). Rockville, MD: Aspen.

Knudson, D.V., & Morrison, C.S. (2002). *Qualitative analysis of human movement* (2nd ed.). Champaign, IL: Human Kinetics.

Landin, D. (1994). The role of verbal cues in skill learning. *Quest, 46,* 299-313.

Lee, T.D., Swinnen, S.P., & Serrien, D.J. (1994). Cognitive effort and motor learning. *Quest, 46,* 328-344.

Magill, R.A. (2001). Augmented feedback in motor skill acquisition. In R.N. Singer, H.A. Hausenblaus, & C.M. Janelle (Eds.), *Handbook of research on sport psychology* (pp. 86-114). New York: Wiley.

Magill, R.A. (2004). *Motor learning: Concepts and applications* (7th ed.). New York: McGraw-Hill.

McCullagh, P., & Weiss, M.R. (2001). Modeling: Considerations for motor skill performance and psychological responses. In R.N. Singer, H.A. Hausenblas, & C.M. Janelle (Eds.), *Handbook of sport psychology* (2nd ed., pp. 205-238). New York: Wiley.

Rose, D.J., & Christina, R.W. (2005). *A multilevel approach to the study of motor control and learning* (2nd ed.). San Francisco: Benjamin-Cummings.

Salthouse, T.A. (1991). *Theoretical perspectives on cognitive aging.* Hillsdale, NJ: Erlbaum.

Schmidt, R., & Wrisberg, C. (2004). *Motor learning and performance* (3rd ed.). Champaign, IL: Human Kinetics.

Shephard, R.J. (1997). *Aging, physical activity, and health.* Champaign, IL: Human Kinetics.

Spirduso, W.W. (1995). *Physical dimensions of aging.* Champaign, IL: Human Kinetics.

Chapter 19

Ashforth, B.E., & Humphry, R.H. (1995). Emotion in the workplace: A reappraisal. *Human Relations, 48,* 97-125.

Carnegie, D. (1981). *How to win friends and influence people.* New York: Pocket Books.

Carter-Scott, C. (1998). *If life is a game, these are the rules.* New York: Broadway Books.

Conroy, D. (2002). Addressing the fear factor: Obstacles to motivation. *IDEA Health and Fitness Source, 20*(5), 38-43.

Dalai Lama, & Cutler, H.C. (1998). *The art of happiness.* New York: Riverhead Books.

Dishman, R. (1988). *Exercise adherence: Its impact on public health.* Champaign, IL: Human Kinetics.

Francis, L., & Seibert, R. (2000) Addressing the fear factor: Obstacles to motivation. *IDEA Health and Fitness Source 20*(5), 38-43.

Gavin, J. (1992). *The exercise habit.* Champaign, IL: Leisure Press.

Goldman, D., Boyatzis, R., & McKee, A. (2002). *Primal leadership.* Boston: Harvard Business School Press.

Heitmann, H. (1989). The learning environment and instructional considerations. In K. Leslie (Ed.), *Mature stuff: Physical activity for the older adult* (pp. 179-204). Reston, VA: American Alliance for Health, Physical Education, Recreation and Dance.

Heywood, K. (1989). Motor skill learning in older adults. In K. Leslie (Ed.), *Mature stuff: Physical activity for the older adult* (pp. 61-79). Reston, VA: American Alliance for Health, Physical Education, Recreation and Dance.

Hoffman, J.H., & Jones, K.D. (2002). Reducing attrition from exercise: Practical tips from research. *ACSM's Health & Fitness Journal 2*(6): 7-10.

Kennedy, C. (2000). Group exercise program design. In D. Green & R. Cotton (Eds.), *Group fitness instructor manual* (pp. 140-176). San Diego, CA: American Council on Exercise.

Maxwell, J.C. (1993). *The winning attitude.* Nashville, TN: Thomas Nelson.

Poole, J. (1991). Seven skills to improved teaching: Enhancing graduate assistant instruction. *Journal of Physical Education, Recreation and Dance 62*(10): 21-24.

Price, J. (2002). Taking a leap of faith: Provide a platform your senior clients can use to confidently spring through exercise anxieties. *IDEA Personal Trainer, 13,* 14-20.

Sonstroem, R.J. (1984). Exercise and self-esteem. *Exercise and Sport Sciences Reviews, 12,* 100-130.

Wagman, D. (1997). Remotivating the motivated. *Strength and Conditioning Journal, (19)*4, 60-66.

Chapter 20

American Senior Fitness Association. (2002). *Senior fitness instructor training manual* (4th ed.). New Smyrna Beach, FL: American Senior Fitness Association.

Annesi, J.J. (1996). *Enhancing exercise motivation: A guide to increasing fitness center member retention.* Los Angeles: Leisure.

Annesi, J.J., & Zimmerman, W. (2001). Group training for increased adherence to regular physical activity. In J. Clark (Ed.), *Contemporary readings in senior personal training* (pp. 59-61). New Smyrna Beach, FL: American Senior Fitness Association.

Clark, J. (1997). Putting wit to work: Creativity pays off for an inventive fitness instructor. *American Senior Fitness Association's Senior Fitness Bulletin, 4*(1), 9-11.

Clark, J. (1998). Older adult exercise techniques. In R.T. Cotton (Ed.), *Exercise for older adults: ACE's guide for fitness professionals* (pp. 128-181). Champaign, IL: Human Kinetics.

Clark, J. (2002, February). The new demand for senior fitness: Gear up and be ready. Paper presented at the annual meeting of the State of Nevada Recreation and Parks Society, Reno, NV.

Clark, J. (2003). *Seniorcise: A simple guide to fitness for the elderly and disabled* (2nd ed.). New Smyrna Beach, FL: American Senior Fitness Association.

Haennel, R.G., Quinney, H.A., & Kappagoda, C.T. (1991). Effects of hydraulic circuit training following coronary bypass surgery. *Medicine and Science in Sports and Exercise, 23,* 158-165.

IDEA Health and Fitness Association. (1999, January). 1998 IDEA industry compensation survey. *IDEA Health and Fitness Source,* pp. 57-63.

Kaikkonen, H., Yrjama, M., Siljander, E., Byman, P., & Laukkanen, R. (2000). The effect of heart rate controlled maximal aerobic power in sedentary adults. *Scandinavian Journal of Medical Science in Sports, 10,* 211-215.

Marx, J.O., Ratamess, N.A., Nindl, B.C., Gotshalk, L.A., Volek, J.S., Dohi, K., et al. (2001). Low-volume circuit versus high-volume periodized resistance training in women. *Medicine and Science in Sports and Exercise, 33,* 635-643.

Schroeder, J. (1995). A comprehensive survey of older adult exercise programs in two California communities. *Journal of Aging and Physical Activity, 3:* 290-298.

Sharkey, B.J. (2002). *Fitness and health* (5th ed.). Champaign, IL: Human Kinetics.

Thompson, S., & Hoekenga, S.J. (1998). Understanding and motivating older adults. In R.T. Cotton (Ed.), *Exercise for older adults: ACE's guide for fitness professionals* (pp. 24-70). Champaign, IL: Human Kinetics.

Valenzuela, J. (2002, April). Tap into the mighty senior market. *IDEA Personal Trainer,* pp. 47-51.

Van Norman, K. (1998). Exercise programming and leadership. In R.T. Cotton (Ed.), *Exercise for older adults: ACE's guide for fitness professionals* (pp. 182-210). Champaign, IL: Human Kinetics.

Ward, K. (1997). Gender and ethnic considerations. *American Senior Fitness Association's Senior Fitness Bulletin, 4*(3), 14-15.

Chapter 21

Aggarwal, A., & Ades, P.A. (2001). Exercise rehabilitation of older patients with cardiovascular disease. *Cardiology Clinics, 19,* 525-536.

Albright, A.L. (1997). Diabetes. In J.L. Durstine (Ed.), *ACSM's exercise management for persons with chronic diseases and disabilities* (pp. 94-100). Champaign, IL: Human Kinetics.

American Diabetes Association. (1998). Economic consequences of diabetes mellitus in the U.S. in 1997. *Diabetes Care, 21,* 269-309.

Aronow, W.S. (2001). Exercise therapy for older persons with cardiovascular disease. *American Journal of Geriatric Cardiology, 10,* 245-252.

Blumenthal, M.N. (1990). Sports-aggravated allergies: How to treat and prevent the symptoms. *Physician and Sportsmedicine, 18,* 52-66.

Bravo, G., Gauthier, P., Roy, P., Payette, H., & Gaulin, P. (1997). A weight-bearing, water-based exercise program for osteopenic women: Its impact on bone, functional fitness, and well-being. *Archives of Physical Medicine and Rehabilitation, 78,* 1375-1380.

Campbell, M., & Colberg, S.R. (2000). Use of clinical practice recommendations for exercise by individuals with type 1 diabetes. *Diabetes Educator, 26,* 265-271.

Campbell, M.L., Sheets, D., & Strong, P.S. (1999). Secondary health conditions among middle-aged individuals with chronic physical disabilities: Implications for unmet needs for services. *Assistive Technology, 11,* 105-122.

Cooper, C.B. (2001a). Exercise in chronic pulmonary disease: Limitations and rehabilitation. *Medicine and Science in Sports and Exercise, 33,* S643-S646.

Cooper, C.B. (2001b). Exercise in chronic pulmonary disease: Aerobic exercise prescription. *Medicine and Science in Sports and Exercise, 33,* S671-S679.

Emtner, M., Herala, M., & Stalenheim, G. (1996). High-intensity physical training in adults with asthma: A 10-week rehabilitation program. *Chest, 109,* 323-330.

Ettinger, W.H., Burns, R., Messier, S.P., Applegate, W., Rejeski, W.J., & Morgan, T. (1997). A randomized trial comparing aerobic exercise and resistance exercise with a health education program in older adults with knee osteoarthritis. *Journal of the American Medical Association, 277,* 25-31.

Gordon, N.F. (1997). Hypertension. In J. L. Durstine (Ed.), *ACSM's exercise management for persons with chronic diseases and disabilities* (pp. 59-63). Champaign, IL: Human Kinetics.

Gregg, I., & Nunn, A.J. (1989). Peak expiratory flow in symptomless elderly smokers and ex-smokers. *British Medical Journal, 298,* 1071-1072.

Groer, M.W., & Shekleton, M.E. (1989). *Basic pathophysiology: A holistic approach.* St. Louis: Mosby.

Hagberg, J.M., Park, J., & Brown, M.D. (2000). The role of exercise training in the treatment of hypertension. *Sports Medicine, 30,* 193-206.

Hill, J., & Poirier, L. (1995). Helping patients manage their diabetes. *Patient Care, 29,* 97-120.

Hochberg, M.C., Altman, R.D., Brandt, K.D., Clark, B.M., Dieppe, P.A., Griffin, M.R., et al. (1995). Guidelines for the medical management of osteoarthritis. *Arthritis and Rheumatism, 38,* 1541-1546.

Hurley, B.F., & Roth, S.M. (2000). Strength training in the elderly: Effects on risk factors for age-related diseases. *Sports Medicine, 30,* 249-268.

Interiano, B., & Guntupalli, K.K. (1996). Clinical aspects of asthma. *Current Opinion in Pulmonary Medicine, 2,* 60-65.

Joint National Committee on Prevention, Detection, Evaluation, and Treatment of High Blood Pressure. (1997). The sixth report of the Joint National Committee on Prevention, Detection,

Evaluation, and Treatment of High Blood Pressure. *Archives of Internal Medicine, 157,* 2413-2446.

Kanis, J.A., Melton, L.J., Christiansen, C., Jonston, C.C., & Khalaev, N. (1994). The diagnosis of osteoporosis. *Journal of Bone Mineral Research, 9,* 1137-1141.

Kohl, H.W., III, & McKenzie, J.D. (1994). Physical activity, fitness, and stroke. In C. Bouchard, R.J. Shephard, & T. Stephens (Eds.), *Physical activity, fitness, and health: International proceedings and consensus statement* (pp. 609-621). Champaign, IL: Human Kinetics.

Lockette, K.F., & Keys, A.M. (1994). *Conditioning with physical disabilities.* Champaign, IL: Human Kinetics.

Lueckenotte, A.G. (1996). *Gerontologic nursing.* St. Louis: Mosby.

Marino, C., & McDonald, E. (1991). Osteoarthritis and rheumatoid arthritis in elderly patients: Differentiation and treatment. *Postgraduate Medicine, 90,* 237-243.

McFadden, E.R., & Gilbert, I.A. (1992). Asthma. *New England Journal of Medicine, 327,* 1928-1937.

Merck manual of geriatrics. (1995). W.B. Abrams, M.H. Beers, R. Berkow (Eds.). Whitehouse Station, NJ: Merck & Co.

Miller, M.E., Rejeski, W.J., Reboussin, B.A., Ten Have, T.R., & Ettinger, W.H. (2000). Physical activity, functional limitations, and disability in older adults. *Journal of the American Geriatrics Society, 48,* 1264-1272.

O'Donnell, D.E., Webb, K.A., & McGuire, M.A. (1993). Older patients with COPD: Benefits of exercise training. *Geriatrics, 48,* 59-66.

O'Grady, M., Fletcher, J., & Ortiz, S. (2000). Therapeutic and physical fitness exercise prescription for older adults with joint disease: An evidence-based approach. *Geriatric Rheumatology, 26,* 617-646.

Ohkubo, T., Hozawa, A., Nagatomi, R., Fujita, K., Sauaget, C., & Watanabe, Y. (2001). Effects of exercise training on home blood pressure values in older adults: A randomized controlled trial. *Journal of Hypertension, 19,* 1045-1052.

Ostir, G.V., Carlson, J.E., Black, S.A., Rudkin, L., Goodwin, J.S., & Markides, K.S. (1999). Disability in older adults: 1. Prevalence, causes, and consequences. *Behavioral Medicine, 24,* 147-156.

Potempa, K., Braun, L.T., Tinknell, T., & Popovich, J. (1996). Benefits of aerobic exercise after stroke. *Sports Medicine, 21,* 337-346.

Reid, W.D., & Samrai, B. (1995). Respiratory muscle training for patients with chronic obstructive pulmonary disease. *Physical Therapy, 75,* 996-1005.

Rimmer, J.H. (1994). *Fitness and rehabilitation programs for special populations.* Dubuque, IA: Brown and Benchmark.

Rimmer, J.H. (2003). Exercise for persons with Alzheimer's disease. In J.L. Durstine (Ed.), *ACSM's exercise management for persons with chronic disease and disabilities* (pp. 311-315). Champaign, IL: Human Kinetics.

Rimmer, J.H. (2001). Resistance training for persons with physical disabilities. In J.E. Graves & B.A. Franklin (Eds.), *Resistance training for health and rehabilitation* (pp. 321-346). Champaign, IL: Human Kinetics.

Rimmer, J.H., & Nicola, T. (2002). Stroke. In J.N. Myers, W.G. Herbert, & R. Humphrey (Eds.), *ACSM's resources for clinical exercise physiology: Musculoskeletal, neuromuscular, neoplastic, immunologic, and hematologic conditions* (pp. 3-15). Philadelphia: Lippincott Williams & Wilkins.

Rimmer, J.H., Riley, B.B., Creviston, T., & Nicola, T. (2000). Exercise training in a predominantly African-American group of stroke survivors. *Medicine and Science in Sports and Exercise, 32,* 1990-1996.

Rosenstock, J. (2001). Management of type 2 diabetes mellitus in the elderly: Special considerations. *Drugs and Aging, 18,* 31-44.

Sato, M., Grese, T.A., Dodge, J.A., Bryant, H.U., & Turner, C.H. (1999). Emerging therapies for the prevention and treatment of postmenopausal osteoporosis. *Journal of Medicinal Chemistry, 42,* 1-24.

Schenkman, M., Cutson, T.M., Kuchibhatla, M., Chandler, J., Pieper, C.F., & Ray, L. (1998). Exercise to improve spinal flexibility and function for people with Parkinson's disease: A randomized, controlled trial. *Journal of the American Geriatrics Society, 46,* 1207-1216.

Shapira, I., Fisman, E.Z., Motro, M., Pines, A., Ben-Ari, E. & Drory, Y. (1995). Rehabilitation in older coronary patients. *American Journal of Geriatric Cardiology, 4,* 48-55.

Shorr, R.I., Ray, W.A., & Daugherty, J.R. (1997). Incidence and risk factors for serious hypoglycemia in older persons using insulin or sulfonylureas. *Archives of Internal Medicine, 157,* 1681-1686.

Stacy, M., & Jankovic, J. (1992). Clinical and neurobiological aspects of Parkinson's disease. In S.J. Huber & J.L. Cummings (Eds.), *Parkinson's disease: Neurobehavioral aspects* (pp. 10-13). London: Oxford University Press.

Stanley, R.K., & Protas, E.J. (2002). Parkinson's disease. In J.N. Myers, W.G. Herbert, & R. Humphrey (Eds.), *ACSM's resources for clinical exercise physiology: Musculoskeletal, neuromuscular, neoplastic, immunologic, and hematologic conditions* (pp. 38-47). Philadelphia: Lippincott Williams & Wilkins.

Stewart, D.G. (1999). Stroke rehabilitation: 1. Epidemiological aspects and acute management. *Archives of Physical Medicine and Rehabilitation, 80,* S4-S7.

Van Den Ende, C.H.M., Vlieland, V., Munneke, M., & Hazes, J.M.W. (1998). Dynamic exercise therapy in rheumatoid arthritis: A systematic review. *British Journal of Rheumatology, 37,* 677-687.

Weir, G.C., & Singer, K. (1995). Diabetes care: It's a whole new ballgame. *Patient Care, 29,* 10-11.

Chapter 22

American College of Sports Medicine. (1997). *ACSM's health and fitness standards.* Champaign, IL: Human Kinetics.

Eickhoff-Shemek, J.M. (2001). Do standards of practice reflect legal duties. *ACSM's Health and Fitness Journal, 5,* 23-25.

Eickhoff-Shemek, J.M., & Deja, K. (2002). Are health/fitness facilities complying with ACSM standards? *ACSM's Health and Fitness Journal, 6,* 16-21.

Martini, E.B., & Botenhagen, K.A. (2003). *Exercise for the frail elders.* Champaign, IL: Human Kinetics.

NSCA [National Strength and Conditioning Association] Professional Standards & Guidelines Task Force. (2001, May). *Strength and conditioning professional standards and guidelines.* www.nsca.com. Accessed on May 17, 2004.

Tharrett, S.J., & Peterson, J.A. (Eds.). (1997). *ACSM's health/fitness facility standards and guidelines* (2nd ed.). Champaign, IL: Human Kinetics.

Index

About the Editors

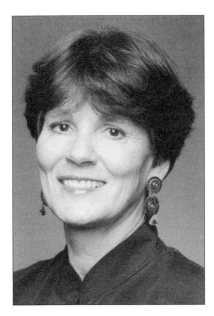

C. Jessie Jones, PhD, is a professor in the division of kinesiology and health science, codirector of the Center for Successful Aging, and past director of the Lifespan Wellness Clinic and Gerontology Programs at California State University at Fullerton. She is a fellow of the American College of Sports Medicine and the American Academy of Kinesiology and Physical Education. Dr. Jones has an extensive teaching and research background in the area of gerokinesiology. Her areas of specialty include assessing functional fitness of older adults, curriculum standards for training physical activity instructors of older adults, and designing senior fitness programs.

Dr. Jones has taught senior fitness classes and conducted training workshops for instructors for more than 20 years. Her national and international reputation for research, program design, and curriculum development in this field has led to her recent appointment as co-editor in chief of the *Journal of Aging and Physical Activity*. Her work has been covered in numerous publications. She is coauthor of the *Senior Fitness Test Manual* (2001, Human Kinetics) with its companion training video and software. The Senior Fitness Test is the only functional fitness test with established reliability, validity, and national norms based on the testing of 7,000 men and women between the ages of 60 and 94.

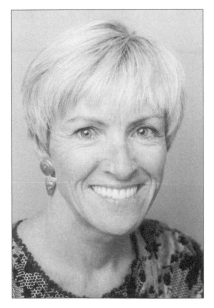

Debra J. Rose, PhD, is a professor in the division of kinesiology and health science and codirector of the Center for Successful Aging at California State University at Fullerton. She is also a professor in the physical therapy department at Chapman University in Orange, California. Her primary research focus is on the enhancement of mobility and the prevention of falls in later years.

Dr. Rose is nationally and internationally recognized for her work in fall risk reduction assessment and programming. Her research in fall risk reduction in the elderly has been published in numerous peer-reviewed publications, including the *Journal of the American Geriatric Society, Archives of Physical Medicine and Rehabilitation, Neurology Report,* and the *Journal of Aging and Physical Activity.* The innovative fall risk reduction program she developed was recognized by the National Council on Aging as one of seven meritorious programs nationwide that promotes a healthy, active lifestyle. Dr. Rose's entire program was published in her book, *FallProof! A Comprehensive Balance and Mobility Training Program* (2003, Human Kinetics). She is a fellow of the American Academy of Kinesiology and Physical Education, former executive board member of the North American Society for the Psychology of Sport and Physical Activity, and co-editor in chief of the *Journal of Aging and Physical Activity.*